Mother's Milk

Mother's Milk

*Breastfeeding Controversies
in American Culture*

Bernice L. Hausman

ROUTLEDGE
NEW YORK AND LONDON

Published in 2003 by
Routledge
29 West 35th Street
New York, NY 10001
www.routledge-ny.com

Published in Great Britain by
Routledge
11 New Fetter Lane
London EC4P 4EE
www.routledge.co.uk

Routledge is an imprint of the Taylor & Francis Group.

Library of Congress Cataloging-in-Publication Data

Hausman, Bernice L.
    Mother's milk : breastfeeding controversies in American culture / Bernice L. Hausman.
        p.   ;   cm.
Includes bibliographical references and index.
    ISBN 0-415-96656-6 (hbk. : alk. paper)—ISBN 0-415-96657-4 (pbk. : alk. paper)
    1. Breast feeding—United States.   2. Breast feeding—Social aspects—United States.
3. Lactation—United States.   4. Mother and child.
    [DNLM: 1. Breast Feeding—United States—Popular Works.   2. Lactation—United
States—Popular Works.   3. Mother-Child Relations—United States—Popular Works.
WS 125 H376m 2003]   I. Title.
RJ216 .H28   2003
613.2′69′0973—dc21   2002156321

For
Rachel and Sam,
who taught me how

Dirt had entered. There was now an abscess. He might have to operate. In any case the child in the future would have to seek its nourishment in tins.

"What?" exclaimed Herr Dremmel.

"Tins," said the doctor.

"Tins? For my son? When there are cows in the world? Cows, which at least more closely resemble mothers than tins?"

"Tins," repeated the doctor firmly. "Herr Pastor, cows have moods just as frequently as women. They are fed unwisely, and behold immediately have a mood. Not having the gift of tongues they cannot convey their mood by speech, and baffled at one end they fall back upon the other, and express their malignancies in milk."

—Elizabeth von Arnim, *The Pastor's Wife*

She was doing "the most natural thing in the world," suckling her young, and for some peculiar reason it was completely unnatural, strained, and false, like a posed photograph. Everyone in the hospital knew this, her mother knew it, her visitors knew it; that was why they were all talking about her nursing and pretending that it was exciting, when it was not, except as a thing to talk about. In reality, what she had been doing was horrid, and right now, in the nursery, a baby's voice was rising to tell her so—the voice, in fact, that she had been refusing to listen to, though she had heard it for at least a week. It was making a natural request, in this day and age; it was asking for a bottle.

—Mary McCarthy, *The Group*

CONTENTS

Preface and Acknowledgments

Mother's Milk: Breastfeeding Controversies in American Culture is a book for physicians and other medical professionals, feminist health activists, breastfeeding advocates, feminist body theorists, and cultural studies scholars in general. It is also, I hope, a book for mothers who seek to understand the cultural influences on their maternal practices. But it is not only a book for those interested in maternity, or even, oddly, breastfeeding. Just as in my first book, I argue here that feminist and cultural studies scholars must interrogate biomedical discourses about embodied sex. There, I wrote that "in a critical return to 'sex' we may find a way to destabilize 'gender' as a normalizing narrative in the twentieth century" (200). The scientific case for breastfeeding is nothing if not a biomedical discourse about embodied sex, and I argue here that we must confront this discourse for its perpetuation of discriminatory views of women, as well as use it to challenge current social practices that work to subordinate mothers' choices and actions. Breastfeeding as an act is no panacea for the subordination of women, but an examination of breastfeeding uncovers central feminist tensions around the meaning of women's bodies, the authority of science, and the social value of maternity in contemporary culture.

I write this book as a mother, breastfeeding advocate, and feminist theorist. Often, those identity positions conflict; writing this book has been an attempt to make them cohere, or at least to become clearer about the contradictions that arise in articulating all three in close relation. *Mother's Milk* is a book that emerges from certain experiences I have had as a breastfeeding mother, but it is not a book that depends on personal reflection. I have tried to link some aspect of each chapter to my own practices or thoughts as a mother, but only in order to ground what I consider a theoretical consideration of embodied maternity in the more mundane experiences of contemporary American middle-class motherhood. Indeed, much of the reflecting that I do about my own experiences in this book has as its purpose the grounding of those thoughts in the specificity of my own position as a middle-class white woman and professional worker. In this way I hope to be better able to identify differences in other women's experiences of breastfeeding, breastfeeding advocacy, and the medical institution.

I want *Mother's Milk* to reach beyond scholarly audiences to convince nonacademic readers about the significance of cultural inquiry and the importance of sustained attention to the way that medicine influences our experience of our bodies and of our social relationships. In the United States, we are bombarded daily with new information about health and the preferred practices with which we can improve our bodies and those of our children. At the same time, we are subject to an avalanche of stories about emerging health risks. For example, during the fall of 2002, as I am preparing this manuscript for publication, West Nile virus has been found in breast milk. This information follows on the discovery that West Nile virus can be passed on through donated blood and organs, and echoes current debates over HIV infection via breastfeeding. The question of whether an infant can contract the virus through its mother's milk has not been answered, but the headline "West Nile Virus Found in Breast Milk" heralds a new risk in the increasingly common perception that toxins make their way from mother to baby through intra- and extra-uterine means.

Breast milk has apparently been a conduit for human viruses for millennia—breastfeeding is not a new mechanism for viral transfer. But the risk, at least in the United States, appears more salient, given recent and fervent public health campaigns to increase rates of maternal nursing and given the apparent relative safety of infant formula as a substitute for breast milk (in the developed world). Yet these kinds of stories about breaking medical news raise a host of questions. How are mothers to make informed decisions about breast- or bottle feeding when the risks of both practices are difficult to identify and assess? How do laypeople interpret medical information, especially since so much of it is conveyed through media sources or advice literature? What are the cultural meanings attached to both breast- and bottle feeding that affect mothers' choices? How do economic circumstances influence feeding practices and maternal embodiment, as well as the familial decisions about infant care that seem to affect them?

Mother's Milk addresses these questions through close readings of public representations of breastfeeding in contemporary American culture. Identifying a set of controversies that emerge in these representations—controversies about insufficient milk syndrome, maternal sexuality, and feeding schedules, to name a few—I demonstrate their complexity and their relation to other, broader controversies about motherhood and gender in the modern world. Public debates about breastfeeding mediate social anxieties concerning motherhood and women's rights; because of this, breastfeeding advocacy needs to become more political, more feminist, in its approach to maternal feeding practices. But feminism, currently articulating a critique of breastfeeding and its advocacy, needs to face head-on the biomedical discourses that support maternal nursing as a health-enhancing practice for both mothers and children. Those discourses do perpetuate stereotypes about maternal sacrifice, but they also provide language to press for women's rights as mothers, especially in a social and political climate in which medical arguments carry significant weight. As a feminist, a breastfeeding advocate, and a mother, I hope that *Mother's Milk* contributes to greater understanding between feminist theorists and maternal activists. Toward that goal, I nudge all sides to be more responsible for the problematic rhetorics that they engender.

I began to think about this project in the year after the birth of my daughter, Rachel, and really got working on it in the years after Samuel's birth. I have been writing this book all of their lives; it is, indeed, a book that could not have been written without them. For this reason, as well as for their infinite patience with their scholar-mother, I dedicate this book to them.

In the early stages of research, I was aided by two able graduate assistants, Siobhan Starr and Terry Pettinger. A Virginia Tech College of Arts and Sciences Pilot Research Grant and a Millennium Grant funded initial research and trips to breastfeeding conferences, as well as the purchase of computer hardware. A Humanities Summer Stipend sent me to my first La Leche League Seminar on Breastfeeding for Physicians, as well as the LLL's international parenting conference in July 1999. The Department of English at Virginia Tech funded seven years of conference travel, most of which was to present research from this book. I particularly want to thank Johann Norstedt, chair of the department during much of that time, for steering stray travel money my way when I needed it most. Judy Grady helped organize that travel, as did Hilary Smith-Ferguson before her. The Provost's Office at Virginia Tech funded a semester's Research Assignment so that I could finish up the manuscript during fall 2001. The reference and interlibrary loan librarians at the Carol Newman Library at Virginia Tech have been consistently helpful in my search for obscure materials. Chris Barber at the La Leche League Center for Breastfeeding Information sent me a copy of the Ross Mothers Survey when I couldn't find it anywhere else. Evelyn Raines, Carol Womble, Tammy Shepherd, Judy Grady, Denise Royal, Dee Hezel, and Terri Whaling made copies for me, answered questions, sent faxes, and otherwise facilitated putting this manuscript together.

La Leche League leaders and members in Blacksburg were, and continue to be, extremely important to this book. They helped me breastfeed my children, conveyed authentic interest in my project, sent me articles and other pertinent materials, and asked me to speak to them about my research. Evalin Trice, Laura Tze, and Jenny Shuster are still leaders in this group. Evalin, Laura, and Marjorie Young were the lactation consultants at the local hospital when Sam was born and we needed a lot of nursing help. I don't think words can describe how important they were to us when he was sick and I was engorged, in pain, and very frightened. Other leaders include Freija

Bergthorsen, who has moved away, and Suzanne Glasson, who walks her dog by my house most days. Morning meetings at Kay Robinson-Beers's house are among some of my best memories of my first years in Blacksburg. I still talk about nursing and mothering with Susan Day and Margaret Radcliffe. Barbara Haney-Cocca, Maureen Campbell Lopina, and Jenny Shuster shared more than just a room at the La Leche League convention in Chicago, 2001; I learned from them to think more fully about the lives of league leaders.

Lawrence Gartner and Katherine Dettwyler provided key assistance with facts and information at important points in my research; I thank them for their generosity. Fiona Giles helped me with titles, suggesting all sorts of outlandish possibilities. Bill Germano had faith in this book while it was still a jumble of ideas. Years ago Linda Kerber suggested that I look at the work of Joan Williams; fortunately, I remembered that suggestion and discovered some of the most interesting contemporary work on gender and domesticity. Carolyn DiPalma and Beth Dolan reminded me of Donna Haraway's "Situated Knowledges."

The David and Rose Hausman clipping service became a reliable source for articles on breastfeeding and infant health, primarily from the *New York Times* and *JAMA,* but more recently from online sources. This service extended even to my mother's friend, Elaine Freeman, who also sent me choice articles and information. Special thanks and recognition go to Sydney and Dawn James, who noticed that a desk in the basement is not particularly conducive to serious scholarly research and subsequently built me an office by enclosing our carport. That they also put in a playroom is all the more reason to thank them, since Rachel and Sam have more space to hang out in while I read and write.

My writing group has included, over the years, Sally Sevcik, Moira Baker, Rita Kranidas, Rebecca Scheckler, Muriel Lederman, Kathleen Jones, Marian Mollin, and Martha McCaughey. Kathy, in particular, keeps me honest as only a historian can. Gretchen Michlitsch read through a number of chapters and offered significant comments before I sent the manuscript in, and Adrienne Berney sent me an e-mail letting me know about her fascinating dissertation, "Reforming the Maternal Breast," which proved enormously useful. Attentive audiences at the University of Pittsburgh, Indiana University, Virginia Tech, a Modern Language Association convention, and numerous Society for Literature and Science conference panels offered feedback on various portions of the book. During July 2002, the participants at the NEH Summer Institute in Medicine, Literature, and Culture at the Penn State Medical College celebrated my publishing contract with champagne, good company, and fine dancing.

Nancy Cervetti reads everything I send her, and talks to me at length about it all, usually late at night and with a lot of humor. I don't know what I'd do without her as a colleague and friend.

And a final thank-you to Clair, partner in love and life, who perseveres through my obsessive commitment to what I call "my work."

Most of chapter 2 and a portion of chapter 4 appeared in "Rational Management: Medical Authority and Ideological Conflict in Ruth Lawrence's *Breastfeeding: A Guide for the Medical Profession*," *Technical Communication Quarterly* 9.3 (Summer 2000): 271–89, and are published here by permission of the Association of Teachers of Technical Writing.

Portions of the introduction appeared in "Between Science and Nature: Interpreting Lactation Failure in Elizabeth von Arnim's *The Pastor's Wife*," *Journal of Medical Humanities* 20 (1999): 101–15, and are published here by permission of Human Sciences Press.

I follow La Leche League practice in the spelling of *breastfeeding* and *bottle feeding*. Quotations from other sources replicate the original spelling.

Introduction

Beginnings

When I was thinking about applying to graduate school in women's studies—as opposed to applying to medical school—I considered how my future career as a university professor might fit with my imagined future as a mother. Humanities professors, I thought, have flexible schedules, and while I knew little about motherhood, I did think that flexibility in one's work life might facilitate having a family. At the time, I wasn't thinking about nursing routines, or mother-infant attachment, or even sleep. I was just thinking about hours spent in an office versus hours spent at home. I thought that since a professor can often work at home (and a doctor usually can't), it seemed reasonable to assume that caring for a family would be somewhat easier on an academic schedule. Babies, I fantasized, slept a lot, and otherwise they were happy and played in their cribs.

As far as motherhood was concerned, I was clueless. After finishing graduate school in 1992, I landed a three-year position as well as a book contract. It seemed like the perfect time to have a baby: I wasn't (yet) on the tenure track, I had a year to revise my manuscript, and I had no professional responsibilities beyond teaching two sections of humanities to first-year students at the University of Chicago. By the time I would have to look for another job, I'd have a baby and published book; no one, I thought, would be able to say that having a baby had slowed my career.[1]

I was at a campus where pregnant women were few and far between; the one mother I knew well was the wife of a colleague, and she was not employed. I got an inkling of what I was in for when, during the final childbirth education class, the instructor encouraged new mothers to breastfeed and then said. "Don't be afraid if your baby seems to want to breastfeed all the time. That's a normal pattern for the first few weeks of life. Breastfed babies don't really have schedules." My teacher was a lawyer who had ample maternity leave after the birth of each child. I had the luxury of a two-month maternity "leave," but only because my baby was due during the summer when I wasn't teaching. By the time I realized that breastfeeding a baby might mean more than a ten-minute interruption every three or four hours, there was no going back. I was seven months pregnant, finishing up my book, and waiting for life as I knew it to end.

Most of my images of life with baby had been produced by formula companies, although I wasn't aware of it at the time. What I was told about breastfeeding—for example, that I should feed on demand rather than on a schedule—did not coincide with the images in my head, those sweet, plump babies that lolled in cribs while mom washed dishes or traded stocks, so I imagined that babies probably didn't demand to feed all that often. Like many other young career-oriented women in our radically age-segregated society, I hadn't spent a lot of time around babies. I hadn't paid attention to those few friends who had babies in graduate school, either; I am one of those people who was not very interested in babies until I had one myself. I hadn't thought about breastfeeding as anything but a superior kind of infant nutrition; indeed, I thought of it as a substitute for bottle feeding.

I was surprised to find myself, a feminist theorist, so little prepared for the experience of breastfeeding. Little that I had read as a graduate student made me aware of the physical burden of being my infant's sole source of nutrition for many months, of the sensual pleasures of nursing, of the exhaustion, or of the odd physiological connection to a dependent other. I had, however, thought about childbirth. As Pam Carter writes, a feminist practice has developed around childbirth, but no such practice has emerged around infant feeding (19). Judith Galtry has made similar observations ("Suckling and Silence" 2; " 'Sameness' and Suckling" 66). While clearly not all feminist mothers follow the same birth practices, women who seek information about how to have a more woman-centered birth experience, or who wish to avoid hospital routines geared toward convenience for the obstetrical staff rather than the mother's wishes, have an ample scholarly and lay literature to sample.[2]

In *Motherhood Reconceived: Feminism and the Legacies of the Sixties,* Lauri Umansky discusses early second-wave feminist perspectives on childbirth that included breastfeeding as a feminist practice. In feminist works that I was reading in the early 1990s, however, I found comments that indicated bottle feeding held the promise of women's liberation, or at least that breastfeeding was not necessary, or even preferred. For example, Nancy

Chodorow writes, "The earliest psychoanalytic theory stressed the importance of the biological feeding relationship in personality formation. Much recent theory, by contrast, suggests that infants require the whole parenting relationship of warmth, contact, and reliable care, and not the specific feeding relationship itself. This theory has been used to keep mothers in the home, *now that biological imperatives are less persuasive*" (217; emphasis added). Sandra Bem writes positively of the potential of "technological innovations such as antibiotics, refrigeration, birth control, and baby formula" to "liberate the human organism from what had once seemed its intrinsic biological limitations" (188). In my last example from what is clearly not an exhaustive list, Carolyn Heilbrun, in an argument against sociobiology, writes, "The history of civilization describes the process by which humans have distanced themselves from nature by inventing and perfecting culture. Traditionalists ignore technological changes, which have made it possible to bottle-feed infants safely and to raise them to adulthood with caretakers other than their own mothers" (20).

If feminists initially saw breastfeeding as part of a feminist practice of motherhood (Umansky, *Motherhood Reconceived*, 52–76), feminist scholars somehow forgot to pay attention to breastfeeding through the 1980s and early 1990s, or, as in the examples above, produced arguments in favor of artificial infant feeding. *Mother's Milk: Breastfeeding Controversies in American Culture* represents my attempt to produce a feminist interpretation of the meanings of breastfeeding in contemporary cultural contexts. It is, significantly, a book about representations, and in it I explore how analyzing representations of infant feeding can lead us to important conclusions about women's place in American society and about some current difficulties of maternal practice. In the United States, breastfeeding represents the complex, often conflicting, set of ideas and ideals about mothers that permeates American culture. There are no answers to most of the questions I explore here. Instead, investigating representations of breastfeeding shows us how deeply conflicted we are as a culture about mothers' practices, authority, and responsibility toward their offspring. What breastfeeding *means* is the result of a complex cultural mediation of many different factors; in this book, I trace some of these factors and their relation to each other. In the end, I suggest that in contemporary culture, a supportive social context for breastfeeding may be an important barometer of women's rights and possibilities.

Central to contemporary ideologies of maternity is the idea of *scientific motherhood*, which, as described by Rima Apple, designates the general cultural agreement that in order to be good mothers women must be guided by scientific advice and subjugate their own perspectives to those of authoritative experts. Apple's careful and convincing study, *Mothers and Medicine: A Social History of Infant Feeding, 1890–1950*, helps us to understand how bottle feeding became the default option for infant feeding in America, but its tight focus on social history tends to read formula advertisements as a reflection of historical developments. Thus, her analysis does not fully address the complexity of meanings produced by the images and discourses about infant feeding that American mothers face today.[3] One scholar who addresses this cultural field, anthropologist Katherine Dettwyler, has demonstrated the ways in which formula companies' advertising negatively portrays nursing mothers and represents breastfeeding as inferior to infant formulas (Dettwyler, "Tricks" and "Promoting"). Yet Dettwyler's analysis, like that of Baumslag and Michels, primarily criticizes the inaccurate and misleading discourses produced by infant formula manufacturers and supported by American social norms; this is only a first step in examining the representational context of infant feeding in the United States today. These powerful indictments of formula advertising and its misrepresentations leave open the possibility of a study that analyzes breastfeeding advocacy and formula promotion *together*, in order to draw a more comprehensive picture of the social and representational contexts of infant feeding and the cultural construction of motherhood in the contemporary United States. *Mother's Milk* thus emphasizes the richness of breastfeeding discourses and their significance as cultural documents.

This introduction briefly touches on many of the themes that I explore in subsequent chapters: the medicalization of infant feeding and the significance of mothering under the expert gaze of the physician; the loss of women's traditional transmission of knowledge about the body, maternity, and infant care; the tensions evident in a culture that reveres scientific medicine and yet wants mothering to be natural. Most significantly, however, I argue that thinking about breastfeeding in terms of representations is an interesting and fruitful approach, because it moves beyond simplifying arguments that currently dominate the field. What is often termed the "breast-bottle controversy" is not just about the rapaciousness of formula companies (a general premise of Gabrielle Palmer's *The Politics of Breastfeeding*), nor the lack of support for breastfeeding from medical personnel (a common lament among breastfeeding advocates), although both of those issues figure prominently in my analysis. Examining a variety of documents that exist in the public domain demonstrates that controversies over infant feeding are embedded in larger social conflicts concerning women as mothers and cannot be understood without detailed, close *readings*.

This cultural analysis partakes of a variety of methodologies. Primarily, I use rhetorical and semiotic readings—close readings of visual and discursive texts, readings that pay attention to the form of arguments and the function of signs—of documents likely to be read by mothers or their health care practitioners. But I also look at the way that other, more socially obscure, accounts of breastfeeding—those in literary texts and medical research, for example—represent the meaning of the practice, especially when such accounts illuminate the meanings evident in more popular sources. In the end, these readings demonstrate that breastfeeding has a signifying function in culture, and that this function must be understood in order to address the overall decline in maternal nursing in the United States that occurred during the first two-thirds of the twentieth century.[4] Current public health initiatives and volunteer efforts have helped to reverse this decline, particularly during the 1990s. To continue this trend, and to extend it to the Third World, which has been experiencing a decline in maternal nursing more recently, it is not enough to educate mothers and prospective mothers about the health benefits of breastfeeding; we must also, as a culture, attend to the meanings of lactation in the modern world.

Feminist attention to breastfeeding has picked up in the 1990s, perhaps in response to enhanced public health campaigns to support nursing, and it has focused on the political meanings of motherhood. British sociologist Pam Carter writes that "breast-feeding in fact represents one of the central dilemmas of feminism: should women attempt to minimize gender differences as the path to liberation or should they embrace and enhance gender difference by fighting to remove the constraints placed on them by patriarchy and capitalism, thus becoming more 'truly' women?" (14). *Mother's Milk* shows why this dualist approach to breastfeeding is nonproductive: by downplaying the biomedical significance of breastfeeding, conflicts about nursing are examined only in the context of strategic arguments concerning the meaning of gender. In contrast, I argue that breastfeeding must be addressed in current conflicts about women's roles and the relation of waged labor to family life because it is a biological caretaking practice that cannot be performed by men: breastfeeding represents, more than pregnancy, women's heavier reproductive burden.[5] When we consider the health advantages to breastfeeding (which I do later in this introduction), even in a First World context of safe water supplies and adequate medical care for many mothers and children, our answer to this reproductive burden cannot be to advocate for formula or suggest that infant feeding method makes no difference except in an ideological sense. Instead, we must make breastfeeding a real choice for women, rather than a practice that two-thirds of women "try" after birth and most often abandon within six months. If the particularity of mammalian sexual difference confers on women a greater biological burden in reproduction, we can choose to ensure that maternity does not hurt women's participation in civil society and the waged labor market; in other words, we can work to ensure that support for breastfeeding does not suggest the need to cloister women among themselves in the home.

Promoting breastfeeding does *not* have to mean promoting an outmoded traditionalist notion of domesticity for women, as some feminist critics suggest (see chapter 6 for this discussion). But such promotion must not shirk domesticity either: whether they do or do not work in the waged labor market, all mothers share some interest in increasing the social value of their work as family caretakers. All mothers would benefit from social recognition of the physical costs (and benefits) of biosocial maternal practices. Whether or not feminists have looked down on women who stay at home to care for their children, the common perception from such women is that feminists do not take their interests to heart. As Joan Williams so persuasively argues, no one (but men?) benefits from such a fracturing of women as an interest group. The social and economic marginalization of mothers is not a problem that can be fixed through technological innovation: we must do *political* work to pursue equality for all women, especially when women's biosocial practices are distinct from men's and involve the capacity to contribute substantially to enhanced health outcomes for both women and children.

As should be clear from the preceding discussion, I approach this study as a breastfeeding advocate. As anthropologist Penny Van Esterik has written, advocacy in the context of scholarly research can be a difficult balancing act (*Beyond* 20–27). I have found through working on this book for almost seven years that my support for breastfeeding—indeed, my enthusiasm and delight in the practice—is both echoed and repudiated as a basis for theoretical speculation by feminists. To be sure, working on this project has taught me to be more circumspect about those aspects of my own maternal practices that are clearly linked to being white, middle class, highly educated, and employed as a professional. Breastfeeding, as I argue later in the book, is an activity facilitated by flexible work, social and financial resources, and supportive professional and kin networks. At the same time, I have become frustrated with feminist collusion with the idea that in order not to induce guilt in mothers who don't or can't breastfeed, we shouldn't argue for its benefits, or even acknowledge that breastfeeding has a biological benefit at all. Surely there is a way to respect mothers' experiences without denying biomedical information about the body, and surely not every practice of white middle-class motherhood is suspect because it is made possible by class and race privilege. Pointing out such privileges, and the specific practices they facilitate, should help us to see why it is important to extend certain beneficial practices to all mothers and children, rather than to condemn those currently made practicable only for a few.[6]

Breastfeeding advocacy, this book will show, is not unproblematic. Its long legacy of collusion with forces seeking to regulate and constrain women's social practices and identities demands an examination. I turn now to a short history of breastfeeding advocacy in Europe and the United States, including in this discussion a consideration of specific historical periods when and regions where maternal nursing fell out of fashion.

Historical Perspectives on Breastfeeding and Breastfeeding Advocacy

Most mothers, throughout history, have nursed their own infants. Mothers who relied on wet nurses, or those who dry nursed their own offspring, have been in the minority, although in certain places at specific times they typified infant feeding practices.[7] France is often cited as an example of widespread wet nursing, as "during the eighteenth and nineteenth centuries the predominant pattern of infant care associated with larger, older cities like Paris and Lyon was rural wet-nursing" (Sussman 2). Indeed, as the tradition of wet nursing began to die out elsewhere in Europe in the eighteenth century, especially among the aristocratic class that had depended upon it almost exclusively in the seventeenth century, France continued with the practice of rural wet nursing (Sussman 6–7). Medical and moral breastfeeding advocacy, until the nineteenth and twentieth centuries, concerned maternal nursing versus wet nursing; as Janet Golden points out, the distinction concerned which woman should nurse one's baby. It is only in very recent history that some women (those in developed countries or the elite in developing countries) could choose against breastfeeding by any woman and expect their infants to survive.

Certain groups have practiced dry nursing exclusively, although, as Valerie Fildes notes, "All the nonbreastfeeding regions so far identified were in Northern Europe, had a cold dry climate, and many were in mountainous terrain"; the cold climate facilitated dry nursing because milk and other foods fed to infants were less likely to spoil ("Culture and Biology" 104). Some cultures abandoned breastfeeding even though the alternatives often resulted in infant death. In seventeenth- and eighteenth-century Iceland, for example, a period during which the infant mortality rate was exceptionally high, infants were breastfed, if at all, very briefly (a week or two), and then fed dairy milk, cream, or fish mixed with cream or butter. This feeding pattern, according to a visiting physician in the eighteenth century, "virtually killed the infants" (Hastrup 96). According to Kirsten Hastrup, the diet was linked to cultural conceptions of women's worth ("farm produce seems to have become a symbol of women's values" [101]), as well as to ideas about national culture in reaction to Danish rule ("Icelandicness had been defined by the domestication of nature. Farming remained the essence of Icelandicness, and in the course of history the stress upon this particular characteristic had more or less fatal consequences" [103]). Yet for *most* populations throughout history, the linkage between breastfeeding and infant survival meant that most infants were fed at the breast. Wet nursing was understood to provide less than optimal nourishment for infants and was undertaken when economic or social circumstances demanded it (the mother needed to work or was obligated by her husband to fulfill specific social duties).[8] The babies of the wet nurses themselves were either nursed along with their charges, put out to nurse with women further down the socioeconomic ladder, or dry nursed, practices that clearly affected mortality rates for poor infants.

Historical approaches to breastfeeding and breastfeeding advocacy pay special attention to periods in which the social meanings of breastfeeding seem to change. Most Western historians see the eighteenth century as a turning point in the transformation of both the practices of maternal nursing and the meanings placed on such practices. For example, in her wide-ranging study, *A History of the Breast*, Marilyn Yalom wraps up her chapter on the "political breast" with the following comment:

> Breasts ... began to take on political significance in the eighteenth century. Since then, women have been asked to offer up their breasts in the service of national and international interests. At certain historical moments, they have been mandated to breast-feed in order to increase the national birthrate, to reduce infant mortality, and to regenerate society. At other times, they have been directed toward bottle-feeding and milk substitutes. In times of war and revolution, they have been encouraged to pad their breasts "for the soldier boys" or to uncover them as symbols of freedom. Breast politics have emanated from a wide spectrum of governmental, economic, religious, and health-care sources—all traditionally male-dominated institutions not known for putting women's interests at the top of their priorities. Not until the late twentieth century would women themselves begin to have a significant say in the sexual politics controlling their breasts. (144–45)

This perspective on the political significance of breasts in the West seems generally accepted in the feminist historical literature. Londa Schiebinger discusses the politics of breastfeeding advocacy in the eighteenth century, arguing that Carl Linnaeus was influenced by the conflict over maternal nursing to name mammals with the Latin word for breasts: "Linnaeus's term *Mammalia* helped to legitimize the restructuring of European society by emphasizing how natural it was for females—both human and nonhuman—to suckle and rear their own children" (74; emphasis in original). Ruth Perry argues that medical breastfeeding advocacy was a "novel phenomenon" in the eighteenth century: "Nothing like it existed earlier," when women were assumed to obtain information about nursing from other women, and physicians were not the repositories of expertise on maternal practices (216).

For Yalom, Schiebinger, and Perry, the politics surrounding the breast are evinced in public discourses concerning its use and purpose. The question of whether breasts are primarily erotic or primarily nurturant is at the heart of these politics; for Perry, this question obscures a more significant social phenomenon:

> The movement to promote breast-feeding in the latter part of the eighteenth century has always been understood as the sane light of reason penetrating the dark corners of superstitious compulsion. Randolph Trumbach has argued that breast-feeding and maternal care lowered the aristocratic death rate in the second half of the eighteenth century and that it was "one of the finest fruits of the Enlightenment." What I have been trying to suggest is that this movement involved an unprecedented cultural use of women and the appropriation of their bodies for procreation. A discourse including sentimental fiction and medical treatises functioned as a new way to colonize the female body and to designate within women's experience a new arena of male expertise, control, and instruction. (231)

For Perry, the ideological ramifications of the eighteenth-century return to maternal nursing in the upper classes, based as it was on a moralistic and misogynistic advocacy campaign, trump the biological consequences of such practice.[9]

As I will discuss in chapter 6, this position typifies the feminist critique of contemporary breastfeeding advocacy. I bring it up here to demonstrate how some historical considerations of breastfeeding in Europe and America similarly advance a perspective on nursing that highlights ideology and downplays the significance of biology.[10] In other words, feminist scholars, and feminist historians in particular, understand the *meaning* of breastfeeding to be about politics; they neglect the biological significance of nursing, which may have contributed to decreased mortality rates among aristocratic infants and mothers in the eighteenth century. Other histories of breastfeeding emphasize the biological at the expense of the political; for example, Valerie Fildes's "The Culture and Biology of Breastfeeding: An Historical Review of Western Europe" offers the following conclusion:

> [I]t does appear that the beneficial effects of breastfeeding for mother and child have been known since time immemorial. Breastfeeding was known to affect the nutrition, the physical and psychological health of the child, and the health and fertility of the mother. As this chapter has shown, the decision to breastfeed or not and the timing

> and type of supplemental and weaning foods have had profound effects on maternal and infant health throughout history. (121)

These competing views represent a significant divergence in historical approaches to breastfeeding and breastfeeding advocacy and, clearly, affect what I can present here as a history of this topic: any history of breastfeeding negotiates a contested terrain with its own sources. Indeed, the conflict between these views pervades almost all approaches to breastfeeding, as contemporary critics are apt to highlight the "exhortation" to breastfeed (emphasizing breastfeeding advocacy as ideological support for maternal regulation; Blum, *At the Breast*, 50), while advocates decry the bottle feeding culture (emphasizing cultural practices that inhibit biologically natural infant feeding). Janet Golden's *A Social History of Wet Nursing in America: From Breast to Bottle* is one source that successfully integrates biological views of breastfeeding with an analysis of its cultural meanings, demonstrating that attending to the political meanings need not entail neglect of biological discourses.[11]

The eighteenth century is considered a watershed in the practice of breastfeeding in the West and the significance of breastfeeding advocacy for several reasons. During this period, male medical practitioners became prominent in advice concerning nursing. Ruth Perry argues that in the seventeenth and early eighteenth centuries, "Women were expected to learn these things [breastfeeding] from other women in a tradition of oral advice and lore. . . . By the middle of the [eighteenth] century, however, motherhood became the focus of a new kind of cultural attention. . . . Both scientists and moralists suddenly had a great deal to say about how women ought to behave as mothers" (214). Enlightenment thinkers like Jean-Jacques Rousseau and Mary Wollstonecraft promoted maternal nursing as a practice of women's virtue. Sexuality and maternity began to be seen as separate functions of women's roles as wives and mothers, and Perry argues that "the desexualization of women was accomplished, in part, by redefining them as maternal rather than sexual beings. . . . the maternal succeeded, supplanted, and repressed the sexual definition of women, who began to be reimagined as nurturing rather than desiring, as supportive rather than appetitive" (213). This realignment contributed to the identification of women with a sentimentalized domesticity in the nineteenth century. American discourses followed the European model, although wet nursing was never as institutionalized in colonized North America as it was in France.

If medical authority over infant feeding helped ground the calls for maternal nursing in the eighteenth century, the nineteenth century saw an intensification of medical views, leading up to the ubiquity of scientific motherhood in twentieth-century representations and experience. Adrienne Berney, in her dissertation *Reforming the Maternal Breast: Infant Feeding and American Culture, 1870–1940*, argues that the nineteenth-century focus on the maternal breast—nurturant center of family life and the home—diminished as the breast became increasingly sexualized (this would be the reverse of the transformation Ruth Perry analyzed in the eighteenth century). Indeed, Berney argues that a husband could "be involved in his wife's lactation" in the nineteenth century, for example, by sucking off excess milk from engorged breasts, but in the twentieth century, "the benefits of breast feeding for mother and child became potentially irrelevant in the face of threats to conjugal affection" (107). During the first half of the nineteenth century, mothers were still considered authorities concerning infant care. In the middle of the nineteenth century, as the social and cultural effects of the Industrial Revolution took hold, American physicians and reformers began to notice what seemed to them a significant decline in maternal nursing, yet the steps taken to reverse this decline had an ambivalent effect. Nineteenth-century concerns articulated skepticism about the "declining stamina of American women" and suspicion about the biological quality of specific women's breast milk (Berney 42). Janet Golden writes,

> A belief that middle- and upper-class women were weak vessels who could not fulfill their biological duties was a distinguishing characteristic of both the popular and the professional medical literature. Doctors had begun to suspect that some middle- and upper-class women lacked the physical stamina necessary to withstand the pain of childbirth and therefore required anesthesia. Similarly, they surmised that well-to-do women found breast-feeding more difficult than did lower-class women. (53)

Yet although developing medical perspectives assumed that poor and working-class women were physically able to breastfeed better than their more affluent sisters, milk depots were first set up in urban centers to lower infant mortality and morbidity among the lower classes, perhaps because these were mothers least likely to be able to pay a wet nurse when their employment or physical status precluded maternal nursing. The first infant health clinics were established in the 1860s, and dispensed "pure [dairy] milk" along with encouragement to breastfeed.[12] Thus the widespread skepticism about certain women's ability to lactate and the dispensing of dairy milk to supplement inadequate human milk production or to compensate for mothers' absence from the home helped to create a context in which practices that encouraged women to breastfeed occurred in tandem with actions that led to its disappearance. As historian Jacqueline Wolf writes, "although physicians continued to recommend human milk over cows' milk for babies throughout the milk campaigns, the unrelenting publicity generated by the clean-milk crusades touted pasteurized, sealed, and bottled cows' milk as safe, palatable sustenance for babies. Soon it was the preferable sustenance as well" (46).

In the early twentieth century, evolutionary discourses encouraged white Americans to think of themselves as "evolv[ing] ... beyond the class mammalia" (Berney 50) and promoted a racialized understanding of women's lactational capacity and practice. Advocates promoted rationalized breastfeeding that mandated scheduled feedings in the context of exclusive nursing for six to nine months; these same advocates criticized foreign, working-class, and nonwhite mothers for irrational breastfeeding that cohered with family or ethnic traditions and that allowed feeding on demand and supplementation with table scraps or other adult foods. Berney states that most breastfeeding women surveyed in the 1920s who did not nurse for the ideal nine months gave "insufficient milk" as their reason, even though they may have nursed into the sixth or seventh month. Clearly the idea of insufficient milk became accepted early in the twentieth century as a convenient and medically resonant rationale for early weaning. This is not to say that some women didn't suffer from milk insufficiency, but that it is unlikely that a woman who could provide milk through the first half of her infant's first year would suddenly be unable to produce enough in the seventh month, unless external circumstances changed her ability to eat enough food, drink enough liquids, and get enough rest. "Insufficient milk" thus became a label women could use to describe a decision to end breastfeeding, for a variety of reasons that we cannot presume to know now but that were embedded in cultural changes around breastfeeding and maternity in general. (I discuss current discourses concerning insufficient milk, which currently usually refers to a condition diagnosed in the early weeks of an infant's life, in chapter 1.)

As part of rational breastfeeding practices, reformers attempted to regulate the age of weaning, arguing that breastfeeding beyond nine months was a health risk for the child. In Berney's analysis, it is not the breast or bottle issue that defined the shift toward bottle feeding in the twentieth century, but the opposition between rational and irrational feeding: rational feeding favored scheduling and other behavioral approaches to infant care (advice not to pick up crying infants, cuddle them, or sleep with them, for example). These rational practices favored by reformers and burgeoning pediatric experts worked against the rhythms of demand suckling that helped women establish and maintain their milk. Thus, even when ideas about infant care relaxed in the late 1930s, breastfeeding rates continued to fall because the notions of schedules and scientifically mediated maternal practices were too strongly entrenched to dislodge. The damage in terms of breastfeeding advocacy had already been done, with women's confidence over the process declining.

In addition, changing expectations about women's roles as wives and household managers conflicted with more traditional breastfeeding lifestyles.[13] This is an important point that cannot be stressed enough. Maternal nursing did not initially decline as a response to women's involvement in waged labor outside the home, although such involvement may have decreased the duration of nursing for many poor, working women in the nineteenth and early twentieth centuries. I agree with Adrienne Berney that much of the decline in nursing was the result of cultural forces that transformed heterosexual women's position in the family—their relationships to children and to their spouses—and mandated that modern women be efficient and scientific household managers. Even if modern mothers breastfed, they were likely to do so under the strictures of scientific motherhood and rational breastfeeding regimes, both of which undermined the physiological success of lactation.[14]

Thus, American women's decline in breastfeeding from the nineteenth century to today results from the following factors:

- their changing roles;
- the rise of pediatrics and the desire to control infant feeding in order to reduce infant mortality and morbidity;
- the popularity of rationalized breastfeeding practices among physicians trying to Americanize foreigners, regulate women, and bring up independent American children;
- changing perceptions of the family and women's relations with children (increasingly distant) and spouses (increasingly close);
- the availability of breast milk substitutes that are relatively safe when augmented by medical support and hygienic maternal practices and environments;
- the fact that breastfeeding advocacy no longer targeted wet nursing (and other women's milk) but formula as the inferior infant feeding practice;
- an emerging taboo on mothers nursing in public; and
- women's desires to operate in a civic world and waged labor force that mandate that they be like men to be accepted as equal.

Recently, laws have had to be established conferring upon women the *right* to nurse in public without being arrested for obscenity. Throughout all these changes, physicians as a group have supported the belief that breast milk is the best food for infants, but have not been able to support breastfeeding itself, either because of a lack of practical knowledge about the normal course of lactation, or because of lingering skepticism about the human female's generic capacity to produce milk.

Moral arguments about breastfeeding tend to dominate biological perspectives for a variety of reasons. Biological meanings of breastfeeding are obscured in the contemporary United States because the medical system and general standard of living tend to mask biological deficits of feeding with formula. As we have seen, medical breastfeeding advocacy has, since the eighteenth century, tended to couple its call for maternal nursing with claims to mothers' duty toward their children and thus a moralistic view of maternal responsibility, although, as Janet Golden remarks, "Nearly every European commentator knew that wet nursing increased infant mortality" (14). The linkage between biological benefit to the infant and mothers' moral duty continues to influence medical conferences featuring breastfeeding advocacy, such as the annual La Leche League Seminar on Breastfeeding for Physicians, although recently such moralistic emphasis has diminished in favor of a view highlighting the struggles women face to breastfeed their infants. Moral ideals of maternal duty continue in contemporary advocates' common assumption of a traditional heterosexual family structure, replete with economic support from the male spouse and an idealized financial dependence on the part of the mother. Breastfeeding advocacy also stakes its claim on the growing body of medical research documenting the health advantages of maternal nursing. Yet, as I show in chapter 6, feminist critics worry that contemporary breastfeeding advocacy is another version of the same story Perry tells, of the political colonization of women's bodies in the guise of improving health and families.

No contemporary feminist approach to breastfeeding and breastfeeding advocacy should simply dismiss, across the board, the information the scientific data offers. Skepticism of scientific claims to neutrality is an established aspect of feminist science studies research, and I am not arguing here for a wholesale refutation of that approach. Throughout *Mother's Milk* I approach biomedical discourses about breastfeeding from a critical perspective. What I want to suggest here is that an engagement with these discourses may provide feminists with a *political* strategy for pressing women's rights as mothers. Feminist critics of breastfeeding advocacy generally fear the essentialist linkage of biological perspectives with traditional ideologies of female domesticity, but the discourses of science are no more essentialist in nature than any other discourse. The key issue is how such discourses are framed politically. As Donna Haraway writes, the "problem is how to have *simultaneously* an account of radical historical contingency for all knowledge claims and knowing subjects, a critical practice for recognizing our own 'semiotic technologies' for making meanings, *and* a no-nonsense commitment to faithful accounts of a 'real' world" ("Situated Knowledges" 187; emphases in original).

The scientific case for breastfeeding, as one kind of "faithful account of a real world," represents a sustained argument about the significance of the mother's body for the infant. Indeed, the argument calls for a different conceptualization of the mother and infant—as a unique subject, a *dyad*, whose indivisibility at a physiological level suggests the inadequacy of contemporary notions of adult personhood to account for it. The scientific case for breastfeeding could initiate a new kind of attention to maternity, if it were to be yoked to a feminist political discourse about women's rights. Historically, as we have seen, medicine articulates a moralistic discourse about maternal responsibility that links nursing with an idealized and sentimentalized concept of the good mother, but biological discourses of maternity need not be framed by misogyny.

That general argument grounds my approach throughout this book, as well as the criticisms I launch against certain kinds of scientific breastfeeding advocacy. There are numerous points at which breastfeeding advocacy colludes with traditional scientific misogyny. What distinguishes this study from other recent feminist explorations of breastfeeding is my willingness to engage with the scientific case for breastfeeding as both discourse and information. I integrate a critical view of science as a site of cultural authority with a consideration of scientific information on its own terms. Further, I analyze the scientific case as a set of stories about mothering and the maternal body, as well as treat it as a data set crucially important to maternal and child health. In my view, infant feeding is a social practice that exemplifies how ordinary people interpret scientific claims about health, and the meaning of medical evidence can never be easily separated from the rhetoric of its presentation. In addition, scientific claims interact with other representations and assertions about infant feeding. But scientific claims for the biological benefits of breastfeeding cannot be dismissed as only discursive, without material effects that can be measured in physiological terms. The trick is to balance the analysis: to note where arguments rooted in biomedical evidence ignore political realities, and to suggest when interpretations of sociocultural conditions should pay attention to biomedical claims about health. In Haraway's terms, we must be responsible for the kind of knowledge that we produce and support.

In order to argue for feminist attention to the scientific case for breastfeeding, I next present an outline of its main features. Following that discussion, I work though the issue of medicalization, which is linked to the scientific case for breastfeeding but is not the same thing. The medicalization of infant feeding constitutes a significant part of the twentieth-century trend of scientific motherhood, a paradigm of maternal practice that subordinates women's agency to the expertise of doctors. This linkage of scientific data to a paradigm of medicalization that diminishes women's authority as mothers makes it difficult, but no less imperative, to argue for breastfeeding as a political right of women.

The Scientific Case for Breastfeeding

What I call the scientific case for breastfeeding is an argument for the biological benefits of breastfeeding over artificial infant feeding and rests on a few general principles: (1) that mammalian milk is species specific, meaning that specific species' milks have characteristics particular to the nutritional needs and evolved practices of those species; (2) that breast milk contains immunological properties unique to the breastfeeding relationship, because antibodies developed in the mother's system are transmitted through breast milk to the infant, whose immune system is underdeveloped at birth; and (3) that the social relation between mother and infant that develops through breastfeeding confers substantial, yet difficult to quantify, advantages on those infants who are breastfed. Artificial infant foods, a term that designates all such foods produced to substitute for human milk, can come close to replicating some of the factors in breast milk (fat content, for example, or ratio of protein to sugar), but cannot, in this perspective, ever exactly replicate human milk or the specific attributes of breastfeeding because those are conferred in the context of the physiological and intersubjective *relation* between nursing mother and child. Indeed, for many breastfeeding advocates, the nursing relationship signifies an intense biological connection that necessitates thinking of the *nursing dyad* as the proper object of analysis, rather than the potentially separable mother and child.

Currently, the scientific case for breastfeeding relies on evidence-based medicine and the mass of statistically significant studies that suggest the biological benefits of breastfeeding. (Historically, as I pointed out above, physicians and others have known the relative mortality and morbidity of breastfed versus nonbreastfed infants, even if the tools to demonstrate the specific biological benefit have not been available.) But a parade of statistics to demonstrate and confirm the scientific case is not, I believe, what is called for here—a blank presentation of statistics can cut short an intellectual consideration of meaning, and they need to be understood in light of their rhetorical propensity to persuade. Yet Donna Haraway writes, "Feminists have high stakes in the speculum of statistical knowledge for opening up otherwise invisible, singular experience to reconfigure public, widely lived reality. Credible statistical representation is one aspect of building connection and coalition. . . . Providing powerful statistical data is essential to effective public representations of what feminist and other progressive freedom and justice projects mean" (*Modest Witness* 199).[15] With this in mind, I want to provide a discussion of the general ideas supported by the scientific case, as a way of demonstrating how practitioners of what is increasingly called "breastfeeding medicine" perceive the uniqueness of human milk and its qualities. Presenting the scientific case in a self-consciously discursive manner highlights its existence as an *argument* rather than a set of facts, what Haraway might call an example of feminist objectivity that she referred to as "situated knowledge" ("Situated Knowledges" 188). In chapter 2, "Rational Management," I consider how the presentation of scientific evidence in a guidebook for physicians is interwoven with ideological perspectives on maternal sexuality and maternal authority. Here, however, I simply want to present, primarily from the advocates' perspective, the scientific bases of the biological benefits of breastfeeding. The scientific understanding of the claims made for breastfeeding needs to be accounted for in any treatment of the politics of breastfeeding advocacy.

Breast milk is a substance; breastfeeding is a practice. Attention to both substance and practice is at the root of scientific approaches to establishing the biological benefit of breastfeeding. For example, studies demonstrating the health benefits of tube-feeding breast milk to premature infants unable to take nourishment by mouth focus on the specific nutritional impact of the substance of breast milk. Other studies, focusing on the relational benefits of early initiation of breastfeeding, document the emotional and developmental benefits of breastfeeding as a practice. Babies who breastfeed suck in a manner appropriate to optimal facial and mandibular development, for example. Because the substance can, at times, be separated from the practice through the use of breast pumps or manual expression and a variety of feeding methods (bottle, cup, or syringe feeding), and because many women in Western society must depend on such arrangements to get breast milk into their infants and to maintain their milk supply while they are separated from their infants, breastfeeding advocates tend, at times, to reify breast milk as a miraculous fluid (liquid gold). But the scientific case for breastfeeding, as a whole, links the practice and the substance together and studies the benefits of the whole package, albeit through disaggregating the relevant factors for analysis.

In this literature, the human infant is often considered an exterogestate fetus (as compared to other mammalian infants) and believed to have specific nutritional requirements for rapid growth after birth, including milk low in protein and high in carbohydrates (Lawrence, "Breastfeeding Advantages"). The low fat content of the milk suggests a need to nurse often, appropriate to a species with frequent or continuous contact between mother and baby and opposed to those species that leave their offspring for long periods in order to procure food (cache species). Generally, arguments about the specificity of human milk to human infants rely on evolutionary discourses concerning species adaptation; while in some human groups adults have developed the capacity to consume large quantities of dairy milk with little ill effect, infants continue to rely on the evolved capacity of human breast milk for what is termed optimal development.

The immunological properties of human milk are various and include immunoglobulins (antibodies to specific microbes), helpful molecules such as lactoferrin (which binds to free iron in the infant's gut so that it can't be utilized by the pathogenic bacteria that thrive on it), and immune cells (white blood cells, or leukocytes, that fight infection and initiate other immune responses).[16] Colostrum, which is the thick yellowish substance produced after birth but before the "true milk" comes in, is especially rich in immune cells. These various factors benefit the infant in numerous ways: some protect the infantile (and immature) lining of the gut, some help the infant ward off infections by transferring antibodies from the mother to the child, and some limit the infectious potential of existing bacteria. Especially significant is the fact that the mother produces antibodies to microbes specific to her environment; because her environment is the same as the infant's, the latter is offered protection from those germs most likely to pose a threat.

All of these immunological factors protect the infant while its own immune system is immature and underdeveloped, and lend scientific credence to the long-known fact that breastfed infants tend to get sick less often than infants dry nursed or fed animal milks or formula. As Jack Newman states, "Until fairly recently, most physicians presumed that breast-fed children fared better simply because milk supplied directly from the breast is free of bacteria. Formula, which must often be mixed with water and placed in bottles, can become contaminated easily. Yet even infants who receive sterilized formula suffer from more meningitis and infection of the gut, ear, respiratory tract, and urinary tract than do breast-fed youngsters" (76).[17] The United States Department of Health and Human Services *HHS Blueprint for Action on Breastfeeding* lists seven specific infections that are lower in incidence or severity in breastfed infants in comparison to formula fed infants: diarrhea, respiratory tract infections, otitis media, pneumonia, urinary infections, necrotizing enterocolitis, and invasive bacterial infections (10). At the core of the scientific case for breastfeeding lies this argument concerning its protective effect against specific acute illnesses in infants.[18]

Less clearly defined in the clinical literature is the immunological protection conferred by breastfeeding against chronic disease. One difficulty in many studies of breastfeeding and morbidity is the lack of a consistent definition of breastfeeding and problems with retrospective analyses that depend on mothers' recollections of their infant feeding practices (see Heinig and Dewey).[19] Breastfeeding advocates claim a protective effect against childhood cancers, Crohn's disease, Celiac disease, type I diabetes, asthma, and atopic dermatitis (eczema), among other illnesses. It is clear from the way that such claims are presented that the evidence is not considered definitive; in exceptionally qualified language, Ruth Lawrence writes, "A *few* epidemiological studies with a *small number* of subjects have produced information to *suggest* that breastfeeding exclusively for four months or longer can provide *some* immunological protection against *some* childhood onset chronic diseases" ("Breastfeeding Advantages" 31; emphasis added). Heinig and Dewey, in their 1996 review of the literature on breastfeeding, are slightly more forceful in their assessment of the protective effect of breastfeeding, but qualify their view nonetheless. According to Lawrence, there is greater evidence for breastfeeding's protective effect against food allergy and allergy-related conditions like eczema and asthma (31). Breastfed babies do seem to respond more robustly to immunizations, as measured in levels of antibodies (Newman 79). Breastfeeding may help prevent sudden infant death syndrome (SIDS), which is "the leading cause of infant mortality after the first month of life, accounting for one-third of all infant deaths" in the United States, and is "the major cause of death for black infants between the ages of one month and one year" (Galtry, "Suckling and Silence," 4), although this is a contested claim (see American Academy of Pediatrics, Task Force on Infant Sleep Position and Sudden Infant Death Syndrome).

One of the most controversial aspects of the scientific case for breastfeeding concerns arguments for developmental advantages—increased IQ (or other measure of cognition) and better bonding between mother and child. Although theories of biological bonding between mother and infant in the first hours after birth have been refuted in the scientific literature itself (see Eyer), Marshall Klaus continues to promote these ideas in influential policy contexts ("Perinatal Care in the 21st Century," *Report of the National Breastfeeding Conference*). While it might seem obvious to maintain mother-infant contact in the immediate postpartum period (primarily because there are no good medical reasons to separate healthy infants from healthy mothers), the rationale of bonding to ward off possible infant abandonment and abuse does not seem to have strong scientific support. Research concerning cognitive development is equally fraught with controversy, given that measures of cognitive development are routinely questioned as to cultural bias.[20] Some cognitive development research concerning breastfeeding has focused on premature infants fed by nasogastric tubing, in order to control for maternal influence and contact during feeding; thus, this area of research is really about the purported "intelligence effect" of breast milk as a substance. In a recent review of the literature concerning infant feeding and cognitive development, Drane and Logemann write that most of the existing studies did not meet specific standards for generalizability, although "Four of the six studies meeting all three standards found an advantage in cognitive development to breast-fed infants of the order of two to five IQ points for term infants and eight points for low birthweight infants." These authors conclude that the research to this point does not offer conclusive answers to questions concerning the effect of infant feeding method on cognitive development. A recent Danish study suggests "a robust association between the duration of breastfeeding and adult intelligence," although the authors do admit that "the question remains whether duration of breastfeeding in our samples was associated with unregistered factors that correlate with offspring intellectual development" (Mortensen et al. 2370).[21]

Thus, even though intelligence testing carries a high risk of ethnoracial bias and confounding factors are difficult to control, some researchers claim that breastfeeding confers a small but significant beneficial effect on intelligence. Jane Heinig and Kathryn Dewey write,

> Taken as a whole, the results of studies on both term and preterm infants are remarkably consistent in showing that breast feeding is associated with enhanced cognitive development. Further research is needed to establish whether this is a causal relationship, and to elucidate the potential mechanisms involved. These mechanisms could include not only the influence of certain breast milk constituents on central nervous system development, but also behavioural aspects related to maternal-infant interaction during breast feeding. (93)

As Katherine Dettwyler suggests, the benefit in terms of IQ is similar to the deficit linked to lead exposure, which provokes a public health outcry (i.e., formula use leads to an IQ deficit similar to that measured in moderate to severe lead poisoning ["Beauty and the Breast" 201]). In addition, Dettwyler has also suggested that, while the incremental increase in IQ might not matter on the upper end of the spectrum, it may well mean the difference between independent living and institutionalization for those individuals on the lower end (e-mail to author). In the end, however, developmental advantages are the hardest to prove because they are based on culturally influenced ideals concerning intelligence and ability, and because other advantages, like those attributed to immunological factors in breastfeeding, are measurable in terms of a clear deficit in formula fed babies: as a population, they experience higher morbidity. Developmental factors are just harder to measure in scientifically credible ways.[22]

There is an emerging discussion in medical circles concerning the benefits of breastfeeding for women, which may include lower rates of premenopausal breast cancer and ovarian cancer, among other illnesses, but the research is relatively new and lacks consensus (Fred Howard). Another condition that interests researchers is osteoporosis. Women seem to lose bone density while breastfeeding but later increase bone density in the period directly after weaning. Interest in the impact of breastfeeding on women's health will clearly add to (or complicate) the scientific case in the years to come.

As I stated above, the viability of this scientific case is a core conflict between feminist critics of breastfeeding and advocacy discourses. I found the scientific case compelling as an expectant mother—but in an abstract, ill-defined way: I decided to nurse because I knew that it was medically recommended, but I couldn't have articulated the specific reasons for that recommendation. In that sense, I was simply following the practice of the majority of women of my race, class, and educational status, who also breast-feed for a host of historically determined reasons we don't usually account for. After further study, I found the scientific case for breastfeeding even more compelling, but I do not think that women who decide against breast-feeding make their decision as a repudiation of this case; other factors, it seems to me, make its arguments not less compelling but less determinative of maternal practice.[23]

One cultural development affects all American women's choices regarding infant feeding: medicalization, in the context of increasing institutional oversight of all maternal practices. The promotion of breastfeeding as biologically beneficial to infants and mothers has occurred in the context of the medicalization of all forms of infant feeding, a process that has contributed to the diminution of maternal authority and also, I believe, to the decline in breastfeeding. But because of medicine's current role in child nurture and development, breastfeeding advocacy has progressed within the context of medicalization, and not against it. Even La Leche League, which seeks to return authority to the mother through breastfeeding, relies on its cordial relationship with medical professionals and its own version of scientific motherhood to promote its cause (see chapter 5 for an extended discussion). Medicalization offers breastfeeding advocacy a complex legacy, which I explore in the next section.

Medicalization and Breastfeeding

As I argue in chapter 5, since the 1950s breastfeeding promotion has increasingly depended on the discourses of scientific medicine. In the early days of La Leche League, the group claimed that breastfeeding was healthful and natural; in the early years of the twenty-first century, complex discussions of the chemical composition of human milk and its unique properties to heal or to prevent disease dominate the discourses of lay breastfeeding advocacy. This progression can be understood teleologically: evidence-based medicine has demonstrated, through its own meteoric development, what it is, precisely, about human milk that makes breastfed babies "more healthful."[24] But this progression can also be understood to indicate the extent to which infant feeding has come under the purview of a medical institution that is increasingly scientific in the kinds of claims that it can make. In this sense, medicine promotes breastfeeding through scientific research studies because that is how medicine makes claims to health; it is also how medicine as a profession keeps breastfeeding (and all forms of infant feeding) under its purview.

The medicalization of infant feeding, as with other aspects of well-baby care, has had profound effects on women's maternal practices (see Apple, *Mothers and Medicine*; Litt), but it has had particularly ambivalent effects on the cultural construction of breastfeeding because medicine both promotes breastfeeding in its official pronouncements *and* often mishandles it in practice. Medicalization is the "transformation of general social problems into technical medical concerns, and the elaboration of medicine as the basis of social control" (Turner 9). In America, infant feeding was medicalized, in conjunction with the development of proprietary infant formulas, beginning in the late nineteenth century.[25] This complex process was the result, at least in part, of mothers' concerns to provide adequately for their infants, in the context of the expansion of their roles as women in modern society. Just as women sought out pain relief during childbirth, ultimately resulting in a diminishment of their control over the experience, mothers wanted safe alternatives to breastfeeding and participated in the overt medicalization of infant feeding (Leavitt; Apple, *Mothers and Medicine*). Thus it would be incorrect to claim that mothers have been victimized by a rapacious medical profession trying to arrogate all authority over infants. Nevertheless, the medicalization of infant feeding, occurring in conjunction with the development of scientific motherhood, has destabilized maternal authority and replaced it with the figure of the doctor. These developments occurred, of course, in concert with the transformation of medicine in the United States from a "weak, divided, insecure" profession with little social power to one that was "powerful, prestigious, and wealthy" (Starr, *Social Transformation*, 7–8), and, significantly, one that claimed increasing authority to manage previously nonmedical social practices. The medicalization of infant feeding and the development of scientific motherhood occurred in concert with the medicalization of American life in general.

Throughout the last century, however, breast milk remained the ideal infant food, even if it was no longer considered the standard (Apple, *Mothers and Medicine*, 157, 166; see also Wolf). Notwithstanding the profound connections between the emerging specialization of pediatrics and infant formula proprietors, the medical community always considered breast milk best for baby, but from the early part of the century through the 1960s, there was doubt as to whether women could actually feed their babies.

Formula was felt to be good enough, or an improvement in those many cases in which mothers were too harried or nervous to provide their own milk (Apple, *Mothers and Medicine*, 150–66). Infant formula was considered the *scientific* method of infant feeding, however, and it was the infant feeding method that physicians received some education about (Apple, *Mothers and Medicine*, 176). Jacquelyn Litt's study of Jewish and African-American mothers' experiences of medicalized motherhood in this century demonstrates that bottle feeding was, at least for the Jewish women in the study, a way to construct an identity as a modern *American* woman whose mothering practices were directed by physicians (109). Today, in the United States, physicians continue to have more experience with bottle feeding, both because it is culturally commonplace and because infant feeding in general isn't a focus for medical school curricula. Breastfeeding advocates in the medical profession continue to decry the lack of understanding concerning breastfeeding in the general population of medical personnel.[26] Physicians and other medical professionals don't know the basic physiology of lactation, often thinking of it along the model of bottle feeding (emptying the breast, for example), and are uncomfortable with the lack of quantifiability in lactation (i.e., they can't tell exactly how much milk the baby gets).

Formula use is bolstered by the medical model of infant care: antibiotics are necessary to cure infections that could be prevented or lessened by the immunities conferred by breast milk. Barbara Katz Rothman refers to this scenario as an instance in which "one technology ... [is] dependent upon another" (*In Labor* 193). (Elizabeth Whitaker has shown that the medicalization of breastfeeding in Italy led to a scenario in which mothers routinely lose their milk because of the regulatory practice of weighing babies before and after their nursing sessions and supplementing with formula.) Mothers are expected to cohere with medically defined feeding regimens: lucky is the breastfeeding mother whose doctor doesn't ask how often the baby feeds, since she might not be able to answer that question, or at least not satisfactorily to a physician who understands schedules to be the appropriate method of feeding infants. Bottle feeding is the normative model for infant feeding, in terms of how infant feeding is approached in routine pediatric practice. Yet as I demonstrated above, medical research has also, in terms of its own standards, demonstrated the health advantages of infant feeding for both mother and child, and doctors themselves are encouraged to press expectant mothers to breastfeed. For example, the *HHS Blueprint for Action on Breastfeeding* states "Providers of maternal and child health care have a special role in the promotion of breastfeeding during the prenatal and postnatal periods. They must be knowledgeable and skillful in counseling women about breastfeeding and lactation, and in providing medical care to breastfeeding mothers and their babies" (14). Mothers are thus caught in the odd circumstance of depending upon professionals who often have little real support to offer. The exhortation to breastfeed may come without practical support, even as nursing is held up culturally as the epitome of devoted motherhood.[27]

Thus the medicalization of infant feeding has had an ambivalent effect on breastfeeding as a practice and on breastfeeding advocacy. Breastfeeding advocates and feminist critics have addressed differing aspects of this ambiguous scenario. Breastfeeding advocacy is caught in the odd position of touting the biological advantages of breastfeeding *while at the same time* pointing out most medical professionals' lack of knowledge concerning lactation. Advocates criticize medical practitioners for not knowing more about lactation and for providing false information to women, but stay within the general medical paradigm of infant feeding. After all, much of breastfeeding advocacy itself is indebted to a medical model of demonstrating the superiority of breast milk as a substance. Feminists tend to focus on the expectation laid out in breastfeeding advocacy materials that all women can and should breastfeed, and demonstrate how breastfeeding as a practice is not always possible or optimal for all women. The expectation that all mothers breastfeed is, for many feminists, a cultural constraint upon each woman's freedom to choose an infant feeding method appropriate to their particular circumstances. Feminist health advocates, like the Boston Women's Health Book Collective, walk a thin line in advocating breastfeeding while acknowledging individual women's right to choose.[28] La Leche League, as we shall see, responds to scientific motherhood by offering scientific information to the mother practicing the womanly art.

Mothers have suffered a diminution in their status and authority in relation to the rise of medical views of infant health and development. The medicalization of infant feeding encourages skepticism about the female body's capacity to nourish infants in an uncomplicated and ordinary fashion, leading mothers to not only seek medical advice about how to most healthfully feed their infants, but to distrust their physical ability to do so (Apple, *Mothers and Medicine,* 166). Mothers, of course, sought and still seek out physicians to provide professional advice and to help them feed their babies, but the development of infant formula was a general solution to a series of problems that should have been more narrowly confined to those infants who needed supplementation or full bottle feeding.

It is not completely clear why, in the middle of the nineteenth century, mothers began to distrust their ability to breastfeed, a pattern that continued to build throughout the latter nineteenth century and through the twentieth. I have discussed the public health practices that promoted breastfeeding yet provided dairy milk to poor women in cities; Jacqueline Wolf argues that one message of such practices was that supplementation or substitution of breastfeeding was a viable, perhaps superior, infant feeding method. Pam Carter demonstrates that the provision of sanitary milk to poor mothers generally undermined their ability to breastfeed, "even though this was not usually their expressed intention" (47), revealing how easily the practice of bottle feeding can overtake breastfeeding in populations of poor, tired, and often unhealthy women.[29] Adrienne Berney focuses on the cultural factors that transformed women's roles, altered sentimental nineteenth-century attitudes about the maternal breast, and encouraged mothers to concentrate on hygiene and efficiency as crucial to good mothering.

The tangle of medicalization in relation to infant feeding suggests why it is problematic for breastfeeding advocates to rely on a medicalized discourse concerning the biological benefits of breastfeeding. Biological arguments are not free from social developments and institutional pressures; that is, they are inflected with ideological meaning. Biomedical research, however, offers information about the body that we cannot simply dismiss as ideologically tainted—as meaningless in a scientific sense because it is ideological. The question is, how do we engage this information—the scientific case for breastfeeding—without simply arguing that it isn't relevant, or, conversely, that it is the most important kind of evidence available?[30] As Brian Turner states, "the problem ... is how to comprehend the historical evolution of the discourse about the body, to acknowledge how our perspectives on the body are the product of social constructions, and to retain an appreciation for the phenomenological nature of the lived body" (8–9). I would add to that "an appreciation for biological perspectives on embodied experience." In this vein, feminist scholars need to figure out a way to approach biological discourses concerning reproduction that resonate with ordinary women's desires to engage in the best maternal practices they can reasonably achieve. We are back again at Haraway's conception of situated knowledge. *Mother's Milk* is my attempt to approach this form of knowledge critically, by attending to the regulatory function of biomedical discourses in conjunction with a reasonable assessment of the body knowledges that biomedical research produces.

It is important to note that the medicalization of infant feeding occurred within the development of American medicine as a private, rather than public, health care system. While the targets of infant feeding reform in the late nineteenth and early twentieth centuries were often poor urban women, and thus the campaigns part of public health initiatives, the privatized structure of medical care in the United States has had a significant impact in terms of the delivery of information about breastfeeding and mothers' access to supportive practical services to promote nursing. Most industrialized countries currently have in place publicly funded health care systems and more extensive maternity leave programs; it is not clear the extent to which these phenomena are linked. It would seem, however, that as long as breastfeeding is medicalized, the differential access to medical care in the United States significantly impacts the actual practice and experience of breastfeeding of mothers and infants across the socioeconomic spectrum. Poor women, African-American women, and women with lower rates of education continue to lag behind other demographic groups in breastfeeding initiation and duration. These are also the groups of women whose access to medical care is compromised by the private insurance system that undergirds medical care in the United States.

Discussions in chapters 1 and 6 consider these issues in greater detail, but due to the scope of this project I am not able to develop a full-fledged consideration of the impact on breastfeeding of private versus public health care systems in the context of industrialized economies. It is crucial, however, to address how race and class, as well as other axes of identity and experience, affect breastfeeding as both representation and maternal practice in the United States today. Interpretation of contemporary rates of breastfeeding is one area where situated knowledge is particularly necessary. Any understanding of racial and class disparities in rates of breastfeeding initiation must illuminate and work through both biological and cultural meanings. In the next section of this introduction I present and briefly discuss this issue, as a way of introducing the chapters that make up the main text of this book.

The Challenges of Breastfeeding Diversity

The Ross Mothers Survey, "Breastfeeding Trends through 2000," includes information about racial and class disparities of breastfeeding among American mothers[31] (see Table 1). These statistics document distinct

Table 1

	IN EARLY POSTPARTUM PERIOD	AT 6 MONTHS	AT 1 YEAR
All women	68.4%	31.4%	17.6%
African American	50.8%	20.6%	12.4%
Hispanic or Latino	70.8%	27.7%	18.4%
White	71.4%	33.8%	18.2%
WIC[32]	56.8%	20.1%	12.6%
Non-WIC	77.8%	40.7%	22.1%
Grade School	54.5%	23.8%	20.4%
High School	59.8%	23.0%	13.4%
College	81.2%	44.1%	23.4%

disparities in breastfeeding rates that can be mapped along the lines of race, education, and class (defined here through WIC participation). In addition, *HHS Blueprint for Action on Breastfeeding* tells us that "in 1998, 54% of low-income Asian and Pacific Islander children and 59% of low-income American Indian and Alaska native children were ever breastfed" (8). Young and less-educated women tend not to breastfeed: "The lowest rates of breastfeeding are found among those whose infants are at highest risk of poor health and development: those aged 21 years and under and those with low educational levels" (Department of Health and Human Services, *Healthy-People 2010*, §16 p. 47). Moreover, in 1997, the infant mortality rate among African-American infants was 2.3 times that of white infants, and African-American women are three to four times more likely than white women to die of pregnancy and its complications (Department of Health and Human Services, *Healthy-People 2010*, §16 p. 7).

But what do these statistics mean beyond descriptive information concerning racialized and class-related health disparities? In the federal public health context, these statistics identify troubling health disparities between ethnoracial and socioeconomic groups. The actions envisioned to end such disparities, however, are confined to a limited arena. The *HHS Blueprint* concentrates its advice for breastfeeding support on educational services, transformation of hospital practices, changes in workplace accommodations for employed breastfeeding mothers, and general "public health marketing ... of breastfeeding as normal, desirable, and achievable" (19). Yet the social context affects women's choices, whether they have a choice, and how they enact what choice they have in everyday practice. Much of what I argue for *is* related to workplace conditions, hospital practices, and medical beliefs, as mentioned in the *HHS Blueprint*. But throughout the book I show how structural constraints on women's reproductive practices are linked to *beliefs*—about women's bodies, contemporary familial arrangements, and women's social roles, all of which are largely ignored in the *HHS Blueprint* and other public health campaigns to increase rates of maternal nursing.[33]

Both the representation and experience of motherhood in the United States are racialized and class-related. What does that acknowledgment mean, however, in the context of presumably biological processes like breastfeeding, or in relation to the information about health disparities discussed above? Judith Galtry comments that "the benefits of breastfeeding potentially ... accrue not only to individual infants, but also the wider society. Yet the dominant American discourse on infant feeding emphasizes personal preference and ... individual responsibility" ("Suckling and Silence" 6). Yet, as Galtry notes, "structural and economic factors significantly determine whether women have any real decision-making power over infant feeding methods" (6). As a result, "the discourse of personal preference serves to disguise . . . the privilege" that allows some women to combine breastfeeding and working while consigning most women to little or no choice—and thus bottle feeding by default (7). The overall effect is a much higher rate of breastfeeding among those women who command greater social and material resources: choice is clearly related to social position and other structural constraints, even if it is articulated as the result of personal decision-making.

Two of the feminist scholars that I examine in chapter 6 address race and class issues attendant to breastfeeding and breastfeeding advocacy, but neither looks at these statistics in relation to health disparities and health advocacy. Indeed, both Linda Blum and Pam Carter argue that poor women and black women have responded to attempts to regulate their maternal experience by not breastfeeding; these scholars suggest that such a response is rational and in a large sense appropriate. Such an interpretation can only make sense in the context of a discussion that disregards the health risks of not breastfeeding, as outlined in the scientific case for breastfeeding. I argue, in contrast, that the statistics on breastfeeding can be mapped onto differentials in women's relations with medical personnel and treatment, as well as to the difficulties of navigating the "normative and logistical constraints on breastfeeding" (Guttman and Zimmerman 1471).[34] To my mind, to understand the meaning of the disparities in breastfeeding initiation and duration, *in the context of structural discrimination,* we need to pay attention both to health risks *and* to political contexts.

I am not trying to suggest that women should simply agree to follow medical advice about breastfeeding at all costs. Rather, I want to frame the discussion of breastfeeding in the contemporary United States so that breastfeeding is understood to be a *biosocial practice.* By using that phrase I emphasize that forms of infant feeding have both social and biological consequences, and that maternal actions constitute a coherent set of activities—a practice—central to maternal agency. In the final section of this introduction I show how each chapter of *Mother's Milk* contributes to this overall goal.

Breastfeeding Controversies in American Culture

The chapters in *Mother's Milk* alternate between examinations of public documents and discourses, on the one hand, and analyses of more academic or medical sources, on the other. The first two chapters demonstrate the complex ways that representations of breastfeeding in public and medical sources are intertwined with contemporary conflicts about motherhood, setting the stage for the following three chapters, which examine specific discursive contexts in which breast- or bottle feeding are advocated. The final chapter concerns recent feminist approaches to breastfeeding and demonstrates why feminist scholars need to rethink the prevailing critique of breastfeeding advocacy that dominates the field today. Although it appears at the end, this chapter contains the arguments that compelled me to write this book.

Public representations of breastfeeding women juxtapose images of privileged and disadvantaged mothers, but convey distrust of all mothers' abilities to care for their children. In the mid-1990s, a famous article in the *Wall Street Journal* expressed great sympathy for "yuppie" mothers who tried to breastfeed their infants but could not make enough milk; a few years later, the *New York Times* carried a series of articles about a young black woman on public assistance who was convicted of criminally negligent homicide when her breastfed baby starved to death. Chapter 1 examines this set of racialized representations of breastfeeding and infant death. I read these representations against images of dead babies from international breastfeeding advocacy campaigns and prime-time television dramas in order to document how concepts of deserving motherhood are inherently racialized at the same time that all mothers are presumed to need supervision of basic maternal practices in order to keep their infants alive. Racialized perceptions of good and bad mothers, however, allow black mothers and white mothers experiencing the same medical syndrome to be represented quite differently in the media.

If chapter 1 concerns the discourses of the public media, chapter 2 examines the ambivalent representation of mothers in literature written for physicians. Specifically, I look at Ruth Lawrence's *Breastfeeding: A Guide for the Medical Profession*—the only guidebook about breastfeeding specifically for physicians—and consider how this text represents the mother's sexuality, her relation to the physician concerning authority over managing infant feeding, and questions of responsibility concerning the mother's ability to breastfeed or decisions about breastfeeding. In this chapter I am interested in interrogating the complex and internally contradictory image of mothers that emerges from discourses within the medical profession, and show that the question of the mother's authority over her breastfeeding experience is centrally at stake in scientific motherhood in the present period.

While mothers themselves were likely to read about (or see on TV) the cases discussed in chapter 1, most mothers only experience the potential effects of representations of mothers in medical literature through encounters with physicians or other health care providers. The health care provider serves as mediator of scientific knowledge about breastfeeding. Chapter 3 returns us to the more public context of infant formula promotion and advice books for mothers—the lay medical literature that provides a discursive link between medical knowledge and maternal practice. In this chapter,

I examine the presentation of breast- and bottle feeding as options for maternal practice; the analysis here comprises close rhetorical and semiotic readings of the formal structures of argument and graphic representations.

Choice is a prominent aspect of the consumer economy of raising babies in the United States—from breast or bottle to the other accoutrements of babyhood, parents face a smorgasbord of potential products and practices to help them cope with their new child. In chapter 3, I look at how choice is represented in the context of pregnancy and infant care advice manuals, as well as formula promotion materials. With regard to the choice between breast- or bottle feeding, serious contradictions arise in the context of writers' attempts to represent both options fairly, with the consequence that the biomedical support for breastfeeding, touted as a significant advantage of this practice, is basically wiped out in the consideration of infant formula. This form of doublespeak demonstrates that the scientific case is easily set aside, even in contexts (such as lay medical guides to pregnancy and infant care, both genres that are generally targeted to new mothers) where one might anticipate its most forceful support. The chapter also addresses how formula companies represent breastfeeding as the superior infant food at the same time that they undermine that information through diagrams linking infant formulas with specific infant behaviors. Ultimately, in this chapter I try to show how breastfeeding is portrayed in the specific contexts most likely to be accessed by ordinary American mothers looking for information about maternity, infant feeding, and basic child care.

Chapter 4 shifts to look at a more specialized discourse that underlies many popular arguments about breastfeeding in breastfeeding advocacy, infant care guides, and medical discussions about infant feeding and sleeping practices. In this chapter I examine how these sources rely on evolutionary theory to support certain views of breastfeeding, family arrangements, and motherhood in contemporary American culture. Racialization is again an important theme in this chapter, as most evolutionary arguments cite specific African groups as examples of the so-called ancestral model of breastfeeding, and thus idealize these groups without acknowledging their status as modern peoples or recognizing their infant feeding traditions as cultural (rather than biologically evolved) practices. In addition, I draw on Sarah Blaffer Hrdy's book, *Mother Nature,* to argue for a feminist approach to evolution that values mothers as agents, as opposed to the general focus on the child's needs that permeates most evolutionary perspectives. Ultimately, in this chapter I argue that advocating breastfeeding through biological arguments based in evolutionary theory is highly problematic because it means ignoring the political perspective on mothering provided by feminist theory, which insists on the mother's subjectivity and rational decision-making practices.

The next chapter moves back into the public sphere of breastfeeding advocacy (as opposed to the more rarified context of academic breastfeeding research). Chapter 5 examines La Leche League, the premier lay breastfeeding advocacy organization in the United States (and internationally), through their publications. This chapter returns to the question of the mother's authority, this time from the perspective of an organization that tries to enhance the mother's authority over child nurture through breastfeeding as both a natural and a scientifically informed practice. Examining the six editions of their breastfeeding manual, *The Womanly Art of Breastfeeding,* I discuss gender stereotypes and how the group portrays fathers in relation to reproductive sexual differences, as well as the perception that La Leche League is an antifeminist organization with conservative social ends. I respond to this perception with a discussion of how League practices, ideas, and advice to mothers relate to both the social position of its founders *and* the cultural climate of the United States in the second half of the twentieth century, which became increasingly hostile to the needs of mothers, regardless of their infant feeding method (see Jones). In the end, this chapter treats differences between maternalist and feminist approaches to empowering women as mothers. Through a discussion of Joan Williams's *Unbending Gender,* I show how the problem of domesticity haunts *both* feminism and La Leche League—indeed, how the problem of domesticity remains a significant problem for contemporary women.

The final chapter of the book concerns feminist approaches to breastfeeding and breastfeeding advocacy. Here I examine the work of recent feminist critics of breastfeeding advocacy—and by extension the practice of breastfeeding—and compare it to the work of feminist breastfeeding advocates. How these two groups read the scientific case for breastfeeding is crucial to understanding their divergent positions on whether breastfeeding is a maternal practice central to feminist aspirations or only contingently related to them. At the end of this chapter, I argue for a feminist health activist approach to breastfeeding, using the statistics on breastfeeding disparities according to race to argue for feminist attention to breastfeeding as an issue concerning racial discrimination in health care. Feminist approaches to breastfeeding need not fear biological essentialism, but should use scientific data to press for better social circumstances for all mothers, including the right to breastfeed with appropriate support.

Throughout the book I expand on the following themes: racialization, women's conflicting roles within a capitalist economy, women's liberation and the idea of choice, and women's relationship to medical authority. The question of the scientific case for breastfeeding as a healthful practice (for both mother and child) is implicated in each of these themes, as is the question of women's right to define maternity on their own terms. I am not so naïve that I believe women will soon (or ever) have that right, and I understand fully that their own terms will always emerge within the discursive constraints of specific cultural formations. I am hopeful, however, that key political struggles over the meanings of maternity may enable a shift in the experience of motherhood toward that goal. Above all, I believe that we must both engage and challenge biomedical discourses about women's bodies and mothers' responsibilities toward their children, in order that feminism not relegate to the realm of private choice a biosocial practice that is central to the enactment of motherhood. We should know by now that technology cannot fix damaged social relations; neither does a repudiation of technology offer us respite from the complexities of modern living. In this book I aim to move debate on the breast–bottle controversy to the issues that emerge when representations of infant feeding are examined in depth, with due respect for their signifying complexity, their collusion with powerful social forces, and their rhetorical capacity to influence behaviors.

CHAPTER 1

Dead Babies

Detective Green: How many of these have you done?
Detective Briscoe: Stake outs?
Detective Green: No, dead babies.
Detective Briscoe: Hey, we don't know the baby's dead.
Detective Green: Right.
Detective Briscoe: To answer your question, too many.
Detective Green: It's my first.
Detective Briscoe: That's too many.

"Mother's Milk," *Law and Order*

Story of a Black Mother[1]

Tabitha Walrond, nineteen years old, African American, and a single mother living with her mother (both of whom were on public assistance) was convicted of negligently causing the death of her seven-week-old son Tyler, who died of starvation in August 1997. The healthy, 7 pound 15 ounce baby boy was born by emergency cesarean section, although the mother had faithfully attended Lamaze classes before the birth (and thus presumably desired a more active role in the delivery of her infant). She had had breast reduction surgery at age fifteen (going from a size 42F to 38DD) and was hospitalized for twelve days postpartum because of an infection. During that time the baby stayed in the hospital and was fed formula in addition to a few nursing sessions.[2]

After discharge from the hospital, Walrond had difficulty obtaining routine well-baby medical care for her son. While accounts of her experience conflict, she testified that she tried to have her child seen for well-baby exams at her health provider, Health Insurance Plan of New York, or HIP, an HMO, but was told she needed a Medicaid card for the baby to schedule a visit. There were difficulties in obtaining the card; two appeared in the mail after the baby's death. The difficulties include being sent by various functionaries from one office to another. Thus, according to Walrond and her mother, they could not take the child to the HIP pediatric clinic (their health care provider) because they did not have a Medicaid card for him and were told that they needed one in order to receive care. When Walrond went to her obstetrician for her postpartum visit, her doctor asked that the pediatric clinic, as a personal favor to him, weigh the baby. Tyler, the infant, had gained only two ounces in one month (an inadequate weight gain by almost all standards; according to La Leche League's *Breastfeeding Answer Book*, "Typical weight gain for the first 3 to 4 months is 4 to 8 ounces ... per week" [Mohrbacher and Stock 114]). But nothing was done at that time: Walrond was told to make an appointment for the infant as soon as possible. There is no indication that anyone told her that he exhibited symptoms of grave illness, and her reported testimony was that he seemed fine.

When Walrond took the infant to a family gathering of the child's father, the paternal grandmother fed the baby a bottle of soy formula, against the wishes of the mother, who, according to newspaper accounts, wished to feed her infant exclusively by the breast (as she had been advised to do by lactation literature and counselors). Her mother, the infant's maternal grandmother, reportedly told Walrond that she herself was small as an infant and that Tyler would fill out in time. Tyler died in a taxicab on the way to the hospital, the morning Tabitha Walrond finally saw that he was desperately ill.

Yuppie Mothers in the News

Shortly before my daughter was born in August 1994, the *Wall Street Journal* published a front-page article on insufficient milk syndrome, "Dying for Milk: Some Mothers, Trying in Vain to Breast-Feed, Starve Their Infants." Fortunately, I never saw the article, and although I ran into some of the most common problems that first-time mothers experience while starting to nurse (engorged breasts, cracked nipples), my daughter thrived. My students that fall, however, seemed to have intimate knowledge of the problems with milk supply that new mothers confront; wasn't it difficult for many women to breastfeed, they would ask, usually on days when I was bleary-eyed from lack of sleep and worrying that my nursing pads wouldn't hold all the breast milk leaking by the end of class. These were first-year students at the University of Chicago; dutifully, they read the *Wall Street Journal* and learned there that many yuppie women were overeducated perfectionists who inadvertently caused irreparable harm to their infants by trying to nurse them.

The twenty or so students I taught that year learned another story about motherhood—that breastfeeding can be a routine aspect of maternal experience, whose defining characteristic (at least in the first year or so) is exhaustion. In the years since, I've been struck by the number of students who subscribe to the view that breastfeeding is difficult and that many women simply don't have enough milk to do it. I'm not referring here to those women who have been told by physicians, erroneously or not, that they don't have enough milk, but to those young women and men who have no immediate experience with newborns but are aware of this popular story about the many mothers who can't nurse. And it's not just my students; women I know in a variety of circumstances talk about *trying* to nurse and *hoping* it will work out. Women who enter into maternity with those assumptions are well-prepared to fail at lactation.

In the *Wall Street Journal* article, the mothers are identified as yuppie. The term seems to be a substitute for the one really intended—white—since the case that receives the most attention in the article is about a woman who was a secretary before she quit to have a baby and whose husband is a clerk at a Food Lion grocery store. These are hardly yuppie professions. This woman and another featured in the article who had insufficient milk (but whose baby did not suffer any identified problems), as well as the unnamed 5 percent of women who can't make enough breast milk, are presented as the victims of a medical establishment that doesn't give them accurate information on their chances of breastfeeding failure. These are women whose problem is being *too educated:* " 'The more intelligence and education the parents have, the greater the danger seems to be,' says Nancy Hurst, director of the breastfeeding program at Texas Children's Hospital in Houston" (Helliker A1).[3] Being too educated also encourages the mothers to depend on experts' advice: Pam Floyd, whose son suffered seizures that permanently damaged his brain, said, "I can't stop asking myself, 'Pam, why didn't you ignore all the experts and give him a bottle?' " (Helliker A1). The women are also presented as striving to excel in mothering: "Some physicians attribute the problem to a generation of perfectionist women" (Helliker A4). In essence, these women are only doing *what they were told to do* (just as Tabitha Walrond argued she had done). They are educated white women following the rules of scientific motherhood. Keith Helliker, the author of the article, presents the problem as a simple biological truism—some women just can't make enough milk to feed their babies.

Pictures of Dead Babies

It may seem irreverent and unfeeling to begin a book on contemporary representations of breastfeeding with a chapter entitled "Dead Babies," but starting out with this discourse will help me to show how significant infant feeding is to contemporary ideas about maternity and womanhood in the United States. When I began research on this book I was struck by how absent breastfeeding was in the cultural context of public representations in the United States; after working on the project for a number of years I am amazed by how many of those representations that do exist link specific forms of infant feeding with death. There is, in fact, a function that the dead or dying baby serves in what has been called "the breast–bottle controversy." Dead babies are used by both breastfeeding advocates and formula promoters. The dying or dead infant works to make arguments for the cause being presented, by visually demonstrating the terrible effect of whatever practice is being criticized in relation to the other, advocated, practice. The dead baby is a record of negligence, ignorance, poverty, or malevolence. Pictures and accounts of dead or dying infants also function semiotically, in that they signify the unconscionable death of the innocent, and are thus understood to convey the meaning "the most awful kind of death that occurs." Finally, representations of dead or dying babies often have a particular racial story to tell. It is this racial story—or, more properly, the racial stories that the discourse of the dead baby refers to—that undergirds its rhetorical and semiotic functions.

This chapter concerns the circulation of one story of a dead black baby, Tyler Walrond, as it made its way through the pages of the *New York Times,* an afternoon session of a breastfeeding conference, and two prime-time television programs. I examine Tyler's story in relation to another story about white mothers and their damaged babies. Both stories rely on representations of breastfeeding as a problematic and potentially dangerous maternal practice, but both stories are, at some level, not really about breastfeeding at all. Instead, they are cautionary tales about contemporary motherhood. These stories teach us to be skeptical about mothers' abilities to keep their children alive, thus suggesting that increasing oversight of maternal practices is necessary to save the children, even as expert advice clearly failed to help the specific mothers featured in the stories. Read separately, these stories seem to be about tragedies associated with breastfeeding failure; together, however, the implied tragedy is that of maternal failure, of mothers who can't be trusted in the simple act of feeding their children.

For breastfeeding advocates, *breastfed* babies who die are often understood to be the victims of a bottle feeding culture that cannot support natural (or healthful) infant feeding, and they argue that the bottle feeding culture is itself supported by consumer capitalism and the unethical marketing schemes of infant formula manufacturers.[4] Their argument is represented in these two famous pictures: a South Asian woman with fraternal twins on her lap[5] (figure 1.1) and a well-known picture used on the cover of a book called *The Baby Killer*, which was produced as part of the boycott against Nestlé (figure 1.2). Yet dead breastfed babies also frequently appear in public representations of breastfeeding in the United States, from popular television dramatic shows like *ER* to public health debates about HIV-positive mothers and infants. In many of these representations, breastfeeding and infant death are linked causally; to a public whose model is formula feeding, it can seem as if ordinary breastfeeding itself results in dead babies.[6] This linkage suggests that infant death can occur anywhere, to anyone's baby, even to those of the most educated and privileged women. Thus, breastfeeding advocates often view contemporary accounts of breastfeeding with increasing alarm and despair and feel that their accounts of the health benefits of breastfeeding and the routine course of nursing for most mother-infant pairs are obscured through the sensationalized presence of the dead infant. Indeed, these representations often portray breastfeeding advocates as rigid believers ("[the breastfeeding movement has] stirred a religious-like fervor in many nurses, breast-feeding consultants, and volunteers for La Leche League International" [Helliker A1]), and present this unflagging belief in lactation as itself a cause infant death. One breastfeeding peer counselor I met, a woman who helps WIC mothers with breastfeeding, said that she is known as the "Breastfeeding Nazi" at the clinic where many of the women she works with go for medical care.

Dead babies are, of course, real. For example, the debates around HIV transmission through breast milk are about preserving the health of mothers and babies in the context of a number of potentially fatal scenarios: HIV-infected mothers dying while their orphaned HIV-negative infants survive, infants infected with HIV wasting away at hospitals with little or no capacity to help them or attend to their specific needs, bottle-fed infants of HIV-positive mothers who die from gastrointestinal illnesses because they lack the immunities provided by breast milk and are exposed to pathogens in their environment through the feeding bottle or unsanitary water, bottle-fed infants who die of starvation because their HIV-positive mothers cannot afford formula and thus dilute its strength to make it last. In the United States and other developed countries, where most infants receiving formula have access to safe water systems (and, in the United States, supplementary formula provisions through WIC), HIV-positive mothers are counseled not to

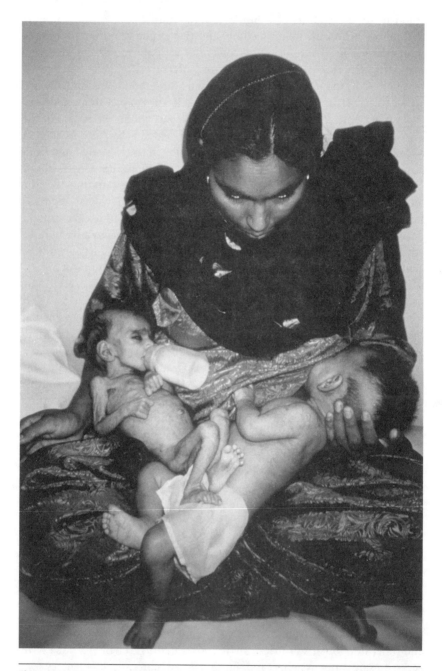

Figure 1.1. This image of a Pakistani mother with fraternal twins appears frequently in breastfeeding advocacy texts, such as Gabrielle Palmer's *The Politics of Breastfeeding* and Naomi Baumslag and Dia Michels's *Milk, Money, and Madness.* Photograph courtesy of UNICEF/HQ89-0049/Khan.

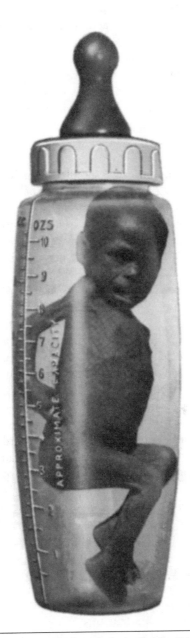

Figure 1.2. This image appeared on the cover of a book called *The Baby Killer,* which was produced as part of the first boycott against Nestlé. Photograph courtesy of War on Want.

breastfeed their infants.[7] In developing countries, the data do not, as yet, clearly indicate a proper course of action, since safe water supplies are not always available and other factors mitigate against formula use.[8] But along with, indeed inextricable from, the medical problems and material conditions that physicians and other health care workers deal with are representational issues concerning how the discussions around these problems are staged and presented, and how they signify in relation to discourses concerning maternal responsibility, the role of biomedical knowledge in regulating infant care and development, and the racialized politics of maternity.

Maternity is always implicitly understood and presented in relation to racial norms and expectations. For example, Jacquelyn Litt argues that the development of scientific motherhood had specific and different effects on mothers of different races. Scientific motherhood "is the insistence that women require expert scientific and medical advice to raise their children healthfully" (Apple, "Constructing Mothers," 90). While the ideology began in the nineteenth century, it has dominated popular views of maternity during the twentieth century, in conjunction with the rise of pediatric medicine and the concomitant increase in medical supervision of healthy infants and children. Litt demonstrates that "scientific motherhood" was one method of dividing women along race and class lines, because the norms of mothering developed in conjunction with "scientific motherhood" are intimately linked to white, middle-class expectations of proper maternal submission to medical authority. When physicians shifted focus from childhood diseases to well-baby care, in the 1930s, more and more of the mother's activities were brought under medical supervision, depriving her of her traditional, personal perspective on her own experiences: "The ideal mother made routine medical visits. And in orienting mothering toward medical standards, mothers were warned to shift away from their own standards of evaluation to ones that gave authority to the observations made by experts" (Litt 34).

In *Killing the Black Body: Race, Reproduction, and the Meaning of Liberty,* legal scholar Dorothy Roberts argues that ubiquitous, negative stereotypes of black women serve to demean black women's mothering throughout contemporary U.S. culture.[9] This occurs partly because the strictures of scientific motherhood set up a standard that many black women cannot accommodate because they lack easy access to medical care or because the medical establishment treats them differently as mothers: "white middle-class women in the early twentieth century began to demand the new medical technologies that male birth attendants controlled. The poorest women, African Americans among them, were actually the most vulnerable to these new medical practitioners, who used them as bodies to practice on. The most and least privileged women were the first to experience medicalized childbirth, but they did so under radically different circumstances" (Litt 29).

The medicalized ideal of maternity today is a social norm that privileges white middle-class women's experiences with doctors, access to medical resources, and attitudes toward medical authority. In contemporary public discourses about proper mothering, evident in debates about family values, child care dilemmas, and the "reform of welfare as we know it" (purportedly accomplished by the Clinton administration in 1996), the norms used to distinguish the good mother from the bad imply racialized ideals of family structure and maternal responsibility; for example, the good mother stays at home and has a male spouse who supports the family on his income while their children are young, but the bad mother needs to work because her children will grow up without a work ethic if they see their mother (dependent on government support) at home caring for them. These images are linked to explicit stereotypes of black women as lazy individuals who need to be forced to be socially productive through work and of white women as appropriately domestic dependents whose nurturant care is necessary for their children to grow up normally. The representations of Tabitha Walrond fit consistently with prevalent stereotypes of black welfare mothers, while the yuppie white mothers of the *Wall Street Journal* article were perceived to be victims; thus, the black teenage mother causes the death of her child while white women are perceived to be duped by medical experts and their own bodies.[10] Race and class are seamlessly conflated in these stereotypes, in which all the black women are poor and all the white women middle class and educated.

The accepted normality of white mothering is evident in breastfeeding advocacy texts. For example, in the first chapter of *The Politics of Breastfeeding*, "Why Breastfeeding Is Political," Gabrielle Palmer juxtaposes two pictures of breastfeeding mothers. On the left is a "Mozambican refugee with all her possessions," lying down and leaning over to nurse one child while a toddler looks at the camera (figure 1.3). The woman and her children are black; she is very thin, but her toddler looks healthy. Her breasts hang pendulously, and the baby pulls at the one he is not suckling. Under the second picture (figure 1.4), "A woman breastfeeding in an English café," the caption reads, "Which image is more familiar on television and in newspapers?" (Palmer 22–23). The woman in the picture is a smiling, young, white mother, whose smallish breast is mostly bared while she suckles her child. In the pictures of dead or dying infants described previously, all the babies and the South Asian woman were dark-skinned. Palmer's comment in the caption is meant to suggest that breastfeeding is too often associated with women in underdeveloped countries who live in squalor and have baby after baby. Breastfeeding is, in this scenario, an adjunct to life devoted to reproductive imperatives, as well as evident maternal depletion.[11] Palmer's implicit point, however, is that breastfeeding *ought* to be associated

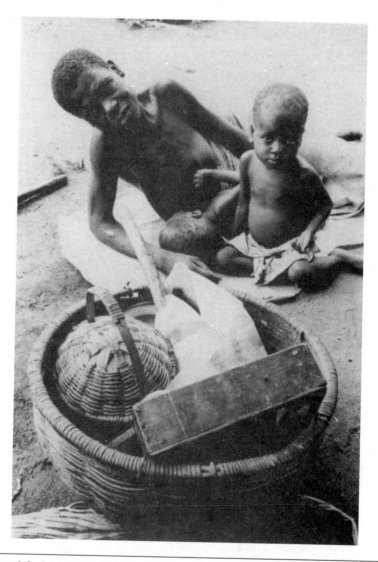

Figure 1.3. Gabrielle Palmer captions this photograph "Mozambican refugee with all her possessions" (22) and contrasts it to the white Englishwoman in Figure 1.4. Photograph by Alexander Joe.

with ordinary middle-class pursuits like going to cafés; in order to imagine breastfeeding as normal, we have to imagine it as something white Western women do. Thus, the explicit purpose of the passage—to expose the political implications of global trends in infant feeding—is undermined by Palmer's rhetorical reliance on the normality of white middle-class mothering.

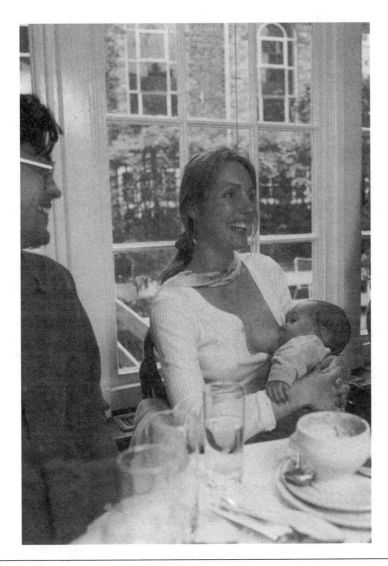

Figure 1.4. Gabrielle Palmer captions this photograph "A woman breastfeeding in an English café" and, comparing this image to that in Figure 1.3, asks the reader, "Which image is more familiar on television and in newspapers?" (23). Photograph by Paul Smith; courtesy of Baby Milk Action.

How do all of these images and discourses fit together? According to breastfeeding advocates, (dark) babies in Africa and Asia die because they aren't breastfed; according to breastfeeding skeptics, (white) babies in America die because they are.[12] One of the reasons the *Wall Street Journal* article ("Dying for Milk") was so astounding was that it targeted yuppie

American mothers, overwhelmingly white and middle class, as those mothers most likely to suffer insufficient milk syndrome without realizing it.[13] This article thus effectively moved the rhetorical hold of the dead baby, usually reserved for the representation of Third World black or brown infants, into the nurseries of the privileged race, class, and nation. Of course, in the United States, breastfeeding is more prevalent among white, middle- and upper-class mothers. The author of "Dying for Milk" suggests that "[s]uch parents are nearly twice as likely as the poor to breast-feed their babies because they read so many books and articles on child-rearing" (Helliker A1).[14] Palmer writes, in a more political tone, "Why is it that whether you were breastfed yourself or whether you breastfeed your own child depends so much on your social and economic class position in your own society?" (20). In the United States, African-American women are among the racial groups least likely to initiate breastfeeding: in 1994 (the year "Dying for Milk" was published) almost two-thirds of white women breastfed at birth, while only one-third of black mothers did so (Ross Products Division, 6). Education is another, perhaps the most significant, indicator of breastfeeding initiation (Lawrence, *Breastfeeding*, 194); the more years of education one has, the more likely one is to breastfeed. While some analysts will argue that the discourses around breastfeeding advocacy target white middle-class women's desires to maximize each pregnancy and optimize their child's intelligence and health profile—and thus are ideological discourses linked to norms of middle-class mothering (Blum, *At the Breast*; Law)—breastfeeding advocates will often counter that poor women of color are the ones who *really* need to breastfeed in order to counteract the health disadvantages their children are born into (inferior housing, poor nutritional profiles, lack of adequate medical attention, etc.).[15]

Linda Blum's *At the Breast: Ideologies of Breastfeeding and Motherhood in the Contemporary United States* argues that African-American women "unsurprising[ly]" and "perhaps even quite rational[ly] . . . reject breastfeeding," largely because their social and historical position in the oppressed underclass of American society offers them a way to resist prevalent discourses linking proper motherhood with breastfeeding (147–79, esp. 169 ff.). In addition, black women's complex relation to sexuality and embodied experience, mediated by hundreds of years of negative stereotyping that connects black women's bodies to exoticism, animality, and service, works against their taking up a practice like breastfeeding (169). The "politics of respectability" articulated by black church women in the Progressive era suggests that black women have long understood their maternal practices to have significant political effects, especially with regard to contesting dominant stereotypes of African Americans: "By claiming respectability through manners and morals, poor black women boldly asserted will and agency to define themselves outside the parameters of prevailing racist discourses. . . . Respectability was perceived as a weapon against such assumptions" (Evelyn Brooks Higginbotham, qtd. in Litt 30). Current stereotypes link breastfeeding to an exhibitionistic female sexuality, and historic stereotypes portray black women as excessively lascivious; put together, these cultural discourses make it difficult for black women to breastfeed even today, should they want to, without risking public censure.[16] Formula feeding emerges as a way to make the culturally perceived sexual status of the black female body a non-issue in black mothering.[17]

Blum's view is that breastfeeding itself can be part of an embodied, feminist practice that "speak[s] back to medical or technoscientific authority" (188), but currently functions that way only for a few privileged white women. She argues that most "public health efforts to promote breastfeeding, even the most well-meaning, have ignored the meanings of *not breastfeeding* for African-American working-class mothers" (193). Blum also believes it is too simple to argue that breastfeeding would offer all women a mode of resistance to an equality paradigm that forces them to be like men in order to participate in civic culture and waged labor. This analysis, she argues, homogenizes women's experiences and expects all women to have the resources and cultural attitudes of white middle-class women. Thus, in Blum's analysis, breastfeeding means different things for women whose class and race identities distinguish both their experience and their social position, and it means different things *to them,* as well as different things *about them.*

This last point was brought home to me when I asked a question at a lecture given by Patricia Hill Collins ("Reproducing Race, Reproducing Nation: Black Women in the Politics of Motherhood"). Her talk focused on social and largely metaphorical dimensions of motherhood for black women. I asked how to approach the issue of race in addressing African-American women's low rates of breastfeeding. I was looking, I said, for a way to understand black women's decisions from their own standpoint, as opposed to medicine's general view that disparaged them and their choices. Collins's response was antagonistic, even hostile; she stated quite clearly that she felt breastfeeding to be a white, middle-class women's issue that black women didn't have time to deal with, given other social priorities and issues of greater concern to them. When she elaborated, she suggested that by breastfeeding in a work setting, black women would risk representing themselves as sexual, which they could ill afford to do. In this way, her views coincide with Linda Blum's and demonstrate the continuing political necessity of a strategy of respectability to combat racist employment discrimination. I had thought I was asking about an approach to analyzing black women's breastfeeding behaviors, rather than arguing that black women should breastfeed more,[18] but it was clear to me that I had articulated my concerns in such a way that I had been perceived as a white woman who was judgmental of black women's maternal behaviors. In the terms of Blum's analysis, I elicited African-American women's resistance to having their motherhood assessed by white norms. Raising the issue of breastfeeding and race *at all* seemed to be political—and racist—for Patricia Hill Collins.

In response to her challenging reaction to my question, then, it seems appropriate to demonstrate that paying attention to race might not end up in a consideration of why African-American women should breastfeed more, nor in a discussion of why they don't breastfeed as much as white women, although I would argue that both topics could be addressed in antiracist ways. Prior to any such assertion, however, there needs to be an analysis of how racialized perceptions of mothering in contemporary U.S. culture relate to discourses about breastfeeding as a practice of maternity. In the service of that latter goal, I am investigating some representational venues where the rhetoric of the dead baby did important cultural work, producing and shaping the cultural construction of racialized motherhood, and of womanhood, in front of our very eyes.

Physicians Talk about Dead Babies

At the La Leche League Seminar on Breastfeeding for Physicians, held at Hilton Head Island, July 2000, a physician and one of Tabitha Walrond's lawyers presented this case and initiated a discussion of "Ethical and Legal Issues that Affect Breastfeeding."[19] Janna Collins, a gastroenterologist, began the presentation with the following words: "I thought it would be valuable for you to hear sort of from the horse's mouth, undiluted by the media, this case, of Tabitha Walrond, which I think is an excellent template for what the problems are in making breastfeeding the standard of care in this country." In introducing herself, Susan Tipograph, a lawyer for the defense of Tabitha Walrond, stated, "I am also not an expert on breastfeeding. I know very little about breastfeeding, although I've learned quite a bit in the last three years, but most of what I know are things I read in the mass media, or things I learned from friends or family members who, in fact, were breastfeeding." Right from the start of the session, then, there is tension around the issue of media representations, which are implicitly criticized as diluting the case or providing misleading or incomplete information about breastfeeding. Among doctors, it seems, some sort of purer flow of information will take place, even though much of the discourse that followed demonstrated the ignorance or negligence of the doctors involved with Tabitha Walrond, that is, their own misleading or incomplete information about breastfeeding.

Significant too is Dr. Collins's comment about "making breastfeeding the standard of care in this country." A standard of care is a specified level of medical treatment that can be expected for a particular illness or condition; it is often distinguished from state-of-the-art treatments that exceed the standard of most communities and experimental treatments that have not yet been proven effective. The standard of care is a measure of a physician's competence and demonstrates the appropriateness of treatment received. What's odd here is the suggestion that breastfeeding itself is the desired standard of care—breastfeeding isn't a medical treatment, it's a method of infant feeding, a maternal nurturant practice. Breastfeeding advocates have tried to represent breastfeeding as the standard or normal *mode* of infant feeding, in order to discuss formula feeding in terms of *deficit* rather than lactation in terms of *benefit,* so Collins's comment may be only a slip from that discourse (breastfeeding as the gold standard[20]). But it's a significant slip, insofar as it represents medicine's perception that infant feeding is (and should be) supervised by physicians, that it is, in fact, a *treatment* for the infant that needs to be monitored by medical expertise.

This sentiment was echoed by one physician, a pediatrician, who spoke during the discussion session following the presentation by Tipograph and Collins. In the midst of a long response to the presentation, she commented,

> Beyond this case, I, what I'm thinking about here is, and the professional responsibilities we have to mother and babies, is, infant feeding is really not considered anything at all until there's a problem. I mean, it's no big deal to feed a baby, is it? Unless there's a problem. And, so, for us as pediatricians, I don't think it's just breastfeeding that we've got to get across to people, it's that infant feeding is a complex thing, and we have to pay attention to it before we get these drastic problems, rather than crisis management.

Another physician suggested that this case showed that there was a need to credential doctors in breastfeeding medicine, demonstrating her view that such a credential would force pediatricians to know something about it. Both statements demonstrate a desire to enfold more of maternal practice within medicine in order to limit bad outcomes, as well as the implication that it is the responsibility of doctors to make sure that infants are fed correctly and sufficiently.[21]

Yet this perception of infant feeding as always already needing medical supervision (discussed in depth as a historical phenomenon by Apple, *Mothers and Medicine*) is linked to a larger question: Was Tyler Walrond's experience the result of medical negligence, ignorance on the part of the health care providers his mother interacted with (itself a form of negligence), and/or the bureaucratic red tape that set up innumerable barriers to access? The physicians' discussion touched on all these issues, coming to rest, finally, on questions of medical responsibility and the difficulty of being an ethical physician in the context of managed care and third-party billing. There was a tacit agreement by responders and presenters alike that many medical practitioners simply do not know what they should about breastfeeding, and that their lack of knowledge disproportionately affects so-called high-risk mothers (who are primarily poor, young, and often of color). But there was also an acknowledgment that bureaucratic policies regarding poor women reflected a negligent, even cavalier, attitude toward their health and the health of their infants. Another physician complained,

> If you look at, for instance, practices, and this one practice really gets me upset in [my state] and I don't know if it's practiced around the country, but all of my low-income patients, those are—I only work with low-income families—they all are sort of almost forced to get Depo-Provera or Norplant on day two after delivery. . . . None of my patients get it because we actually counsel them prenatally, "Do not accept it," and this is happening at a university hospital (I won't say the name of it) and, basically, this happens all over [the state]. And if you look at the Depo-Provera insert, the drug insert, there are three places that it says, "Do not give to breastfeeding women until six weeks postpartum" minimum.

This view, that physicians must struggle with state agencies, insurance companies, and managed care, emerged as a strong theme in respondents' comments, but others clearly sought a medical way to make sense of the tragedy. Lawrence Gartner, a physician and leading breastfeeding advocate for many years, as well as a member of the panel, opened the discussion with a question concerning whether Tyler had experienced jaundice as a newborn. After receiving an answer of "no," he went on to suggest that if the infant had been jaundiced (a condition in which bilirubin is not flushed effectively by the newborn's system), he would probably have avoided the early death. This response suggests Gartner's desire to see a medical way out of the dilemma, expressing the view, "If only he had gotten sick sooner, he might have been saved." Presumably, jaundice would have occurred while Tyler was still in the hospital with his mother, and thus he would have been treated for it then. The treatment, which includes frequent feedings (among other measures), presumably would have required the hospital staff to determine whether Tabitha Walrond was making enough milk for her son (Mohrbacher and Stock 228–35).

For some doctors and other members of the medical profession, ethical dilemmas around the faulty care that underprivileged people get in the United States can be resolved by medicalizing social experiences (like breastfeeding) even more. The alternative interpretation, that this case may demonstrate some of the problems with medicalizing breastfeeding (in particular, and infant feeding in general), was not articulated. Of course, that's not surprising at a medical meeting. Yet medicalizing infant feeding more, rather than less, might exacerbate incidents of lactation failure, in that more knowledge will be concentrated in a group of elite experts, and fewer ordinary individuals will feel competent to interpret their infants' behaviors on their own. The history of breastfeeding in the nineteenth and twentieth centuries suggests that the more infant feeding came under the supervision of physicians, the more likely mothers were to perceive themselves to produce inadequate milk (Berney).

Through the twentieth century, the medicalization of infant feeding and the shift to bottle feeding as the default mode of infant feeding coincided with decreases in infant mortality in the United States. There is no doubt that the provision of well-baby exams for infants and the supervision of infant feeding problems, in conjunction with safe water supplies and improved home hygiene through indoor plumbing, has improved the life prospects for many babies who would not have formerly survived. Yet as Rima Apple so aptly argues, with the "self-conscious promotion of applied science in American life, . . . not all babies received the food best for them. . . . a combination of the ideology of scientific motherhood, confidence in the medical profession, and shrewd media presentation altered the relationship between mothers and physicians and encouraged mothers to seek out commercial and medical solutions to the problems of infant feeding" (*Mothers and Medicine* 182). The mothers she is speaking of, however, do not represent all mothers. Mothers who exemplify scientific motherhood are those with a particular relation to the medical profession—one of appropriate submission to medical authority, yet with the resources to seek out and command medical services when necessary. These are the mothers whose infants benefit the most from scientific motherhood, as traditional folk knowledge transmitted among women no longer operates effectively in modern societies. Scientific motherhood benefits poor and socially marginalized mothers the least, as they are least likely to command respect from medical professionals and more likely to be suspected as problem mothers than those middle-class women who are themselves part of the professional class.

Medicalizing infant feeding benefits medical practitioners and makes them feel better ethically about their relations with the infants they care for, because in making infant feeding physicians' responsibility rather than a mother's, they know exactly whose shoulders carry the burden of infant health and welfare. Yet this conflict over responsibility for infant health is precisely what was at stake in the Tabitha Walrond case. Presumably, as the mother, she should have known that her child was dying and should have demanded emergency medical help earlier. At Walrond's sentencing hearing, "despite the mitigating circumstances in the case," the judge said "'The mother is the bottom line'" (Bernstein, "Mother Convicted"). Tyler Walrond's death, and his mother's conviction for criminally negligent homicide (she received a five-year suspended sentence), illustrate the difficulty of holding a mother responsible for a kind of knowledge that has been given over to the medical profession, at the same time that she faces steep barriers of access to that very knowledge, because of her poverty.

In current U.S. culture, methods of infant feeding are privatized choices, in that they are understood to be made by individual mothers in the privacy of their homes and in the context of their private relationships with their family and doctors. All mothers make such choices in our society, and social contexts are not supposed to interfere with the personal characteristics of such a choice. Other people—friends, coworkers, fellow students—are not supposed to comment on this private choice of infant feeding method, although nursing mothers and bottle feeding mothers alike discuss social pressures to feed their infants the *other* way.[22] For example, nursing mothers comment on the disapproving glances they get when they nurse in public or request break time to express milk while working, and bottle feeding moms talk about the public pressure to breastfeed that sends scorn and nasty comments their way. While both groups probably overestimate the significance of such public disapproval, it is clear that the social context and meanings of infant feeding in contemporary U.S. culture make defensiveness an easy position to take up. Such posturing results from the overdetermined nature of mothering in a society with significant conflicts over women's changing social roles and with few social supports for mothers' particular needs as specific kinds of citizens. Mothers are both too responsible for their children, in that the society not only doesn't provide a context that supports maternal practices but makes the experience of maternity difficult and costly, and not responsible enough, because too much of traditional maternal knowledge has been traded to experts whose guidance of women takes away from their ability to interpret and act on their own.[23] We can see this equation at work in Tabitha Walrond's experience—even though the medical and public assistance system seem to have failed this woman and her child, she was deemed negligent for following what she perceived to be the experts' instructions.[24] Without any local knowledge to counteract the experts' writings,[25] and with no one around her to contradict the expert information (breast is best), she did not see her child dying.

Failure to Thrive and the Problem of Seeing

Does no one notice a starving child? Is the mother a reliable observer of her infant's physical development? These questions are raised by the apparent fact that no one else around Tabitha Walrond saw that her child was wasting away. If they did see, they did not feel that they could comment on that fact. Published news reports record Walrond testifying that neighbors and at least one case worker told her that her son was cute (Bernstein, "Mother Charged"). This seems to speak of a society that either chose not to see failure to thrive or could not see it. Indeed, one physician at the Seminar on Breastfeeding commented that

> You know I happened to notice a long time ago that, you know, we don't look at each other anymore. When you go to the grocery store do you look the person in the eye when you exchange the money? No, nobody looks. When you go to the toll booth, do you look the person in the eye when you give them the money and there's an exchange? Nobody looks at each other, and so it's a possibility that nobody really looked at the baby and noticed that the baby was wasting away because we just don't do that in this culture.

This comment was challenged by another physician, however: "[W]e may not look at each other, but everybody looks at babies. And, even here [Hilton Head Island] when I go to the supermarket, when I'm here, when I'm out and around, everybody looks at babies; they may not see me right away but they always see my baby, so I think we do look at the babies and somebody should have noticed that baby was not thriving." Yet another asked, "Why don't human beings recognize that a baby is starving to death? Why don't they recognize that? Anywhere from people at the hospital to the desk at the Medicaid office to the mother of the baby to the grandmother to my highly educated physician patients whose babies are melting away in front of their eyes? Why don't they see this?" This is a key issue, given that Walrond's conviction depended, at least in part, on the jurors' sense that she should have seen.[26]

How do we know how to interpret what we see? At the Seminar on Breastfeeding, one physician commented that "one of the lessons that I learned when I was in my training from my colleagues who are mid-wives is that there's a difference between physiology and pathology, and the most important or most critical step to take is to recognize when physiology becomes pathology, and we don't teach—at least in obstetrics—we don't teach that fact." This was, I thought, a very interesting comment about *seeing* and *interpreting*. In medicine, a key issue concerns when a process that is physiological (such as pregnancy, childbirth, or breastfeeding) is interpreted to cross over the line into pathology. The shift from physiology into pathology is one thing at stake when diagnosing "failure to thrive," which is defined as "all infants who show some degree of growth failure. It is a syndromic classification that has been used to describe infants whose gain in weight or length or both fails to occur in a normal progressive fashion" (Lawrence, *Breastfeeding*, 366). Part of the problem with failure to thrive—how it appears as a devastating and life-threatening situation—is the caretaker's (usually the mother's) inability to see that the infant is not growing or developing. If the problem is caught early, it's not really failure to thrive, or at least it's not the dangerous condition usually associated with that label. Caught early, it's merely "slow weight gain," and can usually be easily remedied with medical treatment, feeding supplementation, or breastfeeding management.

For example, in *Breastfeeding: A Guide for the Medical Profession*, Ruth Lawrence writes (in a section entitled "Slow Gaining versus Failure to Thrive"), "True failure to thrive is potentially serious; early recognition is essential if the integrity of both brain growth and breastfeeding is to be safely preserved" (367). La Leche League's *Breastfeeding Answer Book*, written to give league leaders specific information and advice on communicating with mothers, states, "It is important to clearly distinguish between slow weight gain and failure-to-thrive. Some mothers whose infants fit into the profile of the slow weight gain baby are sometimes mistakenly told that their babies are failure-to-thrive" (Mohrbacher and Stock 118). What follows is then a symptom-by-symptom analysis of the difference between babies with slow weight gain and those who truly fail to thrive and need "immediate supplementation" (119). But as Lawrence indicates, "The term *failure to thrive* has been loosely used" to describe infants who don't grow as they should (366). The *diagnostic* distinctions between failure to thrive and slow weight gain depend, of course, on interpreting the infant's physical state. The indicators are objective (for example, "still losing weight after ten days, little or no growth in length or head circumference" [*Breastfeeding Answer Book* 118]), but they must be *noticed*. That is, the infant must be seen regularly by a doctor who then observes a problem, or the caretaker (usually the mother) must perceive a problem with the infant's development that causes her to seek medical treatment for her child.[27]

The issue of what we can and do see—and how we interpret what we see—is related to what we think we should see, what we believe could not possibly happen, and what we believe is happening.[28] One of the difficulties in really seeing failure to thrive is that people seem to think that babies will always make their needs known forcefully. In local La Leche League meetings, leaders make sure that expectant mothers understand that sleepy newborns sometimes need to be woken up to nurse. Just as some babies have difficulty nursing for no apparent physiological reason, some babies seem "content to starve" (Helliker A4).[29] While many failure-to-thrive cases are caused by organic illness or poor feeding (either by breast or bottle), there are a number of cases in which the diagnosis is "nonorganic failure to thrive" (or NOFTT). Often associated with psychological deprivation or other environmental causes (such as maternal pathology), NOFTT can present like SIDS (Sudden Infant Death Syndrome), in that no specific cause of the infant's failure to consume enough calories can be found (in SIDS, the cause of death cannot be determined). Ruth Lawrence writes that NOFTT "has been equated with a disorder of maternal/infant bonding and has become synonymous with maternal deprivation. *Reactive attachment disorder* has been the term substituted for the disorder and essentially suggests the mother is guilty until proven innocent" (*Breastfeeding* 372). Thus, in the event that there is no identifiable physiological cause of failure to thrive, Lawrence suggests that the mother will be blamed. She continues her discussion with an extended treatment of the breastfeeding management issues involved with failure to thrive that seem to have maternal milk supply or breastfeeding style as a cause, implicitly arguing that NOFTT in breastfed babies is probably caused by poor breastfeeding technique or undiagnosed problems in maternal milk supply. In Tabitha Walrond's case, the defense argued that she may have suffered from insufficient milk syndrome, caused by her breast reduction surgery.

Still, we might imagine that she would have recognized that her child was losing, rather than gaining, weight. But should we come to that conclusion? There is some evidence that mothers do not always perceive their infants' physical status accurately. One participant at the Seminar on Breastfeeding said,

> I'm an educated mom, breastfeeding mom, and my third baby was a critical failure to thrive, and I didn't see it until there were some severe signs of dehydration. And I think part of it is denial, but I also think part of it is you don't have a point of reference because you're with that baby 24/7, so you go back, months later, and you look at the pictures and you're horrified. But when you're with that baby from birth on, you don't see it because of the changes; it's not like an overnight thing when they're losing that weight. So that can be part of the piece of the puzzle, why the mothers don't see it.

Tabitha Walrond testified that the autopsy photographs of her son—a "severely emaciated child, who had lost 37 percent of his birth weight by the time he died"—were "not how he looked to me. ... Now I see the difference in the pictures, but no, when he was in front of me, I didn't see the difference" (Bernstein, "Mother Charged"). (Indeed, it's unlikely she would have seen precisely *that* difference anyway, given that the pictures of an emaciated infant that she saw were autopsy photos taken a day after his death [Pollitt].) An expert on breastfeeding, Dr. Marianne Neifert, "testified for the defense that failure to recognize even a drastic weight loss is common in such cases because the nursing mother sees the baby every day" (Bernstein, "Mother Charged").[30] At the grand jury hearing of another woman initially charged with criminally negligent homicide in the starvation death of her (breastfed) infant, "important testimony . . . from lactation experts and pediatricians who said many of their breast-feeding patients do not recognize that their babies are not thriving until they are weighed in during a routine checkup" apparently convinced the members of the grand jury to drop charges against the mother (Bernstein, "Prosecutor Drops Charges").[31]

One consistent trend in comments about mothers' failure to see their infants' failure to thrive is the pivotal role of the photograph to establish the reality of the infants' condition. As quoted above, one woman at the Seminar on Breastfeeding said, "so you go back, months later, and you look at the pictures and you're horrified." In "Dying for Milk," one mother comments, " 'Just the other day I developed a roll of film we shot back then, and it makes me cry,' she says. 'At three weeks old he looks like an emaciated fetus' " (Helliker A4). In Walrond's case, the defense attorney "warned the jury that they would be shown 'very upsetting and troubling photographs' of an emaciated Tyler after his death at 2 months. . . . [but that] they would hear evidence from experts that even loving and responsible mothers 'can and do miss these signs' " (Bernstein, "Trial Begins for Mother"). According to newspaper accounts, some jurors indicated, after they had convicted Walrond, that they were sympathetic to "many of the defense's arguments, but felt that the gruesome autopsy photographs of the emaciated child proved that Ms. Walrond was criminally responsible for negligence for failing to perceive that her son was in dire need of medical attention" (Bernstein, "Bronx Woman Convicted"). Clearly the visual rhetoric of the dead baby— the evidence on his body of his mother's blindness (even though, according to Susan Tipograph, "other than the fact that it was grossly malnourished [this baby] was cared for from the clipping of the fingernails to the washing, there wasn't a mark on this child")[32]—was far more powerful than expert testimony about this particular inability to see as a medically recognized experience of mothers.

Given the status of the cute baby photograph in contemporary American culture, and the current emphasis on producing scrapbooks and photograph albums dedicated to memorializing one's children's lives through visual documents, pictures of dead, dying, or malnourished infants take on an enhanced signifying function. They represent the mother's negligence, since they seem to clearly indicate what she should have seen. Yet photographs signify at a certain distance—they are not always what the mother sees or experiences, but what the camera captures. Pictures are *framed,* and as such are always somehow *out of context.* Relying on the photograph to document maternal negligence is necessary in cases of abuse or neglect, but the photograph itself must be understood as not what the mother herself necessarily sees. The fact that in these cases the photograph allows the mother to correct her former perception of her infant demonstrates that for some reason it does not represent what she saw at the time.

In cases of anorexia, women routinely do not accurately perceive their own diminishing embodiment, and one might speculate that a newborn baby (especially a breastfed one) is not always experienced as completely separate from the woman's own body.[33] Other people are not always forthcoming in accurately assessing anorectic women's embodiment. Indeed, in a culture that celebrates thinness as much as American culture does (one look at celebrity award shows like the Golden Globe Awards demonstrates that the cult of thinness in Hollywood is alive and thriving), one could argue that there is a communal inability to observe healthy body size and shape—claims about increasing obesity run rampant in medical news, while everyone, it seems, is on a diet or exercise program, and large numbers of young women routinely starve themselves to achieve the "proper" size. African-American women supposedly suffer less than white women from eating disorders and the cult of thinness, but black babies in the United States are also more likely to be born underweight than white babies, and are thus more likely to be smaller in their first few months of life. Tabitha Walrond's reference points for infant size and development, even though Tyler weighed almost eight pounds at birth (above average for all babies), may have been different from white, middle-class norms.[34] And breastfeeding guidebooks suggest that breastfed babies come in all sizes: "both the quite fat and the very slim baby can be normal and healthy. Neither bigness nor smallness is a reason for concern as long as the baby's food is human milk and nursings are according to his needs. If you feed your baby in the way that is naturally intended for the human infant, his weight gain will be what is natural for your particular child" (La Leche League, *The Womanly Art*, 6th ed., 74–75).[35]

That Tabitha Walrond was not alone in her apparent inability to observe her baby's weight loss was made very clear to the judge in the case, who stated at the sentencing hearing that "he had received about 900 letters from around the world, all supporting Ms. Walrond and asking for leniency": "Among the hundreds of letters, postcards and e-mail messages the judge and prosecutors in the case received, some from as far away as Japan, were many from mothers who said that they, too, had almost let a child starve to death while breast-feeding with the best of intentions." But the judge stated, "misperception 'is not an absolute defense to criminally negligent homicide'" (Bernstein, "Mother Convicted"). Perhaps the key here is the "almost"—the women writing in hadn't lost their babies; they had just gotten close. Thus, their pleas didn't carry as much weight as they might have if their infants had died. These other infants survived because either their mothers, or their doctors, or perhaps even the neighbors or their parents' friends *noticed* that something was wrong and intervened; their babies were diagnosed, not autopsied. Thus, these mothers of infants who barely lived were spared the trauma and suffering that Tabitha Walrond experienced after the death of her son—instead of a trial, they had only the photographs to document their negligent perception.

At the sentencing hearing for Tabitha Walrond, newspapers report that the judge indicated that the psychiatrist who evaluated her for the trial suggested that Walrond "lacked insight into the emotional problems that may have contributed to her failure to perceive that her son was in dire need of medical attention" (Bernstein, "Mother Convicted"). Indeed, Dr. Berger "said Ms. Walrond showed signs of 'narcissistic personality disorder' that may have caused her to react defiantly when her self-esteem was in jeopardy—as when her ex-boyfriend and his mother told her the baby was too thin." This evaluation is reminiscent of the psychological indictment of single white pregnant women in the 1950s, as described by Rickie Sollinger in *Wake Up Little Susie: Single Pregnancy and Race before Roe v. Wade:* "In postwar America, mental illness was considered a universal condition for white unwed mothers, by definition" (87), and "Personality and character disorders [in pregnant single white women who lived in maternity homes] discovered by professionals included masochism, sadomasochism, severe immaturity, psychopathic tendencies, homosexual tendencies, schizophrenia, delinquency, and chaotic personality structure" (90).[36] While putatively about Ms. Walrond's specific case, the judge's view implies that any mother who does not see the reality of her child's embodiment, a reality purported to be accurately caught on photographic film, must be mentally ill.[37]

Insufficient Milk Syndrome

In her presentation at the Seminar on Breastfeeding, lawyer Susan Tipograph said, "it's interesting that the only two people that I know of who were ever prosecuted for this [babies dying of malnourishment while being breastfed] were Tabitha Walrond, who was a young black woman in the Bronx, and Tatania Cheeks, who was a young black woman from Brooklyn, [from whom] the prosecution was withdrawn because they determined that the child had not lost enough body weight for there, for it to [be] obvious to the mother to know [that the baby was failing to thrive]." The only person at the seminar to speak openly of racism (which was otherwise implied by physicians and others through the use of terms like *high-risk moms* and *low-income families*), Tipograph also mentioned that "[t]he prosecutor in the Bronx described the child as being a Biafran baby, which I thought had a little tinge of racism to it, but I won't—but I got a call from a woman who was in fact not an African American who went to the hospital with her child and they told her her child looked like a Biafran baby, but apparently they got over it because she was never prosecuted." If Tabitha Walrond was responsible for her son's death, and Tatania Cheeks at least charged with the death of her infant daughter (although the charges were later dropped), why was the *Wall Street Journal* article "Dying for Milk" so sympathetic to the mothers who tried "in vain to breast-feed" (Helliker A1)? In this piece, the villainy rests with public health campaigns to promote breastfeeding, advice books for parents (like *Dr. Spock's Baby and Child Care,* quoted in the article), and lactation consultants whose mantra is Breast Is Best. Shifting the focus from *failure to thrive* to *insufficient milk syndrome* is partly why the situations differ—the mothers suffer from a syndrome that can cause failure to thrive in infants if not caught early enough. Insufficient milk is a medical condition that, at least in the context of the article, mothers have no control over and do not understand the signs of. Also, in the former cases, the infants who died were five and seven weeks old, while "Dying for Milk" generally looks at babies (purportedly) damaged from an initial lack of nutrition in the first week of life. Another significant factor is Keith Helliker's self-stated support for breastfeeding (Johnson, "Conspiracy Debate"). Although many breastfeeding advocates feel that the article was antibreastfeeding (as testimony, numerous letters supporting breastfeeding were published subsequently in the *Wall Street Journal*), the author, Helliker, does argue that better medical attention to lactation would help eliminate or alleviate problems with lactation failure.

In portraying insufficient milk syndrome and its danger to mothers and babies, representational issues show up similarly to those in the Walrond case, in that the mothers don't see the infants failing until something has gone wrong (a seizure, for example), or only in hindsight, while looking at a photograph. As quoted above, one of the mothers in "Dying for Milk" states, " 'Just the other day I developed a roll of film we shot back then, and it makes me cry,' she says. 'At three weeks old, he looked like an emaciated fetus' " (Helliker A4). Helliker treats this mother's insufficient milk as a straightforward biological issue—she did not have enough: "Wendy Hamilton, 36, wanted intensely to breast-feed. Though she didn't produce nearly enough milk to feed her infant son, she refused to rely solely on formula. Instead, she tried stimulating her milk production by taking medication and by pumping her breasts whenever her son wasn't latched on" (Helliker A4). Anyone familiar with breastfeeding wonders why, with such stimulation, she couldn't make enough milk—lactation, after all, is a supply-demand system. The more the breasts are stimulated, by a suckling baby or by a breast pump (although the former is more efficient), the more milk they make. Other factors do interfere, of course, notably stress, lack of fluid intake, and insufficient calories in the diet. The next paragraph offers a possible answer, however:

"To make matters worse, her son sucked in a terribly painful way. 'Sometimes,' she says, 'I had blood dripping down my chest and tears streaming down my face' " (Helliker, A4).

Blood should never be dripping down one's chest while breastfeeding. (This seems an obvious observation, yet, given the sorry state of public knowledge about breastfeeding, perhaps it's not.) While engorgement and nipple cracking can be a problem in the early days, they should resolve after a week or the mother should seek counseling to improve the baby's latch, position, and suckling. If the baby's sucking continues to be painful after the first minute of nursing, the baby is probably incorrectly latched, which means that he or she may not be stimulating the breast appropriately to produce milk, and most certainly is damaging sensitive nipple and areola tissue. From this account, it seems that Wendy Hamilton couldn't make enough milk because her baby wasn't nursing properly. This is not a biological issue of an innate incapacity to produce milk; it is, instead, an issue of lactation management (in medical terms).[38]

Dr. Marianne Neifert, who testified for the defense at Tabitha Walrond's trial, appears prominently in "Dying for Milk." She also wrote a letter to the *Wall Street Journal* that was published in a special section called "Breast-Feeding Champions" in August 1994 (Letter to the Editor). In the latter text, as in her popular book *Dr. Mom's Guide to Breastfeeding*, Neifert argues that insufficient milk syndrome is a taboo subject among breastfeeding advocates, primarily because it brings negative attention to breastfeeding and implies that breastfeeding success can be difficult. In the chapter of *Dr. Mom's Guide* devoted to "Insufficient Milk Syndrome and Inadequate Weight Gain," Neifert divides insufficient milk into three categories: perceived insufficient milk ("I don't dispute that widespread *misperceptions* about insufficient milk contribute enormously to the early discontinuation of breastfeeding" [319; emphasis in original]), primary insufficient milk ("it describes a low milk supply problem that was present from the outset and that is beyond a mother's control" [321]), and secondary insufficient milk ("The potential to breastfeed successfully is readily apparent to anyone who views the milk-laden breasts on the third postpartum day. . . . If something interferes with regular drainage of milk, secondary insufficient milk can occur" [321]). Further, she admits that "most instances of insufficient milk are due to problems in the management of breastfeeding" (322), and while she presents a number of reasons for primary milk insufficiency (including previous breast surgery, hormone problems, breast radiation, and failure of lactogenesis[39]), the discussion of secondary milk insufficiency is basically a discussion of how to correct common breastfeeding problems by proper management of latch-on, suckling, and feeding routines. Thus, Neifert's discussion of the supposedly taboo problem of insufficient milk is merely what appears in other breastfeeding guidebooks under a different name (for example, "overcoming common breastfeeding problems," or "increasing milk supply").

What we can glean from this section of *Dr. Mom's Guide* is that more women *think* they experience insufficient milk than really do, that many women wean unnecessarily because of this perception, and that most women who actually have insufficient milk do so because of poor breastfeeding management or style. According to Lawrence Gartner, who at the time of writing his letter to the *Wall Street Journal* was professor of pediatrics at the University of Chicago and chair of the Breast-Feeding Work Group of the American Academy of Pediatrics, "In the absence of sufficient knowledge and experience, physicians and others are inclined to offer one of two responses to a breast-feeding problem, either to immediately advise switching to bottle-feeding with formula or to urge continued nursing without assessing whether it is being performed properly and successfully" (Letter to the Editor). Ruth Lawrence, who in addition to authoring *Breastfeeding: A Guide for Physicians* was (at the time of writing the letter to the *Wall Street Journal*) director of the Breastfeeding and Human Lactation Study Center and professor of pediatrics at the University of Rochester, concurs that breastfeeding management is the most significant issue in cases of perceived insufficient milk syndrome: "When an infant does not feed well, the infant should be evaluated by the physician to be sure there is not an intervening reason for the poor feeding. In most cases, minor adjustments in holding, positioning, or latch-on is [sic] all that is required, along with a good dose of reassurance" (Letter to the Editor). No one disputes that cases of true (or primary) insufficient milk syndrome exist—breastfeeding advocates simply tend to question the idea that there are large numbers of women who *physically* cannot make enough milk. When Marianne Neifert claims that as many as 5 percent of the time breastfeeding mothers do not make sufficient milk (Helliker A1), she doesn't distinguish primary and secondary insufficiency, so the figure is a bit disingenuous. After all, as other breastfeeding advocates (and even Neifert herself) indicate, most problems of insufficiency occur because women don't know how to breastfeed and are given incorrect advice to remedy lactation difficulties.

The motivation for the article, it seems, was mothers' guilt rather than infant ill-health. Keith Helliker, interviewed in a story for the *Providence Journal-Bulletin*, "said he became interested in the topic because he knew a couple of women—'yuppies, if you will'—who had tried to breast-feed without success. 'Their babies didn't wind up getting hurt as a result, but there was a feeling in these cases that they could have, that there was so much pressure (on the mothers) to keep trying, and so little concern about just getting the babies fed, that it seemed dangerous.' " He asserted that in the

Wall Street Journal article he emphasized the rarity of cases where infants are damaged by insufficient milk, but that in the cases of his friends "the first two or three months of their lives were essentially ruined by the failure of anybody in the medical profession to enlighten them." The issue is personal for Helliker, because "[a]sked whether his own child was breast-fed Helliker said yes, but added, 'there were problems. Breast-feeding exclusively did not work. He got absolutely as much breast milk as we could get'" (Johnson, "Conspiracy Debate"). Yet certainly it's disingenuous of Helliker to deny that his article is antibreastfeeding, since the second subtitle reads "'Yuppie Syndrome' among Well-Meaning Parents Stems from Bad Advice," and the article itself reiterates that these mothers without enough milk were consistently told that breastfeeding was best for their infants. While it may be that the bad advice was really the advice to keep breastfeeding when there were evident problems, it *seems* as if the bad advice is just to breastfeed. After all, he implies, why begin such an arduous process if you may be one of those 5 percent who simply *can't*, and who thus might be endangering your infant?[40]

In fact, all breastfeeding manuals, as well as most infant care guides, cover the essentials of breastfeeding management, which include information about how to tell if an infant is getting enough milk.[41] The crucial issue is how mothers interpret the signs of adequate milk supply and intake, as well as infant development, growth, and elimination, in relation to advice about the benefits of breastfeeding and the need to persevere in the face of common nursing challenges. All the guides assume, as well, that mothers and infants are under the watchful care of physicians.

Tabitha Walrond's lawyers tried to position her similarly to the yuppie moms in "Dying for Milk"—following the experts' advice, unaware that anything was wrong because she was following that advice and because none of her healthcare providers had identified or addressed the many experiences that put her at high risk for breastfeeding failure (breast reduction surgery, postpartum infection, early bottle feeding). Evidently, in the eyes of the jury, the lawyers were unsuccessful in making Walrond herself into a victim. In the earlier *Wall Street Journal* article, the mothers seemed victimized even when it was their infants who were physically harmed by lack of nutrition. Tabitha Walrond was not at risk because of too much education—although breastfeeding education without practical support seems to have been a problem for her, as well as for the yuppie moms—and she could never be a yuppie, although she did graduate from high school two days before her baby was born. Her main social problems were being poor and black and on public assistance, all of which put her in a category of women at high risk for breastfeeding failure. In all probability, however, her main difficulty in feeding her son was probably physiological, since breast reduction surgery usually involves removing and repositioning the nipple, and often involves cutting through milk ducts. Trauma to nerves can cause problems with milk supply even for women whose ducts are not cut and nipples not repositioned. Most likely, Tabitha Walrond *is* one of those women who suffer from primary milk insufficiency, although, in all probability, it was not a condition she was born with.

But, as the newspaper articles about her trial remind us visually, she is undeniably black. When I was first researching this case, I looked up the articles on LexisNexis, an online database. All I saw was the text version of each article. However, when I looked at the microfilmed newspapers, I realized that each of the three *New York Times* articles about the trial and Walrond's conviction included a photograph of her. Thus, while the articles themselves do not mention her race, the reader is shown it. As with the photographs of dead or dying infants, these images of Tabitha Walrond, black teenage mother, have a signifying function in relation to the articles about her trial. I have no idea what the intent of the newspaper was in including these pictures, or even if it is standard procedure to include a photograph of trial defendants in articles about them. But the *effect* of the photographs is undeniable: they serve to remind the reader that Tabitha Walrond is a black woman, irrevocably different from the white Pam Floyd, former secretary and now mom, who is pictured smiling, with her infant, in a drawing on the front page of the *Wall Street Journal*. This reminder of Walrond's race brings with it all the associated stereotypes of black women as negligent, uncaring, and unfeeling mothers, in contrast to the prevailing image of the white mother as entitled to an idealized, optimal experience of maternity, unfettered by such difficulties as insufficient milk or a damaged baby.

Baby Friendly?

Breastfeeding advocates strive for positive images of breastfeeding in the public media, and become irate at the many depictions that not only get nursing wrong, but misunderstand breastfeeding educational campaigns and public health programs. I have yet to see a TV program that demonstrates even a passing familiarity with the experiences of maternal nursing, let alone the intricacies of breastfeeding management. For example, on NBC's *ER* (one of my favorite programs), a black woman gave birth to a premature baby who was then treated in the NICU (Neonatal Intensive Care Unit) for weeks. When the baby was finally allowed to take nourishment by mouth, the mother sat in a rocking chair and calmly nursed him. There had been no previous discussion or representations of her pumping her breasts, the difficulties associated with establishing a milk supply with a breast pump rather than a baby, or the issues involved with initiating latch-on with a premature infant previously fed intravenously or through nasogastric tubing. The message was "Breastfeeding, no problem!" which, on the one hand, is welcome news, but, on the other hand, is completely inaccurate.

ER also had a head nurse who breastfed twins for part of the 1999–2000 season; she pumped during her breaks on shift. Again, it's a welcome sight to see a breast pump on television and a mother whose use of the pump is no-nonsense and matter-of-fact. There was even one show in which she suggested that the babies wouldn't take a bottle but she had to pump in order to be comfortable while working. (That was a reality I could relate to.) But the representations of her nursing tended to be sporadic and ephemeral—they never depicted the way that breastfeeding can take over the mother's experience of maternity. Pumping enough for twins is certainly possible, but it's no walk in the park; just nursing twins can be a full-time job. When she tells the attending physician, her friend, that she is thinking of weaning her babies at six months but feels a bit guilty about it, he tells her that she can't be a perfect mom and she might as well accept that now. There's no discussion of the health benefits of extended nursing, or her feelings about the nursing experience. It's all about her burden as a mother—and as a single mother, nursing twins can certainly be a burden. In the only other representation of breastfeeding on *ER* that I recall (apart from the resident who pours the nurse's pumped milk on his cereal), a baby dies as a result of amphetamines that the mother was taking in order to stay awake for her job. Another dead baby story.

In October 1998 CBS's *Chicago Hope* aired a program, "The Breast and the Brightest," in which the mothering experiences of one of its primary characters, a doctor, are juxtaposed against those of another mother whose breastfed infant dies due to starvation. In February 2000 NBC's *Law and Order* aired an episode, "Mother's Milk," that also involved a breastfed baby that died of starvation.[42] This latter show was clearly modeled on the Tabitha Walrond case, although specific details (like the race of the mother, her marital status, and her relations with lactation specialists) were changed to fictionalize and dramatize the real events. Both of these shows elicited responses from La Leche League on their web site; these responses were meant to educate mothers and others about the rarity of infants starving because of insufficient milk and to give them important information about how to tell that a baby is getting enough milk. The La Leche League responses also involved repudiating key inaccuracies in the TV accounts of breastfeeding advocacy: the Baby-Friendly contract[43] and villainous lactation counselors.

On both shows, the Baby-Friendly Hospital Initiative (BFHI), a project that "assists hospitals in giving breastfeeding mothers the information, confidence, and skills needed to successfully initiate and continue breastfeeding their babies" (Baby-Friendly USA), is transformed into a contract that the mother signs, promising not to feed her baby formula and to exclusively breastfeed. I suppose it's not surprising that television programs could get breastfeeding advocacy so wrong, given that they can't even get breastfeeding right. I would expect that the shows' writers would do some research, and any sort of minimal research would offer the information that the BFHI is a program to help *hospitals* promote breastfeeding. It is a UNICEF/WHO initiative based on the "Ten Steps to Successful Breastfeeding":

1. Maintain a written breastfeeding policy that is routinely communicated to all health care staff.
2. Train all health care staff in skills necessary to implement this policy.
3. Inform all pregnant women about the benefits and management of breastfeeding.
4. Help mothers initiate breastfeeding within one hour of birth.
5. Show mothers how to breastfeed and maintain lactation, even if they are separated from their infants.
6. Give newborn infants no food or drink other than breastmilk, unless medically indicated.
7. Practice "rooming-in"—allow mothers and infants to remain together 24 hours a day.
8. Encourage unrestricted breastfeeding.
9. Give no pacifiers or artificial nipples to breastfeeding infants.
10. Foster the establishment of breastfeeding support groups and refer mothers to them on discharge from the hospital or clinic. (Baby-Friendly USA)

There is nothing in these ten steps to suggest that mothers themselves sign a contract not to give their infants anything but breast milk—a key aspect of both the *Chicago Hope* and *Law and Order* television programs—and mothers are not prohibited from feeding their infants formula, even in the hospital.[44] These ten steps, the keystone of the BFHI, are about *hospital policies* to promote breastfeeding, not coercing mothers to breastfeed. Moreover, information about BFHI and the ten steps is relatively easy to find—searching the WHO and UNICEF web sites provides a plethora of commentary and discussion. Because of this I can't help but feel that the writers for these two shows simply didn't look for the information and used anecdotal (and erroneous) stories from friends or colleagues or news articles to provide the materials they used in the shows.

The transformation of BFHI into a contract that the mother signs, promising not to supplement feedings with infant formula, allows the television programs to make the mothers into the victims of breastfeeding advocates and public health policies. In this way, these shows follow the "Dying for Milk" model of representing insufficient milk syndrome as a danger attendant to maternal nursing. Instead of highlighting the lack of knowledgeable medical support available for nursing mothers, especially mothers without resources, these shows represent the medical establishment as pushing women to breastfeed and then intimidating them when the mother has problems. In the *Law and Order* episode, the lactation counselor is represented as being more interested in promoting breastfeeding than in the baby who died of starvation. Thus, in these representations, medicine's fault is its interest in lactation and its desire to coerce women to breastfeed, rather than its lack of effective material support for women who breastfeed in a society that doesn't know much about it and doesn't provide a context accommodating to women who choose to do so. These latter issues were, of course, the focus of the "Ethical and Legal" discussion at the Seminar on Breastfeeding after the presentation of the Walrond case.

On *Law and Order* the depiction of the mother is ambivalent: on the one hand she is a teenager who ignored her infant and let it starve because she felt overwhelmed with motherhood, but on the other hand she was breastfeeding her child and trying to do her best as a mother. It is partially her whiteness that allows the program to present her as at least somewhat sympathetic— the stereotypes of black women as always already neglectful and uncaring mothers cannot be invoked to make her seem completely responsible for the infant's death. The show thus manages to indict breastfeeding advocates like the lactation counselor as well as the young mother herself (who is convicted of manslaughter in the second degree and sentenced to 1½ to 4½ years in jail). This leads to a connection between breastfeeding and maternal neglect since, as the prosecuting attorney asks rhetorically at the trial, "babies don't starve to death on [formula], do they?" Of course, a baby *will* starve to death on formula, if it doesn't get enough of it or becomes ill because of unsanitary conditions attendant to bottle feeding—that is precisely what breastfeeding advocacy in the poverty environments of the Third World is all about. In addition, Ruth Lawrence notes that "failure to thrive among bottle-fed babies and babies who are not held is much more common than among breast-fed babies" (MacKeen).[45] But in this television context of unrelieved whiteness (the black characters on these two shows notwithstanding, the mothers with breastfeeding issues or starving children are all white), doing one's best for the baby easily slides into doing the worst, since breastfeeding takes work (the lactation counselor states, "It's just a matter of getting the mother to put the effort into it") and a physical commitment to the baby's interests. Some women have difficulty, and in these shows, society doesn't adequately recognize the suffering of these women: the defense attorney on *Law and Order*, in her closing statement, says, "Only a woman can know the social pressure to breastfeed today and only a woman can suffer the stigma of that failure." As the mother of the dead infant on *Chicago Hope* laments to the breastfeeding doctor, Diane, "Breastfeed; don't breastfeed. Cloth diapers; black and white toys; organic food. God, what difference does it make? The only thing you really have to do is keep them alive. That's all. And I couldn't do it. [Breaking down.] I couldn't do it."[46]

That it is her job to keep the child alive goes unquestioned in both programs, although mothers' responsibility is a conflicted issue in each. Interestingly enough, in most discussions of insufficient milk syndrome and failure to thrive, the father's responsibility does not emerge as a salient issue. On *Law and Order*, it was, although the father ends up helping to convict his wife as part of his plea bargain. On *Chicago Hope* the breastfeeding doctor's husband is a stay-at-home dad (conveniently allowing him to be virtually present through the cell phone conversations during which we never hear his voice), but the mother feels that "He's not the bottom line. I am." When she arrives home to find her daughter being cared for by a neighbor (a black woman who has a daughter of a similar age) because her husband and the neighbor's husband have gone out to see a movie, she finds the baby burning up with fever and, rather than getting angry at the neighbor for not noticing that the infant was ill, or the husband for leaving, gets angry at herself once the baby is out of danger in the emergency room ("I almost killed her, oh my God"). Earlier in the show, when the baby who dies of starvation is brought in as an emergency trauma, she is the doctor who argues that the mother should be arrested because "It's pretty obvious" (her words) what happened. Indeed, it is this sense of responsibility that makes her question her experience of motherhood, not the actual time she spends with her baby: she says to the pediatrician caring for her baby in the emergency room,

> "Billy seems to get it. He likes it. I mean he worries, but he's into it. But that's because he's not the bottom line. I am. It always comes down to me. I'm the one who notices when she's outgrown her pj's, or we need more diapers, or she's going to sleep too late, or she's not napping enough. I mean, somehow I've been put in charge. It's a big mistake. Half the time when I look at her, I feel like, I don't know, I feel like I'm from Mars, and she looks at me like, 'Hey, I'm a baby, I don't know anything. And if you don't know anything then we're lost.' "

This speech comes only a few lines after she has stated, "motherhood: I hate it. I'm no good at it." The other mother's trauma with a dead baby serves as a backdrop for the show's focus on the responsibility of motherhood and the difficulties even privileged women have meeting that responsibility.

In the *Law and Order* episode, the lactation consultant indicates that breastfeeding is successful if the mother "puts in the effort." In addition, the female assistant D.A. prosecuting the case argues that the legal right to choose to be pregnant implies women's responsibility for their infants. In this model, mothers are burdened by their hypothetical right to end their pregnancies. They are the bottom line: "Her lawyer suggests that others are to blame. But are we really at a point where even feeding our babies has become someone else's responsibility?" (Of course, this is what formula feeding allows mothers to do—redistribute responsibility for infant feeding within the family or outsource it to other caretakers—and it is touted as one of the benefits of bottle feeding in infant care guides.) The judge in the case concurs. While castigating the father and the lactation counselor in her remarks, she states, "But ultimately the responsibility for a child must be placed on the primary caregiver, and even today, that still means its mother."

The visible signs of failure to thrive are at issue in both shows. In the *Chicago Hope* episode, the breastfeeding doctor, Diane, says "it's obvious" once during the trauma with the dead infant and then once again while talking to the head ER doctor, although after her experience with her feverish daughter she decides to change her report and indicate that the death might have been accidental. On *Law and Order*, the attorneys cannot empanel a jury because the defense presents all candidates with the autopsy photographs of the dead infant, in order to demonstrate that the defendant can't get a fair trial. Every one of the potential jurors believes the mother knew her baby was dying. The judge asks one, "You understand you haven't heard any testimony," and he answers, "Come on judge, look at this. She had to know." Ultimately, the judge, ruling in a bench trial, agrees. Neither show provides any of the abundant evidence that failure to thrive can be difficult to notice, although the defense attorney on *Law and Order* does get the coroner to agree that long babies can sometimes be deceiving. In these shows, photographs are evidence of what mothers must have seen (and thus known); starvation is obvious, and as a result the infant deaths seem intentional At least on *Chicago Hope* there is a sense that mothers are not all-seeing, that even doctor-mothers can make mistakes and miss the signs of illness (although how the infant's roseola is the breastfeeding doctor's responsibility, since she's been gone all day, is unclear). But even as Diane grants the other woman the capacity to not see and therefore make a mistake, that mother takes on the responsibility herself: "The only thing you really have to do is keep them alive. That's all. And I couldn't do it."

These programs' stagings of infant death resulting from breastfeeding are really targeting contemporary motherhood and its perceived stresses. Both programs' plots hinge on the mothers' responsibility for their infants, their sense of inadequacy in their roles, and the general sense that regardless of others' involvement in their infants' care, they are the "bottom line."[47] Breastfeeding is used as a way to highlight concerns about contemporary

American motherhood (Are all mothers fit to care for their infants? Should mothers work? Does the quality of a mother's care and her commitment to her child's welfare matter? If women consciously choose to become mothers, are they responsible for being good mothers?) because it brings together these concerns in a specific way. A breastfed child depends on its mother, and she is responsible for the child in a way that no other human can be. Breastfeeding establishes a relation between the mother and the infant that goes beyond any other biological relation between humans; physiologically, the two are separate bodies connected in a symbiotic, supply/demand relation of nursing and milk production. This biological relation, in representational terms, absorbs the social concerns about women as mothers (Can they be depended on to be mothers?).

U.S. television stories about breastfeeding infants dying of starvation are about social fears of women's innate inability to mother and nurture their children. The way that public health policy issues are deformed for the purpose of dramatic tension and plot demonstrates that the shows' writers and producers aren't concerned with the real social and medical contexts within which breastfeeding occurs in the United States and elsewhere. Instead, they play off the current social ambivalence about women's relation to children and their responsibility to keep them alive. If women can't be trusted to keep their babies alive, if they can't be trusted to *see* starvation when it's occurring, then they probably shouldn't breastfeed. Indeed, in this scenario, women really can't be trusted to do much of anything that requires their autonomous judgment.

Representing dead babies in America, then, is about managing social conflicts around women—who they are, what they should be doing, and whom they are responsible for. Those women who are perceived to be least reliable and least likely to be governed by an internalized sense of responsibility— black women and other women of color, poor women, young women—are thus at greater risk for being blamed for the terrible things that can happen to any infant, while white, middle-class, educated, older women are more likely to be seen as the victims of their very privilege. This is how the yuppie mothers can come to be the victims of medical experts' discourses on infant feeding. That their risk is directly related to their privilege, at least in these representations, suggests a deep social distrust of *all* women's mothering capacities, a distrust that nevertheless impacts disadvantaged and socially marginalized women in far greater numbers. In the cases of Third World women whose babies die because of illnesses associated with formula feeding—the dead baby images presented by breastfeeding advocates—it is easy to blame formula manufacturers and to see the mothers *and* infants as victims of global capitalism. But, from the perspective of the United States, these women are Third World others whose images do not carry the kind of stigma that images of and discourses about black women suggest in the U.S. context. They are outside the particular racial dynamic that holds Tabitha Walrond responsible for her infant's death, although the use of their images contributes to a racialized context in which breastfeeding is thought to be an exotic maternal practice, as well as a physically depleting one. (Like Tabitha Walrond, however, they are likely to be held responsible for having babies at all.)

The representations of Tabitha Walrond's case and the other cases of infant death in the various media discussed here reveal fault lines around race, class, and education in relation to a mother's perceived culpability in her infant's starvation death. Poor black women, stereotypically perceived to be negligent mothers, can be held responsible for their children's welfare, even in the face of gross medical and bureaucratic negligence. It's not such a stretch to imagine that Tabitha Walrond's perceived responsibility for her son's death derives from a perception of her innate culpability as a black woman (mother of the bio-underclass[48]), whereas white women (mothers of the entitled citizenry) are viewed as having been hoodwinked by medical experts who rigidly adhere to breastfeeding like religious zealots when their babies suffer from the mothers' insufficient milk. But I'm also suggesting that while race and class make a (tragic) difference, there is a clear distrust of *all* women as mothers, a distrust that is both recognized and suppressed in these representational venues. The public staging of dead, starved, breastfed babies is really about the contested nature of contemporary motherhood: its rights, its responsibilities, and the interpretation of its failures.

CHAPTER 2

Rational Management

Some of my feminist students have a story they tell about contemporary medicine and its control of women's reproductive experiences. A long time ago, they write, women gave birth and breastfed in the company of other women. The experience was empowering and joyous. Then men took over, and women were drugged through labor and delivery, and consequently were often unable to breastfeed their children. The experience was no longer empowering or joyous; instead, women experience their most profound disempowerment and loss of agency through these events.

I'm simplifying, of course, and I don't want to demean my students' attempt to grasp the clearly momentous shift in the ordinary experiences of childbirth and infant feeding that have occurred through the last few centuries in many parts of the world. What they would call a woman-centered experience has been transformed into something seemingly controlled by men and the external, technocratic forces of hospitals, health clinics, and health insurance companies. But their simplification often doesn't help them to understand the complexity of women's own involvement in the transformation of reproduction in the modern era—as well as the fact that many women died prior to the discovery of the importance of aseptic and antiseptic protocols during childbirth, and that many infants died during childbirth as well. The simplistic view—it used to be better when women were in control—doesn't account for the ways in which women often ally themselves with modern, technological medicine and its values, and doesn't take account of the profound ignorance that previously accompanied many a woman's birthing experience.

What my students are trying to get at, however, and often don't have the conceptual tools to articulate, are the profound changes that have accompanied the shift of childbirth and breastfeeding from a familial and social domain to one primarily considered medical. Of course, medical history indicates a consistent interest in reproduction and lactation (Yalom 205–40), but for most women for most of the world's history, childbirth and breastfeeding were not occasions for medical intervention except in cases of dire need (and when that care was available). The story of the gradual inclusion of reproduction and lactation into medicine's recognized zone of expertise has been told by a number of other scholars (for example, Apple, Leavitt, Bogdan), and I'm not going to rehearse those arguments here. Instead, I'm going to examine the current context of physicians' interest in and role in what they would call "breastfeeding management," in light of the idea that breastfeeding has not always been (and therefore need not be) considered a particularly *medical* issue.

In this chapter, I examine a medical guide concerning lactation, Ruth Lawrence's *Breastfeeding: A Guide for the Medical Profession* (first edition published in 1980, with a fourth edition in 1994). Through a close reading of Lawrence's chapter on the "Psychologic [*sic*] Impact of Breastfeeding," I show that the medical discussion of the psychological aspects of breastfeeding articulates conflicting ideological views of women and their place in society, demonstrating how medicine reflects and contributes to a cultural context that is ambivalent about women's changing roles and the transformation of their practices as mothers.

The ambivalence about mothers' roles is not specific to medicine, but since medical discourse aspires to a neutrality free of ideological influence (evident in the way that statements are made as conclusions based on scientific data, the result of published research), the intrusion of pointedly ideological statements about mothers in Lawrence's guide is particularly salient. *Breastfeeding: A Guide for the Medical Profession* is unique in the field, as the only such book written expressly for physicians to consult in clinical practice.[1] The discussion of psychological issues attendant to breastfeeding shows how the practice of breastfeeding management in medicine engages some highly charged social concepts about women. Thus, while medical research on lactation continues to provide what breastfeeding advocates consider to be consistent and compelling information about the appropriateness of human milk for infants (and the corresponding inappropriateness of infant formulas in all but a very few situations), the discourse of medical breastfeeding advocacy contributes, through its rhetoric, to the generalized social ambivalence about modern women and maternity.

It's important to remember that Lawrence's guide represents breastfeeding *advocacy* among physicians—a distinct minority position within a profession that only in 1997 returned to a position that fully promotes exclusive breastfeeding for human infants for their first six months of life, and breastfeeding with food supplementation for at least a year (American Academy of Pediatrics). In Lawrence's *Guide,* the medical *management* of breastfeeding is really about managing the mother-infant nursing couple in the context of a society that consistently misunderstands the experience of lactation and its consequences—thus *physicians* who perpetuate this misinformation need to be managed as well. Contemporary infant feeding in the context of medical management provides a particularly interesting example of medicine's involvement with and perpetuation of cultural values, while Lawrence's *Guide* provides an example of a politicized medical discourse that seeks to make the cultural context an explicit aspect of the physician's relation to the mother and infant. Here I concentrate on the rhetoric of a single medical guidebook, and thus cannot claim to show how medical care of nursing mothers is directly influenced by this text; indeed, I resist any simple one-to-one correspondence between rhetoric or representation and the material practice of breastfeeding in contemporary American culture, since the practice is too complex to reduce simply to a unilateral response to medicine. However, in the conclusion I do speculate about certain ways the rhetoric *might* be related to real experiences of maternity. Significantly, Ruth Lawrence cannot avoid repeating cultural prescriptions about maternity, because conceptions of maternity encourage her to represent breastfeeding as a biological role to which women must adjust. This double bind of breastfeeding advocacy—an argument for breastfeeding as an empowering and healthful right of women and infants that typically devolves into an ideological view of proper mothering—has made its analysis by feminists a particularly complex and difficult task. It is precisely this nexus of difficulty, in which interpreting and engaging in specific practices of maternal embodiment are at stake, that has drawn me—feminist theorist, breastfeeding advocate, and former nursing mother—to this project.

Experience in Rational Management Preferred (or, No Mothers Need Apply)

In the preface to the first edition of *Breastfeeding: A Guide for the Medical Profession,* written in 1980 and included in the fourth edition, Ruth Lawrence writes,

> The first part of this book is basic data on the anatomical, physiological, biochemical, nutritional, immunological, and psychological aspects of human lactation. The remainder centers on the problems of clinical management and, I hope, maximizes scientific data and minimizes anecdotal information. The goal is to provide practical

> information for managing individual mothers and their infants. It is also hoped that a balance has been struck between basic science, on which rational management should rest, and advice garnered by experience. (xiii)

Here we can see two pairs of terms—science *versus* anecdote and science *and* experience—in which the staging of the first influences the understanding of the second. If scientific data is held up over anecdote in the first opposition, it is because the physician can only be the champion of the former. Implied is that the source of anecdotal information is women who are not informed by science, "on which rational management should rest." But the second pairing suggests that there is a *balance* between basic science and experience. Here, experience seems to be the territory of the physician—this would be experience in the management of nursing mothers. Any experience of women in this matter seems doubly discounted.

Yet in the foreword to the guide, John Kennell and Marshall Klaus write, "This detailed and well-written book benefits greatly not only from the author's extensive experience running a normal and sick infant nursery but also from her special and unique personal life, rearing and breastfeeding nine healthy children of her own. Thus the author is a veteran in two areas" (vii). The balance referred to above may be a reference to Lawrence's own life. In this reading of the balance between science and experience, the mother has valuable (and unique) experience.

Of course, much of the bad information, the anecdote as it were, is produced *by physicians*, which is an interesting fact in relation to Lawrence's opposition between science and anecdote. That most medical personnel know little about breastfeeding is a claim made by many breastfeeding advocates, both medical professionals and others. Indeed, part of the purpose in publishing the *Guide* is to convince physicians to leave aside the anecdotal, on which they have depended *because they have no experience with breastfeeding*, and be persuaded by scientific data.

This ambivalent opposition between science and anecdote, science and experience, is, of course, gendered, a fact which Lawrence explicitly emphasizes by stating in the preface to the first edition,

> Throughout this book, since a nursing mother is a female, the personal pronoun *she* has been used. In referring to the infant, the choice between *he* or *she* has been made, using the male pronoun only to enhance clarity between reference to mother or child. The physician has been referred to as *he*, although I am thoroughly cognizant of the inordinate injustice perpetrated by this historical usage. (xiii–xiv; emphasis in original)

This pronoun usage is typical in breastfeeding and infant care advice litera-ture and is now almost always preceded by some sort of statement purported to demonstrate the author's understanding of the false universals involved, except in the case of the mother's pronoun, which is indeed accurate all of the time. Usually the caveat will also state that the male pronoun will be used for the baby *always*, in the service of clarity. Rhetorically, however, Lawrence's usage reaffirms the oppositions science versus anecdote, physician versus mother, male versus female.

The Female Biologic Role

Toward the end of the chapter on psychological aspects of breastfeeding, Lawrence writes, "[Niles] Newton has pointed out that a woman's joy in and acceptance of the female biologic [*sic*] role in life may be an important factor in her psychosexual behavior, which includes lactation. She found that women who wished to bottle feed also often believed that the male role was the more satisfying role" (194). Elsewhere in the text Lawrence uses a similar terminology: "Long before our modern society, there were women who failed to accept the biologic role as nursing mothers, and society failed to provide adequate support for nursing mothers"(9); and "[T]he critical impact in the return to breastfeeding in modern culture rests with the issue of the mother's role and her perception of breastfeeding as a biologic act" (180). This terminology—biologic role, mother's role, and breastfeeding as a biologic act—derives from the medical view that "Lactation is the physio-logic completion of the reproductive cycle," which begins with conception, continues with gestation and childbirth, and moves through lactation to weaning (279). In this view, mothering is a set of behaviors defined by a number of biological conditions; the *female biologic role* comprises repro-ductive experiences and capacities understood as natural to human females.

The *Oxford English Dictionary* has a number of different definitions of *role*, two of which seem to be appropriate to understanding this phrase:

> 1. a. The part or character one has to play, takes, or assumes ... b. The typical or characteristic function performed by someone or some-thing ...
> 2. *Social Psychol.* The behaviour that an individual feels it appropriate to assume in adapting to any form of social interaction; the behavior considered appropriate to the interaction demanded by a particular kind of work or social position.

Often when the term *role* is used in its sociological sense, we think of in-dividuals adjusting (or not) to social expectations of their behavior. The use of *role* in sociology carries something from each of the definitions cited above—the idea of playing a part, the idea of a particular function performed by an individual, and the idea of a behavior that an individual engages in because of its propriety in a specific situation. Sociologist Linda Lindsey writes, "The expected behavior associated with any given status [such as 'mother'] is referred to [in sociology] as a *role*" (2; original emphasis). But a "biologic role"? Surely a biologic role is reduced to the second definition of part 1, which deals with functionality. The term *biologic role* recalls mounting behavior in rats, lordosis, or courtship rituals that are instinctive—in other words, the use of *biologic* trumps the essential notion of role as something social, so that the idea of biological functionality is paramount. Indeed, Carolyn Sherif argues that the whole concept of sex roles is problematic since it "uncritically couples a biological concept (sex) with a sociological concept (role)" (392).

In any event, a biologic role is certainly not the same as a social role, which Helena Lopata and Barrie Thorne define as

> a set of functionally interdependent, culturally patterned relations involving duties and personal rights between a social person and a social circle. Thus, it is not a set of expectations but of relations, the culture providing the base for the role by defining who should or should not be assigned or allowed to enter a specific role in a specific social circle and what duties and rights are 'normally' needed in order that the function of the role (again culturally defined) be carried forth. (720)

It is interesting that their example of a *social* role is that of a mother: "An American woman enters the role of mother when she develops, after acknowledging birth, adoption, or fostering, relations not only with a child but with a wide range of members of the circle in order to care for and rear that child. The circle may contain a father, a pediatrician, other children she is mothering, [and so on]" (720). In this sense of role, there is no room for biology; the role of mother is dependent not on the birth itself but its acknowledgment, a social recognition of a particular relation to others.

If lactation is "the physiologic completion of the reproductive cycle," it seems odd to think of it as a role behavior, since pregnancy as part of the reproductive cycle can hardly be spoken of in those terms (although Sheila Kitzinger does, with the phrase "the role of pregnancy and childbirth" [*Experience* 54]). Pregnancy is a biological condition that is part of human reproductive sex differences; it is the result of specific behaviors and involves other behaviors, but is not itself a behavior *per se*. Lactation is also a condition of the reproductive female mammal, but in human societies it functions as a more clearly defined social practice, since its engagement and expression are greatly determined by its specific cultural context, largely because it depends on the conscious behaviors of the mother. If, however, in Lindsey's terms, mothering is the status of which childbearing is an expected role behavior, then "female biologic role" can be understood to reference the expected biological behaviors attendant to mothering. In this view, all the biological aspects of reproduction—conception, gestation, childbirth, lactation, weaning—define a set of experiences, or expected roles, attendant to the status of being a mother, not all of which are engaged in by every mother. In Lawrence's terms, many mothers do not accept the biologic role of breastfeeding; many mothers do not incorporate specific biological behaviors in their engagement of motherhood. Lactation is one such behavior, and it is the only biological behavior of motherhood to be abandoned as a generic practice by a high percentage of American mothers.

Lawrence's passage citing Niles Newton articulates the female biologic role against a putative male role. The suggestion, then, might be that the female role is biological, whereas the male role is social. This would explain the women who bottle feed because of or attendant to their sense that the male role is more satisfying—in this sense their infant feeding practice indicates a refusal of a biological aspect of mothering, and thus a refusal of the female role itself insofar as it is defined as biological. It's hard to say what the male biologic role would be: impregnation? Impregnation is an embodied practice that defines sex differences in reproductive function, but it is also an expected behavior attendant to the status of being a man, and thus a role in Lindsey's sense. Traditionally, however, the male role is defined in social terms—in America, historically, a man is the one who works for the family in the public world of commerce and labor.

It's unclear in this passage precisely what is meant by the phrase *female role* even when it is used without its biologic modifier. Lawrence follows the above quote with a discussion of various regional differences in breast-feeding patterns in the United States, distinctions according to the size of the community in which a breastfeeding mother finds herself, and cross-cultural studies that show "variation in rates of nursing" in large cities, and then writes, "These rates are influenced by education, and in this generation, the higher the education, the higher the incidence of breastfeeding" (194). Surely, however, this contradicts, at least partially, the statement about roles mentioned above, since getting an education, especially a higher education, is not indicative of a strong preference for the female biologic role. Indeed, breastfeeding rates are highest among white, middle-class women with a college education who are older mothers, in other words, women who have postponed childbearing in order to establish a career (or perhaps just in order to enjoy the childless life a little longer). Such women are hardly the standard bearers of the traditional female role.

Lawrence's references in this chapter run from the 1950s to the 1990s, a period during which there have been significant changes in the female role and in women's life experiences generally in the United States. In this context, the following assertion, based on a study done in the 1970s, continues to highlight conflicting ideological views: "Chamberlain studied the differences between mothers who bottle fed and those who practiced unrestricted breastfeeding with their second child. The groups were similar in age, education, parity, intelligence, and socioeconomic status. The breastfeeding mothers were less defensive about their method of feeding, were more oriented toward home life, and had *higher radicalism scores*" (189; emphasis added). Certainly a radicalism score is very culturally specific, and cited like this, without explanation, the comment does not clearly indicate political, social, or spiritual radicalism, or even distinguish between them (and the other sorts of radicalism one might think of). In apparent agreement with Lawrence's view, in the 1970s Alice Rossi stated,

> Good sexual adjustment, positive enjoyment of pregnancy, low profiles of nausea during pregnancy, easier and shorter labor, desire for and success at breast feeding, preference for a natural or minimal-drug childbirth, all seem to form a coherent syndrome. And what of the personality and role profile of women with these characteristics? They can scarcely be traditional submissive women for it takes a high level of assertiveness and unconventionality for an American woman to experience natural childbirth, success at nursing, or gratification in sex. (169)

So perhaps adjustment to the female *biologic* role is not the same as a woman's acceptance of the traditional female *social* role. This line of thought proceeds as follows: Traditional women, who are less likely to be educated, more likely to be younger mothers, and more likely to be submissive in relation to men and male authority, are less likely to succeed at breastfeeding, because it entails the counter cultural (or radical) attitude of embracing the biological aspects of mothering. This view coincides with Niles Newton's claim that "biological femininity is indeed something *different from* cultural femininity—and *in some ways opposite to* cultural femininity." But Newton went on to argue that the culturally feminine women in her study liked the role of modern women and were more likely to "wish to be men" than the women more oriented toward "biological femininity" (99–100; emphases in original). This takes us back to Lawrence's claim (based on Newton's research) that bottle-feeding mothers are more likely to value the male role, but decidedly complicates our notion of what kind of woman—traditional or modern?—is likely to practice the female biologic role of breastfeeding.

Perhaps the problem is in trying to identify any specific factors about a kind of woman who is more likely to breastfeed successfully. Indeed, breastfeeding itself can transform a woman's conception of herself as an individual and as a mother. And certainly, there is more to successful breastfeeding than one's attitude: there are real material issues to be addressed in having the time to breastfeed (whether one works outside the home or not), having resources available to deal with routine physical problems, and having relationships with others who are supportive of maternal nursing (among other issues). In splitting off the "psychologic impact of breastfeeding" into its own separate chapter, the relation of a woman's psychic experience of lactation to these material issues is subordinated to other narratives about the kind of woman most likely to breastfeed and the kind of psychological problems that some women experience while nursing or that keep them from nursing at all.

Throughout this chapter there is a significant blurring between the idea of women's biological capacities and practices and their social roles. In part this is because the idea of a role as an expected behavior can include a biological condition or capacity as a fulfillment of a social status. This is particularly true in the common understanding of "woman's role" because, as anthropologist Sherry Ortner pointed out almost three decades ago, women's nature is perceived to be closer to nature at least partly because their "physiological functions ... may tend in themselves to motivate" such a view (33). Ortner continues the argument:

> not only her bodily processes but the social situation in which her bodily processes locate her may carry this significance [of being closer to nature than men]. And in so far as she is permanently associated (in the eyes of culture) with these social milieux, they add weight (perhaps the decisive part of the burden) to the view of woman as closer to nature. I refer here, of course, to woman's confinement to the domestic family context, *a confinement motivated, no doubt, by her lactation processes.* ... Since the mother's body goes through its lactation processes in direct relation to a pregnancy with a particular child, the relationship of nursing between mother and child is seen as a natural bond. ... Mothers and their children, according to cultural reasoning, belong together (33; emphasis added)

In other words, it is the dominant view of the culture that the female role is a biological one, because women's role in reproduction dominates her life (while men's commensurate role in reproduction is minimal[2]) and her reproductive practices are defined as natural. Ortner aptly cites Simone de Beauvoir as one of the first feminists to articulate an extensive argument against this unjust situation, and comments, "It is simply a fact that proportionately more of a woman's body space, for a greater percentage of her lifetime and some—sometimes great—cost to her personal health, strength, and general stability, is taken up with the natural processes surrounding the reproduction of the species" (Ortner 31). Lawrence writes, in the same vein, "The function of the mammary gland is unique in that it produces a material that makes tremendous demands on the maternal system without producing any physiologic advantage to the maternal organism" (78). Ortner consistently argues, however, that it is the cultural interpretation and articulation of women's physiological functions in terms of reproduction that create the association of women with nature, and not any simplistic biological determinism.

One problem with "female biologic role" is thus the way the terminology tries to reduce breastfeeding to an involuntary function of the body, the physiological completion of the reproductive cycle, that is nevertheless culturally embedded. As Lawrence herself writes, "In the human . . . there is a strong voluntary nature to nursing behavior" (76). Another problem involves the sense that roles must be adjusted to (or not), and that adjustment, if insufficiently accomplished, can be used as a judgment against a mother: she can't breastfeed because she can't accept her (biologic) role as a mother. (In a chapter called "The Psychology of Pregnancy," Sheila Kitzinger includes a subheading entitled "Inability to adjust to the role of pregnancy and childbirth" [*Experience* 54]). While the psychological dimensions to lactation cannot be underestimated, such views themselves underestimate the material dimensions of breastfeeding, the embodied experience of breastfeeding. Representing breastfeeding as a practice rather than a role behavior might mitigate against some of the significant ideological pressure toward proper mothering as a reflection of natural femininity.

There is another sense in which Lawrence's use of Niles Newton's research, and Newton's specific wording of the idea about the female biologic role, is troublesome. The term *psychosexual behavior* is the larger category of which female biologic role is a factor. Lactation is also included in psychosexual behavior. The *OED* definition suggests that the social psychological understanding of the word *role* includes or subsumes the category of behavior: "The behavior that an individual feels it appropriate to assume in adapting to any form of social interaction." Thus to me the whole sentence would make more sense if it read "Newton has pointed out that a woman's *psychosexual behavior* may be an important factor in her *joy in and acceptance of the female biologic role* [whatever that is], which includes lactation." That sentence, even with the problematic terminology, at least suggests that breastfeeding (as a practice) is part of the female biologic role, and that psychosexual behavior is the larger category of which the female biologic role (perhaps not her whole role, just a part of it) is a smaller aspect. But either way, the terminology raises a bothersome issue concerning the nature of the overarching psychosexual behavior of which the biologic role, and lactation, are a part. And the problem is this: Is breastfeeding a sexual activity or not?

To Be or Not To Be Sexual

It is a commonplace among breastfeeding advocates to find the Western view of the breast as a sexual organ and object of erotic fixation at fault for many women's distaste for even the idea of breastfeeding (for example, Dettwyler, "Beauty and the Breast"). Indeed, Lawrence refers to two such studies when she comments, "Hendrickse . . . states that the biggest block in the minds of women relates to feelings of shame associated with breastfeeding. More than half the women in the Newcastle survey were prevented from breastfeeding because of a sense of shame. The shame is a result of relating the breast to concepts of sexuality" (198). Yet on the previous page, she states, "Mothers are made to feel intellectually stagnant and uncreative while breastfeeding. Indeed, they are also made to feel asexual at the peak of their sexual cycle" (197). The implication in this last statement is that breastfeeding is part of this peak of the sexual cycle. Thus, the sexual cycle peaks with reproduction; indeed, the sexual cycle here is a reproductive cycle (see also La Leche League, *Womanly Art*, 6th ed., 111).

It seems odd, to me, to think about breastfeeding as part of a sexual cycle that has at its peak procreation, even though other scholars who write about childbirth and breastfeeding argue this very point. Kitzinger's *Experience of Childbirth* has a full chapter called "The Climax of Labor" (181–217) and additionally discusses erotic aspects of breastfeeding (229–33). In the field of gender studies (where I have done most of my research) there is a tendency to separate sexuality from reproduction as a way of undercutting heterosexism (see especially D'Emilio). Perhaps I have internalized the Western view of asexualized motherhood, promulgated by psychoanalysts and others, as discussed by Susan Contratto. Many cultures, however, have sexual taboos concerning breastfeeding women, the most common being a taboo on sexual intercourse with a breastfeeding mother. If childbearing and breastfeeding represent the peak of a woman's sexual cycle, the taboos on sexual intercourse with a lactating women might be interpreted as recognizing that her sexuality is bound up with the child. Alice Rossi supports this view:

> In societies in which childbirth and lactation are handled in a relaxed and open manner, mothers are also permitted and encouraged to take sexual pleasure in their infants. This pleasure may be enhanced by the frequently associated pattern of prolonged postchildbirth sexual

abstinence in many such societies. Social anthropologists have tended to view such sexual abstinence as serving a child-spacing function and assuring the adequate nurturing of one child before the onset of a second pregnancy, and medical research supports the view that breast feeding is a natural, if unreliable, form of birth control.

But an awareness of the intimate connection between genital stimulation and lactation suggests that such sexual abstinence may strengthen the bond between mother and child by permitting sensual gratification in maternity which our society officially denies to mothers. (166)

Recently, some feminist scholars have embraced maternal sexuality as a concept and concentrated on breastfeeding as one of its experiential and representational modes (Iris Young; Blum, "Mothers, Babies, and Breastfeeding"; Contratto; Sichtermann; see also Giles, *Fresh Milk,* for direct accounts of lactational sexuality). In this understanding of maternity, breastfeeding and other maternal practices can represent an alternative sexuality (in Blum's words, embodiment) that is not caught up, necessarily, in service to a man or to capitalism, but which has another focus (her child, herself) as its object. As Susan Contratto argues, "The [dominant psychological] belief is that good mothers do not have sexual feelings in relationship to children, that good mothers are generally asexual" (226). If there is sexuality in the relation of mother and child, it is experienced by the child and in that sense is healthy and normal (228–29). Other feminist scholars have questioned this belief.

Both Niles Newton and Alice Rossi argue for maternal sexuality itself as natural and normal, with Rossi going so far as to argue that maternal satisfaction in reproductive practices works against the interests of dominant males (167), but as biologically-oriented researchers, Newton and Rossi believe that what's good for the mother (sexually) is also and necessarily good for the child (nutritionally and psychologically) (see also Riordan and Rapp, qtd. in Dettwyler, "Beauty and the Breast," 184). Barbara Sichtermann, on the other hand, suggests that feminists should emphasize maternal sexuality in breastfeeding regardless of the child's needs: "[W]hat women would have to bring about would be a cultivation of the eroticism of the breast and of breastfeeding. By that I don't mean adequate feeding of a baby (which, happily, coincides with it but which should not be of paramount importance). What I mean is the art of love, the expression of female sensuality, intermingling of bodies, or even ecstasy" (64). It is interesting to note that her emphasis on a maternal eroticism that disregards the child's nutritional needs is based upon the idea that "Today there are no longer any (serious) 'biological' reasons for a mother to nurse her child at the breast" (62). It is precisely because breastfeeding is voluntary that it makes itself available, in Sichtermann's view, as an erotic practice for women.

Yet advocating maternal sexuality is a tricky issue. In the introduction to the revised edition of her *Breastfeeding Your Baby,* Sheila Kitzinger, who has elsewhere advocated for understanding childbirth and lactation as sexual processes, writes, "Breastfeeding is a psychosexual process. I do not mean by this that it produces genital sensations or that it is sexually exploitative. In the United States a few years ago, a four-year-old girl was taken away from her mother by doctors, psychologists, and social workers because she had been in 'mouth-breast contact.' The idea that to breastfeed is an erotic indulgence or an exercise in power over a child is a perverted view of the breastfeeding relationship. Happy breastfeeding, whether with a baby, a toddler, or an older child who has an especially close 'going to bed' time, which includes breastfeeding, can be deeply satisfying for you both. Like other psychosexual experiences, it needs to be based on confidence and a sense of self-worth" (6). In this passage, arguing for lactation as an aspect of maternal sexuality requires strict distinctions between perverted views and happy breastfeeding. Other scholars (Lawrence, *Breastfeeding,* 321; Dettwyler, "A Time to Wean," 56–58) discuss problems with public views of children nursing longer "than they should," views that are tinged with perceptions of sexual deviation in the nursing relationship and that can have legal ramifications for nursing mothers. Lauri Umansky's discussion of a 1991 case in which a two-year-old child was removed from the mother's custody because the mother called a community hotline to ask if it was "normal to feel aroused while nursing" demonstrates that breastfeeding an older child conjures up a whole host of sexually questionable acts, including child molestation and orgies ("Breastfeeding in the 1990s").

In the United States, because most women do not publicly nurse toddlers or older children, a routine complaint lodged against women who breastfeed for more than a year is that they are sexualizing these children; this view sees the mother's breasts as inherently sexual in an adult sort of way, and suggests that the experience she has of her breasts as sexual is itself transmitted to the child through breastfeeding.[3] Separating sexuality from reproduction might circumvent this charge of inappropriate sexual relations with children through breastfeeding and seeing mothers as asexual might allow them a respite from sexual encounters, which some or many might see as a welcome change in their experience as adult women. (Many nursing mothers experience the feeling of being "touched out" and seek, in their free time, periods of isolation rather than sexual encounters with adult partners. Indeed, this feeling is common enough to be included as part of *The Womanly Art of Breastfeeding,* La Leche League's guide to nursing [6th ed., 111], and it was mentioned during my own childbirth education classes as a possible consequence of breastfeeding in the early months postpartum.)

Some feminist scholars have perceived the separation of sexuality from maternity to be connected to a culturally inscribed dichotomy between male and female sexuality. Elizabeth Grosz argues that "Women's bodies do not develop their adult forms with reference to their newly awakened sexual capacities, for these are dramatically overcoded with resonances of motherhood." Her analysis suggests that puberty for boys is culturally understood to anticipate adult sexuality as pleasurable, while "the onset of menstruation is not an indication at all for the girl of her developing sexuality, only her coming womanhood," understood as potential maternity (205). Thus Grosz understands the separation of sexuality from motherhood to begin with the cultural values associated with and giving meaning to the differential embodied changes that girls and boys experience at puberty, and states, "given the social significance of these bodily processes [menstruation and lactation] that are invested in and by the processes of reproduction, all women's bodies are marked as different from men's (and inferior to them) particularly at those bodily regions where women's differences are most visibly manifest" (207). In this reading, the question of sexuality or maternity as a reading of women's embodied experiences is always already implicated in a political understanding of the hierarchy of sexual difference. Whether breastfeeding is understood as sexual or asexually maternal depends upon the cultural context and a comparison to male norms of sexual behavior and embodiment.

In a move designed to counter the predominantly Euro-American and masculinized view of the female breast as sexual, Katherine Dettwyler espouses a conceptual and experiential separation between maternity and sexuality centered narrowly on breast functionality. She argues that the belief in breasts as inherently sexual organs (for men's pleasure) is a culturally circumscribed and problematic view of female sexuality and embodiment: "Are mammary glands *intrinsically* erotic in humans? The ethnographic evidence clearly says 'no'" ("Beauty and the Breast" 181; original emphasis). Throughout the essay she engages an evolutionary argument: for example, she writes, "Whether breastfeeding was pleasurable to the mother or not is a moot point. As long as breastfeeding conferred a reproductive advantage, the behavior would have been selected for, whether or not it was pleasurable to the woman" (185). In this view, breastfeeding is the universal, natural, biological function of the human breast and "sexual pleasure from manual or oral manipulation of the breasts" is "learned behavior, learned in a particular cultural context" (202) because "breasts were designed, first and foremost, to feed children" (205). For Dettwyler, critiquing the culturally specific, Western view of the breast as primarily sexual will encourage a view of breastfeeding as a normal biological behavior of reproductive human females. Her complex and comprehensive treatment of the issue argues for a separation of maternity from sexuality only because she believes the cultural significance of breast eroticism to significantly impede the more important function of the breast as a source of nourishment (broadly conceived) for the child. In this view, breasts are sexual only insofar as they are connected to sexual activity through reproduction and its embodied practices.

Indeed, for the large majority of the world's women, embodied reproduction (involving pregnancy, childbirth, lactation) continues to be a result of sexual activity. In a sense, theoretical calls to analytically and experientially separate sexuality from maternity[4] repudiate the nexus of sexuality and childbearing that is the reality of many (if not most) women around the globe. For women who are actively engaged in reproductive behaviors and experiences, sex is not just for pleasure—it can and often does have the result of procreation either in mind (as an intention) or in the material result of the sexual encounter. It may be that perceiving the mother as asexual is only possible in the modern developed world, where most women's adult lives are not defined by the reproductive "cycle of conception, pregnancy, birth, nursing, weaning, and conception . . . that would occupy most months for . . . twenty to twenty-five years of their lives" (Bogdan 105).

On the other hand, this view does not suggest that reproduction and its attendant practices (breastfeeding, for example) represent the peak of women's sexual cycle. Susan Contratto argues that there is no research supporting the notion of a female sexual cycle, either keyed to the menstrual cycle or equated with childbirth or nursing: "Inherent in the procycle position are questions about the normalcy of women who do not have children; who make homosexual, as distinct from heterosexual, object choices; and who do not form families. . . . I would suggest that the die-hard proponents of the cycle-syndrome picture of normal female development are trying to scientifically prove cultural attitudes about appropriate female gender roles" (231–33). Lawrence's representation of breastfeeding as part of women's psychosexual behavior is a way of normalizing it as an acceptable aspect of reproduction—"See, it's just a part of the female biologic role, just like childbirth." Breastfeeding advocates note that, generally, lactation is *not* perceived as a reproductive activity, it is merely a mode of infant feeding, a social choice. Thus, because of the social emphasis on female breasts as sexual, the choice to breastfeed appears to represent an inappropriate sexuality on the part of the mother toward her children. This perception of breastfeeding as expressing an already inappropriate maternal sexuality fits with Lauri Umansky's analysis of the Karen Carter case, where authorities connected the mother's nursing of a two-year-old child with her supposedly excessive sexual encounters with men (all previous to her daughter's birth;

"Breastfeeding in the 1990s"). Socially, reproductive sexuality is good sexuality, so anything that is a part of that kind of sexuality is perforce positive, although it needs to be performed within heterosexual marriage in order to insure its legitimacy.

The shame attendant to breastfeeding (or not breastfeeding because of shame) concerns the breast as a part of bad sexuality—sexuality that has as its goal not procreation but pleasure. Breastfeeding is perceived to be the peak of the sexual cycle insofar as the breastfeeding woman feels no shame and experiences her breasts as functioning biologically. Indeed, breastfeeding is the peak of the sexual cycle when the nursing mother is not impeded in her breastfeeding by her (always already bad?) sexuality.[5] Thus Lawrence aligns breastfeeding with sexuality only insofar as that sexuality is the good kind of female sexuality, one which understands and accepts the satisfactions of the female biologic role.

The Blame Game

Another issue in the chapter that involves an interesting set of contradictions concerns the reasons why women do not breastfeed. Lawrence is at pains to let her professional colleagues off the hook, but she is ambivalent about the source of the problem, which can be defined as large numbers of women who never breastfeed as well as many women who begin to breastfeed but give up or experience lactation failure within a few weeks or months of parturition. Lawrence writes, "Before the trend toward bottle feeding can be reversed, one has to understand why some women do not breastfeed. It cannot be blamed on society or the medical profession when a woman cannot accept this as part of the biologic role of a mother" (197). Here again we have the specter of the biologic role and the attendant sense that the woman does not breastfeed because she has not adjusted to this role properly. Oddly enough, however, Lawrence goes on to explain a number of social reasons that influence women's failure to breastfeed or even failure at breastfeeding, including the social devaluation of motherhood, the lack of appreciation of mothers' intellectual experiences while mothering, "beliefs and attitudes toward breastfeeding" (which can't be conceptualized apart from culture, it would seem), and the shame some women feel in relation to their breasts that prevents them from feeling comfortable with breastfeeding. And, at the end of the chapter, Lawrence has strong words for physicians who do not provide adequate and scientifically up-to-date information about breastfeeding to their patients for fear of making mothers feel guilty if they feed with formula. She argues that women need to be given enough information to make informed decisions:

> There are no studies in the literature that support this position
> [denying mothers information about breastfeeding in order to avoid

inculcating guilt]. In the dozens of reports on efforts to increase breastfeeding among many cultures, there is no report of producing guilt feelings. Women interviewed in open-ended questionnaires have not mentioned guilt feelings in response to the questioning. The only individuals who ever mention guilt are the older generation whose daughters are now choosing breastfeeding. The grandmother feels guilty because noone [*sic*] ever told her her; noone [*sic*] ever encouraged her to breastfeed. (199)[6]

So then the physicians *could* be at fault for relying on anecdotal evidence rather than science. Indeed, while Lawrence explicitly says that neither society nor physicians should be blamed when a woman does not breastfeed, she provides ample evidence that it is precisely society and the medical profession that make successful lactation difficult for many women. And female physicians may be worse than male physicians. In an earlier passage, Lawrence reports that in a study concerning the correlation of rates of breastfeeding with the office practices and advice of pediatricians, "the female physicians were more apt than the male physicians to discredit what . . . lay mothers could do to help other mothers" (194).

Of course, these female physicians, unless they were all like Lawrence with her nine offspring, might have admired the male role. Indeed, in their discrediting of lay mother's groups, they are establishing their allegiance to science and devaluing anecdote (even experience) as the source of valuable information about breastfeeding. Perhaps the problem is that the female physicians couldn't breastfeed because their commitment to their careers compromised their adjustment to the female role, or at least compromised their time. Ruth Lawrence is surely the anomaly in this case: after all, how many female physicians have nine children, let alone nine breastfed children? Without this experience, they have nothing to balance with scientific data, and so they may distrust such experience. On the other hand, they may have plenty of clinical experience managing nursing mothers, which they may feel is experience enough to balance with basic scientific information. In any event, in siding with science against the anecdotal and experiential knowledge of mothers, the female physicians in Lawrence's study are relying on science and its gendered authority (rational management), just as Lawrence encourages them to do.

Conclusion

Currently, pro-breastfeeding physicians take an activist role in promoting maternal nursing. At the 1999 La Leche League physicians' seminar on breastfeeding, the predominant view was to counsel pregnant mothers extensively about the benefits of breastfeeding, their plans for infant care after birth, their career plans (if they are working or plan to work after the baby's birth), their specific breast anatomy, and any lifestyle issues that the physician feels might interfere with successful nursing. Physicians attending the meeting considered whether the mother's lactating breasts are the pediatrician's or the obstetrician's responsibility, and there was some sentiment (although not universally shared) that it was appropriate to discuss personal financial matters with women planning to return to work, and to suggest to such women that if their income was to be spent on so-called luxury items rather than necessities, perhaps they could stay at home with their babies. Subsequent meetings, in 2000 and 2001, did not exhibit the same paternalistic attitude about women's decisions about finances and waged labor, but focused on the struggles women face to breastfeed in a variety of social and economic situations.

Education and reinforcement are the key terms in the physician's lexicon as a breastfeeding activist—education to convince the mother of the value of breastfeeding and breast milk, and reinforcement to bolster her self-esteem and confidence in the context of physical problems or social pressures. At a number of points in the *Guide*, Ruth Lawrence writes that women felt their doctor's views and advice to be an indispensable part of their feeding choice: "The [WIC] mothers said if only their physician would tell them it was important, they would do it for as long as the physician said" (16); "Many [mothers] decided [to breastfeed] long before the pregnancy, but those who chose bottle feeding admit they could have been persuaded if only someone had cared enough to tell them how important breastfeeding is to the infant" (224). Lawrence is highly aware of the cultural impact of breastfeeding education and support: "Pediatric literature reinforces pressures on women regarding their infants and leads pediatricians to a role of shaping public views of infancy, motherhood, and humanity in general" (268)—and believes fervently in the physician's activism: "The physician can help support mothers and fathers seeking to fulfill parental, occupational, and personal needs in a rapidly changing society" (389), even though she also knows that many physicians routinely give the wrong advice when managing breastfeeding: "Many physicians suggest to mothers that a supplementary bottle can be added at any time. Actually, when lactation is going well, it is not needed, and when it is not going well, a bottle may aggravate the problem" (268).

Increased maternal education concerning breastfeeding is supposed to counteract the view that mothers should not be put in a position that promotes guilt about an infant feeding choice; indeed, many breastfeeding advocates, while labeled fanatics by non-advocates, claim merely to want to balance the scales by offering what they consider to be truer medical information about the benefits of breastfeeding and the detriments of infant formula (e.g., Dettwyler, "Promoting Breastfeeding"). It's an argument that makes a lot of sense, especially given that there is no corporate sponsor for breastfeeding, and no company that will make a lot of money from a woman's choice to nurse. Because medical research has, since the 1970s, documented health disadvantages for formula-fed infants, it also makes sense that physicians should be the ones promoting breastfeeding, especially since their profession is at fault for promoting bottle feeding (however inadvertently) throughout much of this century.

But the educational efforts to inform women about the benefits of breast-feeding, emblematized in the slogan Breast Is Best, highlight some of the problems attendant to physicians' involvement in breastfeeding advocacy, what Linda Blum implies is a hegemonic "exhortation to breastfeed." Often education and emotional reinforcement are plentiful, while material support—household help, methods of personally managing breastfeeding difficulties, even money to extend maternity leave or rent a breast pump—are less available or nonexistent, even though they might be more crucial to successful lactation. That is how educational efforts can be experienced as exhortations, especially by non–middle-class women, since the information can be presented without any practical method of following through to achievement. The data on educational attainment and breastfeeding rates, presented in the introduction, suggest that educational campaigns to increase rates of maternal nursing are most effective for those mothers who are already educated in other areas *and* who have the resources to make postsecondary education a reality, that is, middle-class women.

Whether educational campaigns work as well for mothers whose relation to educational institutions and protocols is more tenuous remains to be seen.[7] Emily Martin suggests that middle-class women are more likely to be influenced by medical models of female embodiment; this would suggest that educational campaigns promoting breastfeeding that emphasize medical issues would be more successful with middle-class mothers than with working-class or poor mothers. Poor mothers especially are more likely to have their mothering experience supervised by state or local authorities, and thus their relationship to such educational campaigns is different from middle-class mothers, whose relation to their physicians is usually more voluntary.

The rhetorical conflicts in this chapter demonstrate the strained nature of medicine's authority over breastfeeding, partly as a result of the difficulty of Lawrence's task—to write a guide to breastfeeding that doesn't offend physicians, who have been some of the worst perpetrators of misinformation about infant feeding through their collaboration with infant food manufacturers (Apple, *Mothers and Medicine*; Baumslag and Michels; Palmer). The conflicts show that breastfeeding can never be rationally managed by scientific medicine, because as a biosocial *practice*, breastfeeding is enmeshed in webs of social meaning. Those webs (and their knots of overdetermined signification) enter into and complicate what the author tries to present as a relatively straightforward account of the "psychologic impact of breastfeeding," an impact that raises questions about the relationship of biological reproduction to the expected roles that women take up in modern societies. And lurking within these discourses is the ever present question of who really has the authority to manage breastfeeding—the physician, whose rational practices are founded in basic science and the experiences of clinical medicine, or the mother, whose reproductive activities engender experientially-based knowledge and the circulation of anecdotal advice.

As Lawrence herself suggests, "Breastfeeding is a very different activity when it is carried out by a small minority compared with breastfeeding when it is commonplace in the community" (186). Perhaps when a majority of women are again breastfeeding, and breastfeeding for an appreciable length of time, this tension over the physician's authority will become moot. Even though almost 70 percent of women leave the hospital breastfeeding, it is still a minority choice in terms of the culture's understanding and acceptance of it and because by six months the number of women still nursing hovers at just over 30 percent nationally. And these numbers are different for different groups. As long as breastfeeding is a minority choice, certain members of the medical profession will perceive the need to be activists about breastfeeding, because there will be no widespread cultural base of knowledge about lactation as a social practice. And since medical professionals are still most likely to be consulted by mothers about infant feeding problems, the more information about breastfeeding available to medical personnel the better. The problem of medicine's authority over infant feeding is embedded in other changes in modern life in developed countries, where professionals provide information about motherhood that used to be available from within the family and lay community (Apple, *Mothers and Medicine;* Grant). Until there is a resurgence of community-based forms of information exchange, exemplified in this instance by La Leche League, whose influence seems to be greatest on middle-class, white mothers who do not work outside the home, mothers will still turn to physicians with questions about breastfeeding and infant care.

It is unlikely, however, that any medical campaign to promote breastfeeding will succeed in convincing the majority of women to lactate for the recommended twelve months (or even at least six months) if physicians convey the notion that breastfeeding is the mode of infant feeding proper to the female biological role. That medicine promotes a normative view of mothering should not surprise anyone; it is an essentially conservative profession.[8] But physicians should also understand that this conceptualization of breastfeeding as a biological behavior that is related to a woman's proper acceptance of her female role can impede their advocacy of maternal nursing, in the least because it brings more and more of the woman's body and experience under medical management and scrutiny. Many women resist this surveillance, and one could argue that such attention impacts poor and nonwhite women most negatively, because their mothering practices have historically been treated with suspicion and as contingent upon state approval. One can only hope that the success of breastfeeding socially will eventually lessen medicine's role in its management, since, as Ruth Lawrence writes, "A normal full-term infant can usually be breastfed with only minor adjustment, even without the support of medical expertise" (406).

Until then, rhetorical analysis shows that medical discussions of breastfeeding can be as permeated by social ambivalences about women's behaviors as other public discussions of infant feeding and care. The point is not, of course, to propose that we can rid medical language of ideological influence or conflict. Rather, the point is to make medicine face up to its real conflict—its uncertain relation of authority over the lactating mother. Some scholars have suggested that, historically, regulating women is usually at stake in public breastfeeding advocacy (Perry; Yalom). Rima Apple has aptly demonstrated, from the 1890s to the 1960s, the growing reliance of American mothers on scientific expertise to guide infant care; this trend coincided with the development and widespread use of infant formulas as breast milk substitutes (*Mothers and Medicine*). Medical management was essential with artificial feeding in the early period of proprietary development, as the physicians fine-tuned specific formulas for their patients, and the growth of pediatrics in this period is due, at least in part, to this necessity (Apple, *Mothers and Medicine*). But breastfeeding presents the medical profession with an ambiguous patient, given that it is the mother's body that provides the nutrition for the infant. In managing the nursing infant, medicine must also manage the mother; thus medical professionals tap into unspoken social fears about contemporary maternal behaviors.

It may be that successful breastfeeding depends upon material support that is infrequently and unevenly available to women in contemporary American society. After all, attainment of education can mask other demographic differences that may contribute to educated women's higher rates of nursing. In the 1990s, St. Joseph's Regional Medical Center in South Bend, Indiana, started a lactation program to promote breastfeeding. The main components of their program include support from lactation consultants at the hospital, the opening of an outpatient lactation center, and an onsite breast pump rental program. They also give all maternity patients a "Breastfeeding Discharge Kit" that includes "an Ameda One-Hand Breast pump with Flexishield, six washable cotton breast pads, a 1/4 ounce tube of Lansinoh [pure lanolin], and a packet of breastfeeding information. . . . the kit is offered regardless of ability to pay." Their rates of maternal nursing, documented July through September 1998, were that "75% are still breast-feeding at 3 months and 51% at six months," well above the national and state averages at that time (Baskerville). This data suggests that attending to the material realities of breastfeeding in contemporary society may be the ticket to raising rates of maternal nursing, especially rates of long-term nursing.

Ruth Lawrence has been immensely important in advocating breastfeeding among members of the medical profession, and this chapter is not meant to diminish her commitment or contribution to breastfeeding medicine. I do think, however, that physicians would benefit themselves by thinking through the relation of rhetoric to practice. Lawrence never suggests that breastfeeding is only—or predominantly—a psychological issue, but there is an implication in much breastfeeding advocacy, medical and nonmedical alike, that if women would get over their hang-ups and "just do it," rates of maternal nursing would increase terrifically. In spelling out, albeit covertly, why medicine thinks women *don't* "just do it," Lawrence's discussion of the psychology of breastfeeding demonstrates many factors that keep mothers from successful lactation, especially the overdetermined ideological significance of lactation itself.

CHAPTER 3

Breast Is Best

I was born in 1962 and breastfed for about three months; my only younger sibling, similarly nursed, is twenty-two months younger than me. Thus, I don't remember my mother nursing us at all, and I don't recall having been around nursing infants as a young child. After all, it was the sixties—I was lucky to be breastfed at all. Yet when I was pregnant with my first child, I never really made a choice about breastfeeding, unlike the other choices I felt I consciously made, such as maternity care (midwife in a hospital), childbirth education (Bradley method), or my desire for unmedicated childbirth. I just never thought twice about bottle feeding. No one that I knew started out feeding their infants that way, or if they did, I didn't know about it. This was the nineties, when nursing, after picking up in the 1970s and then dropping off again in the 1980s, began a resurgence. Still, most American women who do nurse only do so for half a year (or less); more than two-thirds of all mothers in the United States are not breastfeeding when their infants are six months old.

It was only after I began reading about breastfeeding, after, in fact, my daughter was born, that I realized how out of the norm some of my infant feeding practices were. I nursed my daughter until she was 21 months old and I was seven and a half months pregnant with her sibling; I nursed my son until he was past three years of age and I was tired of lugging a breast pump to conferences. Many of the women in my La Leche League group breastfeed longer than I have. Doing the research for this book has been a process of relocating my own experience (prolonged nursing in the midst of a community of other long-term nursing mothers) to the more general

American context of limited nursing or no nursing at all. Most of all, I've tried to understand how choices about infant feeding are informed by a variety of social and cultural factors, including the focus of this chapter, infant formula promotion materials and pregnancy and infant care guidebooks.

Specifically, I want to explore how formula feeding is represented in relation to the seemingly ubiquitous information that "breast is best."[1] Thus, I ask, what kinds of discourses support formula feeding in the context of public information that breastfeeding is the best way to feed babies? I also analyze how choices about infant feeding and ways of overcoming difficulties in the practice of infant feeding are presented in popular advice materials that ordinary women might seek out or have sent to them when they become mothers.[2] The choice to feed with formula might seem so obvious to some that it doesn't merit attention, but in my circles formula feeding is largely perceived to be a shame or, by some, a tragedy. And, I will admit, I am often saddened when I see infants, especially newborns, fed with a bottle, although I feel this less viscerally now that I am no longer nursing myself. These are my own biases, and I recognize that because of them I need to work harder to understand infant feeding decisions and practices that go against my sense of what is appropriate, healthful, and right. Breastfeeding advocates often can't see why most American women eventually feed their babies with infant formula. It's often perceived as an irrational choice, a selfish or uneducated behavior, the result of a mother just not trying hard enough. Yet mothers who feed with infant formula do not make that choice because they are stupid or lazy; according to medical analysts, they know the purported health benefits of maternal nursing (Gabriel, Gabriel, and Lawrence). They make their decisions based on *other* ideas about child care, nutrition, and the maternal body, as well as on life priorities and material constraints that may preclude breastfeeding.

I remember long hours at a local bookstore, both while I was pregnant and after my daughter was born, leafing through various guidebooks. After her birth I was mainly trying to get information about how to encourage her to sleep, but as the idea for this book took hold of my thinking, I became interested in the representations of breastfeeding. As I developed ideas for this project further, I began collecting pregnancy advice books and infant care guides, buying them from local commercial venues like Books-a-Million, Waldenbooks, and my university's off-campus bookstore specializing in trade books. When I became pregnant with my second child, I collected all formula promotion materials that came my way and stashed them in a file.

What I demonstrate in this chapter, as a result of examining these texts, is that a common format and message pervades their presentation of infant feeding choice. Significantly, the representation of a choice of infant feeding method sets out an equivalence between breast- and bottle feeding that overrides any specific information about the health advantages of nursing. In addition, information about infant feeding tends to correspond to hegemonic American ideas about infant behavior, maternal behavior, and ideal personhood that value autonomy and an internally developed ability to regulate oneself. This unspoken set of values contributes to the undermining of breastfeeding within the structure of equivalent choice because nursing seems to lead to dependency on the part of the child and a lack of autonomy on the part of the mother. Finally, the formula promotion materials explicitly link infant behavior with what I designate a "symbolics of ingestion," which is a formal structure that interprets infant behavior according to what the baby eats. The symbolics of ingestion is explicitly tied to a consumer mentality and market economy, that is, to the purchase of the right formula to correspond to the baby's actions.

In short, I argue that representations of formula feeding convey powerful, culturally sanctioned, ideas about the body and the self. These ideas make formula feeding seem to be more natural—more comfortable within customs, practices, and ideas common in American life. Bottle feeding, which would seem to be—and is represented in this literature as being—an artificial infant feeding method that is modeled on breastfeeding and is secondary to it, actually becomes *the* model for all infant feeding in the developed world. It does so because it more closely resembles the dominant values and ideas in America concerning how persons behave. In this claim I am following the analytics put forth by French theorist Roland Barthes in *Mythologies*. In that text, Barthes shows how dominant cultural myths work as systems of meaning that come to be seen as natural when there is no public understanding of their historical emergence. Thus, once a culture loses its common memory of breastfeeding as the ordinary and expected method of feeding infants, through the abandonment of breastfeeding by only one or two generations of mothers, bottle feeding becomes not only normative, but the paradigm from which accepted ideas about maternity, infancy, and development emerge. No one really remembers when breastfeeding was ordinary, and equally obscure are the social values that supported its practice. Further, and from a more Foucaultian perspective, one could say that bottle feeding is the inevitable result of Western ideas concerning self-regulation and individual autonomy—its invention was not just the outcome of technological expertise and development, but at least partially the result of conceptual necessity. In this view, bottle feeding answered a specific social need to realign the relation of mothers and infants according to emerging values about mother–infant separateness and the mother's companionate relationship with her spouse.[3]

To be more specific, while "breast is best" is the clarion call of any contemporary discussion of infant feeding, mothers are also presented with the idea that formula feeding is an appropriate alternative that is just as good. Thus, the representations of infant feeding I examine present the paradox of claiming that breast milk is best for human infants but manufactured infant formulas are fine too.[4] Moreover, breastfeeding appears to present the mother with a number of problems of embodiment that bottle feeding does not, and infant behaviors that American mothers have been led to perceive as important to regulate—amounts of crying and sleeping, developing independence, and time between feedings—all present problems to the breastfeeding mother that are solved by recourse to a model of personhood defined through bottle-feeding norms. Indeed, I will argue that representations of breastfeeding tend to accommodate the practice to Euro-American notions of scheduling that may do more than just inhibit successful nursing—they make it seem inferior to bottle feeding because in all of these categories breastfeeding constrains the mother's ability to regulate the infant. And infant formula ends up as the default choice for infant feeding because figuring out the right one for your baby is a consumer activity (what should I buy?) that fits into other structures of living in contemporary America.

In large part, popular representations of infant feeding in marketing materials and advice literature promote bottle feeding over breastfeeding through oppositions aligning bottle feeding with those behaviors and practices (both infant and adult) that match expectations espoused in American society at large.[5] Breastfeeding no longer represents values that match up easily with the American cultural landscape, and it seems dangerously close to other values that Americans specifically repudiate, such as a lack of defined boundaries between individuals, the uncertain regulation of the infant into cultural values, and an ambivalence about the mother's body as simultaneously a reliable source of nourishment for her baby and a site of sexual excitation. This may be why older, educated, middle- and upper-class white mothers are most likely to breastfeed in American society—privileged by their class position and racial identity, and further bolstered by the added value (real and imagined) of postsecondary education, these women have little to lose by participating in a practice that no longer fits neatly into national practices and ideals of infant care.[6] Like me, they also might not perceive their decision to breastfeed as a choice, especially one enabled by their social position. This is the group of women most likely to know other women who breastfeed, and thus the group most likely to perceive breastfeeding as normal.[7] Yet reading infant feeding discourses in popular sources meant to educate expectant and new mothers demonstrates how deeply bottle feeding provides a model for infant feeding and, more profoundly, for the hegemonic ideas of the culture within which the infant feeds.

The Big Sell

In 1981 the World Health Organization adopted the International Code for the Marketing of Breast-Milk Substitutes. The Code "applies to the marketing and practices related thereto, of the following products: breast-milk substitutes, including infant formula; other milk products, food, and beverages, including bottlefed complementary foods, when marketed or otherwise represented to be suitable, with or without modification, for use as partial or total replacement of breast milk; feeding bottles and teats" (World Health Organization 8). In addition, "The Code stipulates that there should be absolutely no promotion of breastmilk substitutes, bottles and teats to the general public; neither health facilities nor health professionals should ever have a role in promoting breastmilk substitutes; and free samples should not be provided to pregnant women, new mothers or their families" (UNICEF, "Breastfeeding: Foundation for a Healthy Future," 9). The United States voted against the Code when it was originally ratified by the World Health Assembly, and, while it ratified the Code during a reaffirmation vote in 1994, the U.S. government generally refuses to enforce compliance with its requirements. In the early 1990s the Baby-Friendly Hospital Initiative (BFHI) became a worldwide movement to support the Code; one of its ten baby-friendly steps is to ban free supplies to the hospital from formula companies. The Unites States has also refused, at the national level, to implement practices to encourage compliance with the BFHI, although some U.S. hospitals have independently done so. Women in the United States thus usually give birth in environments that promote formula use, even when lactation consultants are on staff and when rooming in (generally understood to promote breastfeeding) is made available. Since the early 1990s, formula companies actively promote their products to the public through advertising (which, like the advertisement of prescription drugs, has not always been the case [Lawrence, *Breastfeeding,* xi; Palmer 273–74]). Even OB/GYN offices that explicitly support breastfeeding may engage in practices that allow formula companies to directly market their products to pregnant women.

My experiences with my second child are probably typical of most U.S. mothers who see obstetricians or certified nurse midwives in private practices, even though my reasons for inviting direct formula marketing were connected to my research, and not about making a choice about infant feeding. When I was pregnant with my first child, I was intent on a pregnancy free from as much technology and intervention as possible. I tried to ignore all promotional literature. When we left the hospital after Rachel's birth, we took home a nice diaper bag and some other freebies like A&D ointment and a nasal syringe. I did not bring any formula home. But by the time I was pregnant with my second child I had started research on this book, and so I sought out promotional literature, formula give-aways, and the like. When I got a rebate coupon for Natalins prenatal vitamins, made by Mead Johnson (makers of the Enfamil Family of Formulas™), I enthusiastically sent it in, along with information about my baby's due date, my age, the number of children I already had, and whether I was intending to breastfeed. When I left the hospital, I took home the large can of premixed Similac, and I sent in a coupon, with similar personal information, to Ross Laboratories (makers of Similac).

Information, more rebate checks, promises of free gifts, a whole carton of Similac, and a teddy bear showed up in the mail. I have never been so heavily targeted in a direct marketing campaign in my life. I dutifully sent back questionnaires indicating that I breastfed my first child past the age of one and was exclusively breastfeeding my second; I expected this information to stop the flow of advice and promises of gifts, but I was wrong.

A recent study published in *Obstetrics and Gynecology* indicates that while exposure to formula promotion materials does not seem to affect rates of breastfeeding initiation, such exposure does seem to result in increased breastfeeding cessation in the first two weeks (Howard et al. 302).[8] This suggests that although all of the promotional materials dutifully state that breast milk is best for babies, that information is overwhelmed by the persuasiveness of the rhetoric for formula use in the context of early postpartum nursing experiences. Other scholars have discussed the ways in which formula companies use subtle signals to push their products: for example, breastfeeding women in the advertisements are likely to be brunette and unsmiling, while formula feeding moms are both more cheerful and blonde (Dettwyler, "Tricks of the Trade"). However, few scholars have paid attention to how formula promotion is formally presented. I argue that formula promotion materials are persuasive, in part, through the specific formal arrangement of options within which "choice" is presented. These materials introduce formula choice—that is, choice between kinds of formula made by an individual company—as the most significant decision mothers make in responding to infant behaviors. My analysis focuses on what I call the mythology of infant feeding—a systematic way of organizing the meanings associated with infant feeding choices.

Promotional materials from formula companies create a model of infant care in which choosing the correct formula is crucial. Thus, while there is routine lip service to the superior biological qualities of breast milk as infant *nutrition,* the various formulas are represented as solving key problems that parents of infants routinely face: colicky crying, babies that refuse to sleep, general fussiness, and gas. Identifying the cause of these problems and then solving them is conceptualized as a consumer issue—buying the right formula—in the context of a choice that is possible because of the variety of formulas made by the particular company producing the literature. Formally, these ideas are presented in charts printed in the pamphlets and informational materials sent to expectant and new mothers. Significantly, breastfeeding and its attendant practices (nonnutritive suckling, co-sleeping, babies being held for long hours each day) never show up on the charts that match up formulas with baby behaviors and their possible causes.[9]

Three months pregnant with my second child, I first went to my caregiver, a certified nurse-midwife, in February 1996. At the office I received a prescription for Natalins prenatal vitamins with an offer for a rebate check. In mid-March I received a letter from Mead Johnson along with my check; the letter assured me that "At Mead Johnson, infant health and nutrition have been our focus for nearly 90 years." On May 22 I received a free sample of Keri Silky Smooth body lotion, a coupon for money off on any Keri lotion product, and a pamphlet entitled "Head-to-Toe Advice for You and Your Baby." The envelope for the next mailing includes the following alert: "Four moms talk about what labor and delivery are really like." The pamphlet about birth includes cheery stories that minimize pain (the mom who admitted her back ached "threw together a casserole" while in labor[10]) and encourage women to relax, complete with pictures of smiling moms, babies, and an occasional father (none of the people pictured as parents were the actual authors of the four scenarios). Following that I received the first coupons for formula, a reminder to ask at the hospital for a Peter Rabbit diaper bag, and the first formula chart. The envelope with this material has written on it "Who will you depend on once someone small is depending on you?"; it arrived June 18, 1996.

The chart appears under a lengthy caption, headed by the title "The Enfamil Family of Formulas" (figure 3.1). Using the chart proves to be an easy matching exercise—formula brand name in the left column, type (milk or soy, for example) in the middle column, and the right-hand column indicating which type of babies such formula is "designed for." Breast milk itself seems not to be designed for any particular babies, or perhaps there are simply no babies truly designed to receive breast milk.

However, a new chart appeared in the next mailing, July 5; this mailing also included the old chart as well. The new chart reverses the order of the first (figure 3.2). Reversing the order of the chart has an interesting semiotic effect, because this chart, entitled "Your Guide to the Enfamil Family of Formulas," begins not with formula but with specific behaviors exhibited by the baby

THE ENFAMIL FAMILY OF FORMULAS

The following guide will help determine the formula that best fits your baby's needs.
Ask your baby's doctor which of the Enfamil Family of Formulas is best for your baby.

Our infant formulas are designed to provide nutrition appropriate for full-year
feeding. Experts agree on the many benefits of breast milk. If you decide to use
formula, you need good, nutritious choices.

Brand	Formula Type	Designed For
Enfamil	Milk-based	Most babies
Lactofree	Milk-based; lactose-free (no milk sugar)	Babies with common feeding problems (such as fussiness, gas, diarrhea) when due to lactose sensitivity
ProSobee	Soy-based; milk-free; lactose-free	Babies with a family history of allergy or with milk sensitivity
Nutramigen	Hypoallergenic protein; easy to digest; lactose-free	Babies with colic or other symptoms, due to milk protein allergy

Our toddler formulas are alternatives to cow's milk specially designed for toddlers.

Enfamil NextStep TODDLER FORMULA	Milk-based alternative to cow's milk	Most toddlers
Enfamil NextStep Soy TODDLER FORMULA	Soy-based alternative to cow's milk	Toddlers with milk sensitivity

Figure 3.1. The Enfamil® Family of Formulas™. Arrived June 18, 1996. Matching baby type with formula type.

or its family. Entitled "My Baby Has," the first column includes categories from "No ongoing problems interfering with feeding" to "Colic signs, such as: Prolonged irritable crying for more than three hours each day." While the chart has three columns, as in the first one, the middle column is interpretive rather than descriptive. Entitled "Which Could Mean," this column suggests a reason for the baby's behavior, such as "Trouble digesting lactose (milk sugar)," which then moves the reader to the next column, "This Could Be The Formula That Fits." This final column names the specific formula brand and its ingredients or special benefits (such as eliminating lactose); thus it collapses the two left columns of the first chart into one. If the first chart simply matches baby type with formula type in a simple one-to-one correspondence, this second chart, which was included in all the subsequent materials sent to me by Mead Johnson, uses typical baby behaviors and matches those to formula type. Thus, interpreting baby's behaviors is about

Your Guide to the Enfamil® Family of Formulas™

My Baby Has	Which Could Mean	This Could Be The Formula That Fits
❑ No ongoing problems interfering with feeding	An ability to easily digest and be nourished by a milk-based formula	**ENFAMIL®** • Milk-based • Has a blend of essential fats close to breast milk
❑ Common feeding problems such as: • Fussiness • Gas • Mild diarrhea	Trouble digesting lactose (milk sugar)	**LACTOFREE®** • Milk-based • Only brand that eliminates lactose but keeps milk protein • Looks, smells and tastes like other milk-based formulas
❑ A parent or parents with allergies	A risk of developing an allergy to the cow's milk protein found in milk-based formulas – or other milk sensitivity	**PROSOBEE®** • Soy-based • Lactose-free • Eliminates milk protein • Contains easy-to-digest carbohydrate • Only major soy formula with no table sugar, to avoid unnecessary sweetness
❑ Colic signs, such as: • Prolonged irritable crying for more than three hours each day ❑ Cow's milk protein allergy symptoms, such as: • Skin rash, sneezing, coughing, diarrhea, vomiting	Colic due to milk protein allergy An allergy to cow's milk protein	**NUTRAMIGEN®** • Hypoallergenic protein formula • Eliminates lactose (milk sugar) • Easy to digest

Ask your baby's doctor which of the Enfamil Family of Formulas is best for your baby.

Figure 3.2. Your Guide to the Enfamil® Family of Formulas™. Arrived July 5, 1996. Matching infant behavior to formula type: establishing the symbolics of ingestion.

choosing the right formula—and, needless to say, breastfeeding is never a choice on the chart.

Thus, in a mailing about infant sleep that I received on July 12, the personalized introduction letter states, "Of course, if you're bottle-feeding or supplementing, finding the formula that agrees with your baby will help you *all* sleep better. That's why Mead Johnson created the Enfamil Family of Formulas—a whole range of choices that takes each baby's unique needs into account." The following mailing, which I received July 18, includes a pamphlet entitled "Figuring Out Feeding." The chart inside has a headline, "Since every baby's different, we've created a Family of Formulas." The caption to the side reads, "Experts agree on the many benefits of breast milk. If you decide to use formula, you need good, nutritious choices. And no one gives more choices than the Enfamil Family of Formulas. So if your baby's fussy or her feeding needs change, you and your doctor may decide to try switching the type of formula you use."

Whose baby isn't fussy? Implicit in the information is a semiotic approach to reading a baby's behavioral symptomatology in relation to a range of product choices. Breast milk is a living substance that is itself always changing in relation to the mother's diet and also in coordination with the baby's needs (watery foremilk at the beginning of a nursing session and creamy hind milk at the end; differently composed milks at the beginning and end of the day; different milk for weaning infants than for newborns). Significantly, it is presented as what the experts agree is best for all babies but not what is uniquely suited to your baby. It's sort of a one-size-fits-all garment, and can't be altered when a baby exhibits the symptoms of, well, being a baby.

In this model, common infant behaviors are represented as both expected and problematic: thus crying, in the pamphlet "Coping with Crying" (received August 1, 1996), is something a baby does to communicate a number of different messages (discomfort, thirst, excess gas, a jabbing pin, surprise or fear, or a "more serious problem"). Of course, babies cry when hungry, but the pamphlet never suggests simply feeding a baby when hungry (perhaps since formula-fed babies usually eat on a schedule); instead, the suggestions include swaddling, strolling, taking the baby outside, playing music, or turning on a rhythmic background sound (among other options). The caption next to the chart with the headline, "Finding the right formula can help quiet things down," states that "*Any* baby will cry when it's hungry, having trouble digesting food, developing allergies, or colicky" (emphasis added). *All* babies get hungry, of course, but the percentage experiencing the rest of the causes of crying listed is far lower. But by linking hunger to developing allergies, having trouble digesting, and colic, this Mead Johnson pamphlet replicates in its text the message in the chart on the same page: "No ongoing problems interfering with feeding" is structurally the same as "Colic signs, such as . . . " since both behaviors merely indicate different types of formula. Ordinary hunger is like developing an allergy or having colic; all three make babies cry, and each requires a particular kind of infant formula.

The pamphlet has advice about all sorts of ways to respond to infant crying, and doesn't stress feeding. That's a good thing. Yet the chart, which is the centerfold of the pamphlet, suggests that choosing the right formula is essential to taming the crying baby. Anthropologist Meredith Small writes,

> Traditionally, parents in Western culture think there must be something wrong with the baby's diet or digestive tract; perhaps they are feeding it the wrong formula, or it has excessive gas. But studies show that there's really no relation between food and the far end of the crying continuum. Most Western babies are adequately fed, and all-night crying is clearly not caused by hunger. It is also not the result of food type. There is no difference in the number of infants reported as excessive criers among bottle-fed or breast-fed infants. . . . Only about 10 percent of all infants have some sort of milk protein intolerance

and even fewer have trouble with carbohydrates. Contrary to what most parents believe, distended bellies and gas are most often the result of swallowing air during crying rather than incompatible formula. *And yet 26 percent of formula-fed infants go through a formula change in reaction to parental complaints about crying.* (149; emphasis added)

Apparently, the idea that crying is connected to the composition of infant food is convincing to about a quarter of the American parents who bottle feed their babies.

Small suggests that European and American babies cry more often than babies in other parts of the world, or at least that they are allowed to move from the initial stage of whimpering to full-fledged wailing more than children in other cultures:

In a study comparing the amount of crying by babies from America and Holland with crying by infant !Kung San, Ronald Barr found that babies in all three cultures cry with equal frequency—that is, they begin to whimper at the same rate. All the babies, regardless of culture, also produce a similar curve of crying over time with a peak at about two months. But there is a dramatic difference in the duration of crying across cultures; Western babies cry much longer per bout, and the total amount of time spent crying each day is longer in both Holland and America. (153–54)

Small cites studies in Mexico and Korea that also suggest that the amount of infant crying and colic are effects of different cultural parenting styles; for example, in Korea, one-month-old babies spend about 8 percent of their time alone, while American infants of a similar age spend about 67 percent of their time alone (Small 154). It's not surprising, of course, that such information doesn't make it into the formula promotion literature—these ideas are only rarely represented in the most responsible baby care guides—but knowing that infant crying is, at least in part, subject to cultural views and practices makes the connection between crying and types of infant formula all the more intriguing. If breastfeeding advocates are right that formula companies are disseminating Euro-American views of parenting as they try to expand their markets in the Third World, then these corporations are effectively creating the infant behaviors that their products are supposed to address (see Palmer for discussions of the effect of Euro-American infant-feeding paradigms in developing countries). Formula-fed infants are most often fed on a schedule, since formula takes longer to digest than breast milk and because making up an entire bottle when the baby just wants a little sucking is a waste of often scarce resources. Infants in traditionally breastfeeding cultures are more likely to be put to breast quickly when they cry, so they spend less time crying and are held more often. As Euro-American views of infant behaviors, including the appropriateness of scheduling and regulating the infant's intake of foods, become more common in Third World contexts, infant formula becomes easier to accommodate because it fits into these newly established values about babies. Infant formula then becomes as much of a conceptual necessity as a material reality, as Euro-American views of the body and infant behavior colonize body consciousness in other parts of the world.

After receiving a packet about toddler formula, NextStep Soy, on May 14, 1997, my contact with Mead Johnson promotional materials ceased.

The materials I received from Ross Laboratories, which makes Similac and related products, seemed more informative about breastfeeding than did those from Mead Johnson. Formula companies know that mothers who breastfeed are more likely to use formula than straight cow's milk when they supplement, so support for breastfeeding is not a wasted effort for these corporations.[11] Indeed, since fewer than half of mothers who breastfeed in the hospital are still nursing at six months postpartum (in 2000), advocating breastfeeding and promoting infant formulas are not mutually exclusive endeavors. The materials from Ross tended to include more information about breastfeeding and to acknowledge my personal choice to breastfeed— for example, the "Birthgram" I got after I had requested my case of premixed Similac states, in part, "You've made a great choice to breastfeed, because there's nothing quite like feeding your own milk. But if you do decide to supplement, you can trust Similac with Iron and Isomil Soy Formula with Iron—the 1st Choice of Doctors."[12]

This mailing also included a pamphlet with what I perceive as positive and helpful information about breastfeeding, including a picture of a happy mother nursing her baby. This mother was blonde and white, with a conspicuous wedding band.[13] (Often the pictures of nursing mothers suggest they are single by showing a left hand that is ringless, implying that breastfeeding is the choice of less-than-respectable mothers [Dettwyler, "Tricks of the Trade"].) The Ross information about formula feeding is often couched in terms that suggest that formula is most appropriate as a supplement to breast milk. But on the back of the pamphlet, there's a familiar chart (this one with two columns) with Ross infant formulas on the left and a column on the right with the heading "Doctor Recommended," with statements such as "If your baby has milk allergy or intolerance" (for Isomil Soy Formula with Iron). Another mailing includes a pie chart that divides up babies into "Most Babies," "Babies with Feeding Problems," "Babies with Diarrhea," "Babies with Food Allergies/Colic," and "Premature Babies," and provides each category with the appropriate Ross infant formula.

Interestingly, when presenting the recommendation of the American Academy of Pediatrics (AAP), the text reads: "Iron-fortified infant formula is the only acceptable alternative to breast milk," and "Cow's milk or low-iron infant formula should *not* be fed" (emphasis in original). After this, we read "During the first full year, you'll want to feed your baby an iron-fortified formula, such as . . . " Thus, even though the AAP recommends breastfeeding as the most appropriate mode of infant feeding, Ross can technically convey that sentiment while at the same time promoting its own products. The next pamphlet I received includes the same pie chart, although the text around it concerns other feeding issues.

Some of the information in these promotional materials is incorrect, and some of the truthful information is twisted so as to make infant formulas seem superior to breast milk (the representations of infant iron needs are marvelously effective at making breast milk seem insufficient), but erroneous information is not the only way, or even the major way, that formula is promoted. As Gabrielle Palmer and Saskia Kemp write, some Mead Johnson materials represent breastfeeding as a matter of surviving a variety of conditions, such as nipple pain, breast infection, overabundant milk, lopsided breasts, and depression (11). Yet I am most intrigued by the semiotic persuasiveness of the charts, which advocate specific consumer products for particular baby situations or behaviors. The persuasiveness of specific rhetorical constructions that seem to advocate breastfeeding while really showing the ease, efficiency, and nutritional parity of formulas should cause concern. But the interpretive semiotics of the charts seems more powerful to me. In these diagrams, infant feeding is both the basis for parenting practices *and* the answer to all problem baby behaviors. This suggests that the existence of infant formulas creates a new semiotic context for infant behavior, whereby interpretation attends to what I have called a *symbolics of ingestion*. The charts, matching up infant behavior with a possible digestive cause and the specific formula to meet such a challenge, constitute and enforce this semiotics of baby care, and they suggest that anxiety about one's baby can be calmed and cured in the consumer marketplace.

It is true that breastfeeding advocates also often see maternal nursing as the basis for parenting practices, yet they do so by presenting lactation as a response to infant needs that involves nutritional and emotional requirements in the same activity. Breastfeeding is never just nutritional, and babies who are allowed free access to their mother's breasts clearly nurse for a variety of reasons. In the formula materials, infant feeding is the process of getting the right substance into the baby, and doing so involves a complex interpretive process of matching the baby and her actions to the consumer chart. All issues—sleep, crying, proper growth and development, and so on—come down to determining the right substance going into the baby. And the substance must be bought.

In some ways, breastfeeding advocates have appropriated the structure and content of this discourse, describing breast milk as "liquid gold," and focusing on breast milk (as opposed to the whole package of behaviors involved in maternal nursing) as what's best for baby. Breast pumping is the usual way for American women to manage waged employment and maternal nursing—pumping focuses on the aspect of providing maternal milk for the child. In breastfeeding promotion materials, the fact that pumping milk allows a mother to maintain breastfeeding during those times when she is with the child is often subordinated to the issue of providing the breast milk itself, thus reducing the practice of breastfeeding to the delivery of human milk from mother to infant.[14]

Advocates' promotion of breast pumping is clearly pragmatic in a political climate hostile to maternity leave, but it also fits with the current symbolics of ingestion that organizes ideas about babies' needs and maternal experiences. Breast pumping makes mothers separable from babies in a way that promises mothers freedoms previously available only to men and childless women, and focuses mothers' (and others') attention on what goes into baby, not on the kind of experience that babies have while feeding or on what it means to interpret nursing as the delivery of a nutritional substance. Pregnancy and infant care advice literature is much more likely to pay attention to distinctions between breast- and bottle feeding than is the formula promotion literature, but these sources also end up promoting bottle feeding, albeit through other rhetorical complexities of the "choice" paradigm.

Breast Is Best

Infant formula promotion materials emphasize a choice of products within a brand, setting up within each brand a *semiotic* field linking infant behavior and product differences. Pregnancy and infant care advice manuals, on the other hand, utilize a *rhetorical* structure of choice in their discussion of infant feeding methods. To introduce just a few examples, *The Complete Idiot's Guide to Bringing Up Baby* has a chapter entitled "All You Can Eat: Breast-Feeding and Bottle-Feeding," which has as its subtitle, "Breast-feeding vs. bottle-feeding—and how to do whichever you choose" (Larson and Osborn). Anne Blocker's *Baby Basics: A Guide for New Parents* presents the following options as choices: "Breastfeeding," "Formula Feeding," and "Combination Breastfeeding and Formula Feeding" (141–56). *Dr. Spock's Baby and Child Care* does not present infant feeding as a matter of choice in the overall structure of his chapters and discussion, but has this to say when introducing bottle feeding: "we know that there are real health benefits to mother's milk and that formula should be used only when breast-feeding is not an option. If you are choosing a formula, there are several different brands to choose from" (Spock and Parker 141).

In a society where commercial infant formulas exist, mothers do choose between breast- and bottle feeding, although many (like myself) don't register the choice as one at all. All pregnancy and infant care advice books include a section on infant feeding that presents the method—breast or bottle—as a choice. Breastfeeding guidebooks eschew the rhetoric of choice by presenting only methods for nursing and for feeding infants expressed breast milk. At this writing, there is only one guidebook exclusively about bottle feeding, *When Breastfeeding Is Not an Option* (formerly *Bottlefeeding without Guilt* [Robin]), but even this book includes a chapter entitled "More Than a Simple Choice," suggesting that even in a book solely devoted to bottle feeding, that decision needs justification (or at least representation as a valid choice).[15]

How does the existence of a real choice in infant feeding (i.e., the expectation that babies will live with either method) affect what women do? Obviously, when commercial alternatives to breast milk were few and far between, women nursed their own infants, hired other women to do so, or fed them something else. Infant mortality rates followed accordingly, and, as I discussed in the introduction, only in countries where the climate was rather cold did children who were hand fed stand a chance of surviving in appreciable numbers, although their survivability was severely compromised by not being breastfed. Once pure dairy milk became available and safe methods of bottle feeding were devised, American mothers began turning away from breastfeeding in large numbers. Proprietary infant foods were once scorned by physicians, who promoted their own formulas as specific prescriptions for each individual child, but the medical establishment eventually came around when it was clear that mothers preferred the ease of prepared products. Once it was endorsed by the medical establishment and individual doctors, bottle feeding took America by storm: between the last years of the nineteenth century and past the midpoint of the twentieth, the majority of American women chose not to breastfeed their infants. During this period general standards of living, including the provision of safe water and indoor plumbing to large numbers of Americans, improved, and infant mortality decreased even though large numbers of infants were no longer breastfed. Clearly, when not breastfeeding does not seem to automatically or obviously compromise the health of babies, bottle feeding becomes a compelling option. When choice is available, many women choose against breastfeeding.

In a discursive analysis of contemporary pregnancy advice manuals, Helena Michie and Naomi Cahn discuss the rhetoric of choice as it appears in those texts. The rhetoric of choice is not, of course, the same thing as making a real choice. The authors quote Joan Williams: "[T]he rhetoric of choice diverts attention from the constraints within which an individual choice occurs onto the act of choice itself" (Michie and Cahn 70). In their reading, choice is a problematic concept in pregnancy advice literature. In that context, it usually refers to choices of doctors, hospitals, and medical practices during both prenatal care and childbirth; while pregnant women are advised again and again to make *informed* choices, the social context and meaning of those choices in the larger world outside the immediate pregnancy is ignored. The choice is personalized and made to seem about one's own pregnancy, body, and fetus, rather than about the structures of medical care that make such choices about pregnancy care seem normal. Indeed, the fact that pregnancy and childbirth are defined as medical conditions necessitating a certain level of care and expert attention means that the specific choices presented to pregnant women and their partners are rarely understood or experienced as *political* or related to a social field of competing forces (see Treichler). Michie and Cahn continue: "With choice comes a sense of personal responsibility and, with that, often socially induced guilt. As [Robin] Gregg puts it, 'One of the paradoxical things about prenatal tests and other procreative technologies is that their existence has created a situation where choices *must* be made.... In many ways, subtle or not so subtle, choice turns into pressure'" (71). The authors conclude: "'Choice,' then, links the discourses of individualism and consumerism in downplaying the role of social forces and making reproduction into private enterprise" (72).

Michie and Cahn's analysis of choice in prenatal treatment and childbirth practices aptly introduces the "breast or bottle" discussions in pregnancy and infant care advice literature. Represented in relation to the choice that all mothers will make, the two methods of infant feeding are presented in terms of advantages and disadvantages to both mother and baby. Breastfeeding is almost always discussed first, and its health benefits to the infant are always extolled. What follows is usually a discussion of proper technique, nutritional issues for the mother, common myths about nursing and the mother's ability to produce milk, and, finally, the ubiquitous and lengthy presentation of possible problems that might arise (plugged ducts, perceived insufficient milk supply, breast infection, for example). Bottle feeding will usually merit less discussion, although there is sometimes extended attention paid to preparation and formula types. The bottle-feeding section usually concerns the how-to's of choosing, buying, preparing, and administering infant formula.

Just reading the chapters, it's easy to see that the breastfeeding sections seem to devolve into negativity, because the last pages of each discussion of lactation concern problems that can be experienced by the mother as a result of her choice to breastfeed. Because bottle feeding removes the mother's body from the picture, there is no commensurate section in the bottle feeding discussion—indeed, here the mother's body is conspicuously absent. In the end, the problem with the "choice to breastfeed" is that the mother's body becomes, through that choice, the site of potential problems that are unfamiliar, apparently uncomfortable, and possibly overwhelming (especially to new mothers or mothers-to-be). Because the rhetoric of choice sets up each option symmetrically, once we are past the required "breast is best" statement, the presentation of bottle feeding suggests that in not breastfeeding the mother can also choose not to deal with her own body in the context of feeding her infant.[16]

All pregnancy and infant care advice books have to include bottle feeding as a choice that is commensurate with breastfeeding, because the statistics on maternal nursing suggest that to ignore bottle feeding would lead to a disastrous decline in sales. Thus, even William and Martha Sears, staunch advocates of breastfeeding and medical consultants to La Leche League, include a chapter "Bottle Feeding with Safety and Love" in their popular *The Baby Book*—although, to be honest, they have *two* chapters on breastfeeding and only one on bottle feeding, and they begin the chapter on bottle feeding with a discussion of the risks of artificial baby milks (which is quite unusual in the genre). Books solely devoted to breastfeeding have their own market niche. But general guides always present breast- and bottle feeding as symmetrical choices, even though they always contain the message breast is best.

What to Expect When You're Expecting (2nd edition) the most popular pregnancy advice book currently on the market, begins its section entitled "What It's Important to Know: Facts about Breastfeeding" with "why breast is best."[17] The authors present information about the biological superiority of breast milk and the general health benefits of nursing (for example, "breast milk is more digestible than cow's milk," "nursed babies are almost never constipated," "breast milk contains one-third the mineral salts of cow's milk," "breastfed babies are less subject to illness in the first year of life [because of the protection] provided by the transfer of immune factors in breast milk and in the premilk substance, colostrum," "nursing helps speed the shrinking of the uterus back to its prepregnancy size"[251–52]) as well as other factors that make breastfeeding pleasurable ("breastfeeding brings mother and baby together, skin to skin, at least six to eight times a day. The emotional gratification, the intimacy, the sharing of love and pleasure, can be very fulfilling" [253]). But this discussion is immediately followed by a subsection entitled "Why Some Prefer the Bottle," which includes the suggestions that "bottle-feeding doesn't tie the mother down to her baby," "bottle-feeding allows the father to share the feeding responsibilities and its bonding benefits more easily," "bottle-feeding doesn't interfere with a couple's sex life," and "bottle-feeding may be preferable for a woman who is squeamish about having such intimate contact with her infant" (253). Each of these arguments for bottle feeding concern the mother's embodied relation to her baby or her husband (the assumed adult partner); indeed, in the discussion of sex the authors write that "leaky breasts during lovemaking are a turn-off for some couples. *For bottle-feeding couples, the breasts can play their sensual role rather than their utilitarian one*" (253; emphasis added).

Most women in American society grow up with the idea that breasts are primarily sensual in function, as Katherine Dettwyler argues in "Beauty and the Breast: The Cultural Context of Breastfeeding in the United States," even though this idea is generally limited to Euro-American cultures and thus is anomalous in most of the world (see also Yalom). Dr. Miriam Stoppard, in *The Breast Book*, has a chapter on "The Sexual Breast," and one on "The Nurturing Breast."[18] The neat division of breast usage into "sensual" and "utilitarian" roles divides women's experiences of their bodies into two categories: sensual with reference to sexuality, and utilitarian with reference to infant feeding.[19] Yet as I explored in the previous chapter, the relation of reproductive activities like lactation to sexuality is not so easily categorized, and it is still sex that leads to pregnancy and childbirth (most of the time). And since women in American society are unlikely to perceive their breasts as having a so-called utilitarian role until they need to make a choice about infant feeding, it's hard to see how such a choice could be made freely, given years of embodied experience with breasts perceived to be primarily sexual. The division of breast function into "sensual" and "utilitarian" categories suggests a neat compartmentalization that is not only unusual in embodied experience but indicative of American responses to the female body—a desire to separate sexuality from reproduction, a fear of blurred boundaries between maternity and sexuality, and an attempt to regulate women's experiences into socially acceptable functions.[20]

The discussion about breast- and bottle feeding in *What to Expect When You're Expecting* continues through the subsections "Making the Choice," "When You Can't or Shouldn't Breastfeed," and "Making Bottle-Feeding Work." This latter discussion begins with the admonition, "Though breastfeeding is a good experience for both mother and child, there is no reason why bottle-feeding can't be too. Millions of happy, healthy babies have been raised on the bottle" (255). In two sentences, the entire discussion of breastfeeding's benefits—previously presented in largely medical terms—are reduced to a good experience that bottle-feeding mothers can replicate. Indeed, bottle feeding is associated with health in this passage, while breastfeeding only confers a positive *experience* for mother and infant. The text continues, "When you can't, or don't wish to, breastfeed, the danger lies not in the bottle, but in the possibility that you might communicate any frustration or guilt you feel to the baby" (255). This seems to argue against previous information presented about the health benefits of breastfeeding, some of which linked formula feeding to conditions such as Sudden Infant Death Syndrome (SIDS): "Beta-lactoglobulin, a substance contained in cow's milk, can trigger an allergic response and, following the formation of antibodies, can even cause anaphylactic shock (a life-threatening allergic reaction) in infants—which some suspect could be a contributing factor in some cases of sudden infant death syndrome (or crib death)" (252).

My point here does not concern whether the information presented about the benefits of breastfeeding is true or not, but points to the fact that the presentation of bottle feeding as a valid choice for infant feeding necessarily negates the representation of breastfeeding as the biologically preferred and medically-approved form of infant feeding. The last word on infant feeding in this section of *What to Expect* allows the mother-to-be to imagine that the most important thing about infant feeding is the experience, which suggests that the presentation of the health benefits of breastfeeding is only so much discourse. Interestingly, the last sentences bring bottle feeding back to breastfeeding as the infant feeding norm, but suggest that bottle feeding can replicate what is most important about maternal nursing, which is mother-infant closeness: "Know that, with but a little extra effort, love can be passed from mother to child through the bottle as well as through the breast. Make every feeding a time to cuddle your baby, just as you would if you were nursing (don't prop the bottle). And when it's practical, make skin-to-skin contact by opening your shirt and letting the baby rest against your bare breast while feeding" (255). Of course, the mother who doesn't nurse because she is squeamish about intimacy with her baby may have just as hard a time baring her breast while bottle feeding.

Anne Blocker's *Baby Basics: A Guide for New Parents*, which gets highly positive reviews from readers on Amazon.com's web site, emphasizes the symmetry of breast- and bottle feeding. Blocker writes, "There is no right or wrong way to nourish baby during her first months of life. You and your partner need to select an option that works best for you. . . . Milk is baby's first food. It offers complete nourishment for your baby's early months of life. Your choices in the milk department are breastmilk, formula, or a combination of both. The American Academy of Pediatrics recommends breastmilk or formula be provided until age 1" (140). The first subsection in this chapter ("Feeding Made Simple") is called "The Choices: Breastfeeding," and it presents a number of advantages to breastfeeding, the first being that it is an "optimal economic choice," followed by "special bonding time with baby," "helps the uterus contract," "uses extra calories," "convenience," "colostrum ... is packed with antibodies and other protective substances," "breastmilk is rich in infection-fighting white blood cells that help destroy bacteria," "breastmilk is easier for babies to digest than formula," "breastmilk stimulates maturation of baby's intestinal tract," and "breastmilk does not stain baby's clothing like formula does" (141–42). The chapter then follows with an extended section on "Breastfeeding Success Tips" and a section entitled "If You Do Experience Breastfeeding Problems ... " (143–52). The next section, "Formula Feeding," is only two pages long, and includes the following advantages: "Freedom for mom from being baby's sole food source," "Anybody can feed baby," "Convenience," "No need to worry about mom's diet or any medications she may be taking," "You know exactly how much formula the baby is taking," "Because formula takes longer to digest, bottlefed babies do not need to be fed as often as breastfed babies," "You can still experience feelings of closeness during feeding times similar to someone who is breastfeeding" (152–53).

The symmetry of advantages listed for each mode of infant feeding is interesting: "convenience" is listed for both breastfeeding and bottle feeding, although with breastfeeding the reason for convenience is detailed ("Breastmilk is always ready and at the right temperature" [142]), while the reason for formula's convenience is absent. Breastfeeding is listed as "being easier for the baby to digest," while the same issue is also entered as an advantage for bottle feeding—because formula takes longer to digest (i.e., is more difficult to digest), baby doesn't need to eat as often. Prominent among the advantages to formula feeding is the freedom enjoyed by the mother because her body does not need to be present or regulated in order to feed her baby, although formula feeding can still lead to the closeness experienced by the breastfeeding couple. Finally, the length of the section on breastfeeding can be attributed to the necessity of providing a lot of tips to ensure success, followed by the delineation of possible problems that lactation involves. These all have to do with the mother's body or the baby's health. In the formula section there is no discussion of the possibility of ill-health associated with artificial baby milk, and the mother's body is, as I have already noted, out of the picture. As presented, formula feeding seems the choice of infant feeding method with fewer problems associated with it, for both mother and baby.

Dr. Spock's Baby and Child Care is one of the most well-known infant care guides.[21] The seventh edition, "now fully revised and expanded for the new century," was published in 1998. *Baby and Child Care* follows the same model as *Baby Basics* in presenting breastfeeding as more challenging for the mother's embodied experience. For example, in a section titled "The Mother's Diet," Spock states, "Some mothers hesitate to nurse their babies because they have heard that they will have to give up too much. ... [T]he nursing mother can usually continue to eat a balanced diet" (113). Later in this section, however, Spock warns the nursing mother away from cow's milk, recommending "a nondairy beverage and high-calcium foods, such as green leafy vegetables and beans.... The nursing mother's diet should include the following nutrients: (1) plenty of vegetables, especially green leafy vegetables like broccoli and kale, (2) fresh fruit, (3) beans, peas, and lentils, which have vitamins and plenty of calcium, and traces of healthful fats, and (4) whole grains" (113).

Whose normal diet looks like that? This certainly isn't the ordinary diet of most Americans, and yet it is presented as if eating this way wouldn't require regulation and change.[22] In *Baby and Child Care* the nursing mother is also warned that animal meats and milks tend to concentrate pesticides and other chemicals, which can get to the baby through her breast milk. There is no information in the corresponding section on formula feeding that toxic chemicals can find their way into (and have been found in) infant formulas, either through the ingredients themselves or the manufacturing process. Thus, the mother's body is represented as a possible conduit for unwanted chemicals and as a necessary repository for "good" chemicals (vitamins and minerals) through a closely regulated diet that does not resemble the social norm. Gabriel, Gabriel, and Lawrence write that "women believe there is a direct relationship between what they take into their body, the food they eat, and the breast milk they produce.... Women who are guided by the cultural values of self-reliance, who see themselves as capable of following certain dietary and other related prescriptions and proscriptions, are the ones most likely to breastfeed" (501). Spock's doublespeak (don't worry about what you eat; this is what you should eat) enhances the idea that nursing necessitates special care of the mother's body—regulating attention and care—that many women resist or feel they can't live up to. Dietary regulation is also a way for women to demonstrate the purity of their bodies, to assure the purity of the substance coming out of their bodies, but there is no corresponding discussion of the possible contaminants in formula, or only an occasional mention of the strict industry standards to regulate formula content.[23]

Spock's presentation of bottle feeding begins with the following discussion: "Not so long ago babies were raised on infant formula as a matter of routine. Today we know that there are real health benefits to mother's milk and that formula should be used only when breast-feeding is not an option. If you are using formula, there are several different brands to choose from" (141). Spock goes on to recommend soy formulas (this emphasis against dairy is very interesting and anomalous in the literature). The discussion of bottle feeding is about one-third the length of the discussion of breast-feeding, and involves an extended section on the preparation of formulas (including sterilization, washing, and mixing). There is no discussion of the risks of formula feeding, but neither is there a presentation of the benefits of formula feeding to balance the benefits of breastfeeding. The benefits of breastfeeding are presented in the same matter-of-fact tone that Spock uses throughout the text, emphasizing immunity factors in breast milk, the purity of breast milk, and mothers' satisfactions about the breastfeeding relationship. Indeed, in Spock's *Baby and Child Care* there is no suggestion of a symmetry of choice as it occurs in the other texts, although the general presentation of infant feeding conveys the sense that breastfeeding is difficult, that it requires special care and regulation of the mother's diet, and that it isn't as matter-of-fact or obvious as bottle feeding.

Penelope Leach, who may be surpassing Dr. Spock's popularity as the current baby and child care guru, offers the more conventional advantages/disadvantages discussion in her *Your Baby and Child: From Birth to Age Five*. In a chapter entitled "Feeding and Growing," she includes "Immediate advantages of breast-feeding," "Advantages of longer-term breast-feeding," "Advantages of bottle-feeding," and "Getting the best from both breast and bottle." The section on the advantages of breastfeeding includes the routine health information detailed in other books, and the advantages of bottle feeding include the convenience and ease of feeding at the beginning. Significantly, Leach writes that "If you are neither pregnant nor breast-feeding, your body is no longer enmeshed with your baby's well-being, so it can belong to you again. Instead of soul-searching about whether your body can adequately nourish his, you know that almost anyone can feed him" (58). Leach also includes two "Parents Have Their Say" inserts, one about breastfeeding ("Nursing mothers seem enslaved" [because they can't leave their infants at home]) and "Bottle-feeding is treated as taboo" [there is so much pressure to breastfeed that bottle-feeders like the author are subjected to nasty looks in public] [57, 78]). Leach gently chides both parents with a commonsense tone: is it so terrible, she writes, that nursing mothers don't leave their babies for even a short time in the first three or four months; is that really equivalent to enslavement? And to the bottle-feeder she remarks that "only a minority of babies are breast-fed for more than a week or so after birth, and only a tiny minority are given nothing at all except breast milk for several months," so cool off—bottle-feeders really are in the majority (78). In the end, her discourse supports breastfeeding as the biologically appropriate infant food, but the structure of her discussion tends to minimize the health benefits of breastfeeding by *not* mentioning the health hazards of formula use.

Thus Leach, like the other authors, offers her readers a choice in which the explicitly preferred option is devalued to a position of mere equality through the structure of the opposition itself. She even suggests that the choices that parents make are not the ones that they end up achieving: in a special section entitled "Breast, Bottle, or Both?" Leach presents the stories of three women,

Angela, Maria, and Jessica. Angela planned to breastfeed for three months during her maternity leave but then feed with formula; she ended up nursing exclusively for five months and then continuing, with supplementation, for almost a year. Maria wanted to breastfeed for a year or until the baby weaned but used supplementary bottles from two months on and weaned her baby from the breast at four months. Jessica wanted to breastfeed for as long as the baby wanted, but the baby was bottle fed from her third day of life (60–61). Interestingly, it is the women who wanted to breastfeed the longest who found themselves, for whatever reason, unable to; the woman who anticipated nursing the least was able to persist for the longest time period. Leach introduces the women's experiences with the following comment: "Plans are good, but plans that don't work for you and your baby aren't good plans, so have no qualms about letting them go" (60). Of course, letting go of breastfeeding is usually a one-way street; one can always go from breast to bottle, but the reverse is quite a bit more difficult. Leach's matter-of-fact acceptance of the "letting go of breastfeeding," the implied meaning of the stories, suggests her own endorsement of the difficulty of fitting nursing into one's life expectations and practices, which is the narrative provided by Maria and Jessica. This story is very similar to the historical narrative outlined by Rima Apple in *Mothers and Medicine,* where she discusses the midcentury advice to mothers that even if they breastfeed, they'll eventually "count on bottles" at some point (so they might as well learn how to use them [150–66]). The message from Leach is that breastfeeding will probably be more difficult than you expect, unless you are the lucky woman with an easy baby.

The general tendency in representing infant feeding in pregnancy and infant care guides thus creates a symmetrical choice between methods that are presented as equivalent. Even though these texts identify breastfeeding as more healthful for infants, the medical evidence that supports the "breast is best" advice is downplayed or directly contradicted in the discussion of bottle feeding. Even a text like Richard Feinbloom's *Pregnancy, Birth, and the Early Months: A Complete Guide,* which presents bottle feeding in a half-page discussion as opposed to the full eleven pages devoted to breastfeeding, begins the discussion of bottle feeding with the following sentence: "Even though formula lacks some of the special features of human milk, such as germ-fighting antibodies and white blood cells, babies do very well on it" (263). Thus the initial arguments for breastfeeding that Feinbloom provides ("From a nutritional point of view, [breastfeeding] has never been equaled let alone surpassed" [253]) are negated by the notion that "babies do very well on" formula. Both sides of the argument seem to present equivalent information, meant to assure mothers that either choice is medically approved and socially appropriate.

As I discuss in chapters 4 and 5, breastfeeding advocacy took on the challenge of the "breast is best but formula is really just as good" discourse by promoting breastfeeding and breast milk as an optimizing experience and substance: babies grow on formula but thrive (and are smarter!) on breast milk. It is only recently that medical and lay breastfeeding advocates have questioned the wisdom of representing lactation as an optimizing maternal practice, because in doing so formula feeding remains the standard or norm that defines the experience of infant feeding. In representing lactation as optimizing, breastfeeding advocates seem to be arguing that all children deserve the "Cadillac" of infant foods, rather than the "Chevy," but in this scenario infant formula remains an option that offers the basic nutrition for infants in the face of life obstacles or choices that make breastfeeding difficult. Thus, lactation becomes the preferred option for well-off women with leisure or the kind of jobs that can accommodate nursing or pumping, or women who are accustomed to intense self-scrutiny and self-regulating conduct, that is, mostly women who can afford to give their children the best already.

Breastfeeding advocates would argue that these advice books misrepresent the risks of feeding with formula, and I would have to agree. While the benefits of breastfeeding always include its healthful biological characteristics, the discussions of bottle feeding rarely discuss the symmetrical dangers associated with infant formula use (such as higher risks of chronic illnesses, etc.). Ostensibly, this pattern will help mothers not feel guilty if they cannot nurse or choose not to nurse, but it also runs the risk of patronizing mothers by not providing accurate medical information.[24] The question of whether the information provided is accurate is significant in the context of the symmetrical opposition of choice that is set up in relation to infant feeding. Lots of the information about breastfeeding is wrong, but the most significant misinformation concerns the equivalence of the two infant feeding practices. That is, the structure of choice, available because of the technological development of breast milk substitutes, overdetermines any specific comment that may convey patently wrong ideas about infant feeding.[25]

Feeding Schedules

Another significant aspect of the representations of infant feeding in these guide books appears in the references to each feeding as a discrete event. Most infant care advice books replicate this concept of infant feeding, whether referring to breast- or bottle feeding, a concept that demonstrates the extent to which infant feeding is currently conceptualized on a model that is likely to undermine breastfeeding (Millard; see also Stoppard 86). Early in the twentieth century, even breastfeeding advocates like Truby King were advising British and Australian mothers to feed their babies on a strict schedule, but it is clear that in many other societies an infant feeding schedule is simply not part of the cultural imaginary of infant care.[26] In traditional !Kung San society, infants are fed semicontinuously. The advice about feeding in American infant care guidebooks teaches mothers, even breastfeeding mothers, to regulate their infants according to the cultural norms of food consumption by assuming that infant feeding naturally occurs according to some sort of plan that is divided into discrete nursing periods or "feeds." Even those books that are generous in the number of nursing sessions they suggest (eight to twelve in the immediate postpartum period) convey this idea that the infant will organize his or her hunger into separate and measurable feeding experiences.

Ann Millard argues that in the early part of the twentieth century, "regular times for feeding were seen as crucial to infant health, and even survival." Scheduling infant feedings, whether women were nursing or using the very early formulas, was part of a larger social view that saw women and infants "as needing discipline and professional guidance in the form of schedules." Today, however, medical authorities see a feeding schedule "as physiologically crucial to the maternal milk supply" and as "an innate characteristic of normal infants" (218). Millard's research involved examining medical textbooks concerning infant feeding published from the turn of the twentieth century to the 1990s. Her discussion reveals that while there has been in the last twenty years a return to the idea of demand feeding, where the infant is fed upon specific cues the mother (or caretaker) learns to interpret as signs of hunger, "the expectation of a feeding schedule has been maintained" (216). She writes that most contemporary medical texts assume that "regularity in the timing of feeding is a normal part of infant behavior" and argues that "demand feeding is an ambiguous concept necessitating maternal interpretation of infant demands in order to maintain a regular sequence of feedings spaced well apart" (217).

In this way, Millard suggests,

> pediatric authorities generally view the nature of the infant as driving the process of breastfeeding, [such that] their advice [is] no longer opposed to but congruent with human nature.... The issue of control has been disguised as advocacy of what is normal for infants and maternal lactation. In a sense, the clock has moved from the realm of culture, including science, training, and discipline, to that of nature and organic processes—from outside to inside the human body. The absence of a regular schedule is thus taken as a sign of abnormality on the part of the infant, the mother, or both. (219)

This view is absolutely congruent with the representations of feeding routines or schedules in the pregnancy and infant care guides. For example, in *Having Your Baby: A Guide for African American Women*, Hilda Hutcherson writes, "In the first few weeks, the baby should nurse at least eight times a day. Some babies may nurse as often as fifteen or more times. After the first month, infants usually nurse every two to four hours. *But each baby will have an individual, preferred schedule of feeding*, and what might work for one will not work for another" (328; emphasis added). Sometimes the embedded notion of a schedule is quite subtle. Richard Feinbloom first offers advice to feed on demand—"Babies nurse best when they are hungry.... [Mothers] should follow the baby's lead, not the clock's. During the first few weeks many babies nurse as often as twelve times in twenty-four hours. Some of the nursings may occur as often as an hour apart. There may be a bunch of nursings during one part of the day, while at other times they may be spaced out" (254)—but then offers the following advice: "Once breast-feeding is well established—ideally, after two to three months—*and the frequency of feedings begins to space out*, it is often possible to introduce the baby to bottle feeding" (261; emphasis added). The implication in both these texts is that the baby will naturally space out its feeding demands.[27] Hutcherson assumes that such a spacing out is related to the baby's *personal* schedule, while Feinbloom suggests the notion of a schedule with the idea that once feedings space out bottle feeding can be introduced (although it's unclear why the breastfeeding mother would want to do so).

Other advice books reiterate this basic approach to an infant's feeding schedule. Anne Blocker writes that "Smart Parents Do ... Feed baby on demand instead of following a strict schedule. Feed her based on *her* schedule, and let her eat until she tells you that she is full. Before you know it, baby will settle into his or her routine" (163; original emphasis). Dr. Spock provides a lengthy discussion that sporadically touches on frequency of infant feeding. In answer to the question "How often can you nurse?" he writes, "So in one way the answer is to nurse as often as you wish. But in another way I think it helps the inexperienced mother to protect herself by generally trying to keep at least two hours between feedings.... But when your nipples have shown they are invulnerable and when you feel confident about your milk supply and your ability to judge your baby's hunger and other discomforts, nurse as often and for as long as you decide it's sensible" (126–27). Simpkin, Whalley, and Keppler write, "Breastfeeding on demand means feeding the baby when she is hungry rather than on a schedule. It probably means feeding every one to three hours" (274). Even those texts that just suggest a time frame for feedings are using the idea of appropriate feeding intervals not found in other cultures. Thus, demand feeding means that there is no schedule but yet there is one.

Only Dr. Spock speaks directly to the issue of the mother imposing a schedule on the baby, and he does this, as he mentions elsewhere in the text, in order to recognize the mother as an individual with needs apart from her baby. DeLoache and Gottlieb state that "Dr. Spock is credited ... with relaxing the emphasis on rigid scheduling that was so pervasive in American infant care when he began writing [in the 1940s]" (21), yet we see in his writing an implicit acceptance of the notion of a schedule—of the mother watching the clock to determine whether it's time to feed or not. Thus, even in the context of a relaxed view, the idea of a schedule, of timing the infant's feeding, comes through.

Finally, presenting infant feeding as an issue of discrete experiences that have a beginning and an end and can be timed is itself a cultural imposition. Other cultures in which infants are fed semicontinuously do not understand infant feeding to be about the number of feeds in one day (see Stoppard 86–89). This is not to say that those societies have devised a better method of infant feeding, although it may be true that such a pattern is more conducive to breastfeeding success, but rather that all patterns of infant feeding are cultural impositions on babies. The fact that cultures differ on this issue demonstrates this point. Robbie Pfeufer Kahn distinguishes between "agricultural time" and "industrial time"—the latter, of course, distinguishing a time of scheduling and linearity.[28]

American culture tends to favor infant feeding patterns and descriptions that follow what we might call the formula pattern, which is not to say that advice about feeding schedules and feeding times emerged only with the development of infant formula, but rather that infant formulas fit in with American attitudes about regulating the body and the experience of nutritional ingestion. Feeding according to a schedule, whether it is perceived to be imposed by science on the mother and baby or to emerge from the baby's own developing internal regulation, is more like American notions of healthful adult eating: a few defined meals per day with long periods of non-eating in between. Feeding on a defined schedule fits into most patterns of waged labor, and thus can be taken up by mothers who must leave their children for external employment.[29]

Thus, scheduled feeding allows mothers to more quickly regulate the baby into the cultural norm, just as having the baby sleep alone from birth initiates the cultural norm of physical independence, spatial separation, and autonomy prized in Western societies. Feeding from the mother's body can frustrate the regulation of the infant into these normative behaviors—because human milk is more digestible and thus the infant wants to feed more often; because the mother can't regulate the baby's intake (she can't measure it or force more into the baby); because the infant may nurse for a variety of reasons and consequently demand to nurse far more often than would seem necessary for nutritional reasons. The mother's body thus can become the site of problems manifested in her infant's culturally anomalous behaviors—demand for semicontinuous feeding, demand for physical closeness at night and at other times, lack of a defined schedule, and so on—and breastfeeding can seem the cause of a child's maladaptation to social rules and expectations. Breastfeeding then seems to be against what is normal—sleeping alone, sleeping through the night, scheduled feedings—and thus *bad for infants.* Or at least it does not promote the regulation that is good for infants, so that they will grow up to be good sleepers and good eaters, according to the way that American culture defines these social practices. Indeed, as implied in the medical literature analyzed by Ann Millard, which is echoed in the advice books discussed here, breastfeeding only makes for "good babies" when the infant regulates him- or herself into the appropriate pattern of spaced feedings. The description of what babies do is always already a prescriptive statement about what they should be doing, and ultimately it is the mother who is responsible for enforcing that behavior on her child.[30]

Conclusion

One of the main purposes of this book is to investigate and analyze the culture of bottle feeding that breastfeeding advocates claim is a main cause of the inability of breastfeeding promotion to raise rates of maternal nursing above a certain level. There are, of course, many factors that lead to low rates of maternal nursing. But as this chapter has shown, part of this culture of bottle feeding concerns the representational mode of infant feeding choice as it appears in formula-promotion materials and pregnancy and infant care guidebooks. Presented as, above all, a choice, representations of infant feeding flatten differences between breast- and bottle feeding into a symmetry of options that devalues nursing and overvalues infant formulas. In these representations, the mother's body becomes the site of problems, a potential conduit for forbidden chemicals, and the subject of specific regulatory regimens. These regimens are concerned with the mother's diet and the regulation of the baby into a schedule, as well as with a conception of adult female sexuality strictly separate from reproductive nurturance. The cultural specificity of these representations is nowhere commented upon, as the baby's behaviors are presented through scientized language that suggests an inherent developmental teleology toward American norms of behavior. Biomedical support for maternal nursing, however, is presented only to be occluded by all the possible ways to make bottle feeding like breastfeeding, as well as by the consumer possibilities of a symbolics of ingestion that defines the representational strategies of infant formula promotional materials.

It is no wonder that nursing mothers in the United States often feel at a loss when interpreting their infants' behaviors; the narratives and representational structures that define infant feeding all lead from breast to bottle.[31] Mothers with options and resources can resist the prevailing norms by educating themselves, relying on an idealized "maternal instinct" or attachment to their babies, and/or seeking alternative medical care to refute the established paradigms, but most mothers in American society face the bottle-feeding paradigm each time they take their baby to the doctor's office or clinic for a well-baby visit and are asked how often the baby nurses and how the baby is sleeping.[32] They clearly confront this paradigm when they reach for a general guidebook for advice about infant feeding. Regardless of what the American Academy of Pediatrics might say about the many benefits of breastfeeding, medical practice in the United States is still largely ignorant of the way that the bottle-feeding paradigm structures its views of infants, mothers, and the relations between them.

For many, many mothers, it is clear that infant formula offers a choice that is a relief from the strangeness of breastfeeding as an embodied practice and from the difficulties of maintaining such an embodiment in the face of its ambivalent representation in popular promotional literature and guidebooks. For every challenge that babies present to mothers, it seems that what they (the babies) eat is at the root of the problem; thus, changing what they eat seems a reasonable solution, given what is available as reason in the context of these representations. Embodied practices like breastfeeding are not separate from cultural expectations and other practices; rather, they are sustainable only through widespread social recognition, acceptance, and affirmation of their value. The guidebooks clearly value maternal restraint and regulation in relation to diet, and the idea of the infant feeding schedule transfers these values onto the infant (who, if he/she nurses "too much," is often accused of treating the mother as a human pacifier, which again demonstrates how a technological mythology has overridden nursing practices and discourses—it's hard to imagine a !Kung San infant being accused of treating his/her mother as a human pacifier). For mothers who find personal restraint and regulation difficult (and who doesn't—especially in a culture intent on instant gratification?), within the representational context of feeding advice materials, bottle feeding seems to allow an emphasis on the transmission of these values to their infants without the intervening problematic of their own bodies.

The structure of infant feeding choice and the importance of regulating the infant's feeding practices, as presented in both the formula promotion materials and the pregnancy and infant care advice books, reveal a myth about technological advancement and the value of science as an arbiter of social practices. Indeed, these texts elaborate a mythology of reproductive practices removed from the body through the scientific development of consumer products. Through the widespread use of infant formulas, infant feeding has become both more public and more private—more public as it has emerged as a significant consumer market, but more private because it is conceptualized as an individual choice made by the mother in consultation with her (presumed male) partner and the baby's physician. In reality, it is a choice usually made in a completely market-driven context, especially now that formula companies advertise directly to the public, which is why formula companies are so happy to provide free samples to new mothers. Significantly, the ubiquity of formula feeding has meant that infant feeding is no longer conceptualized as a reproductive practice at all, but is defined as a "domestic arrangement" that organizes the "social-reproductive" issue of "child-raising" as opposed to childbearing, which, it seems, is irremediably biological (Law 408–9). Robbie Davis-Floyd would argue that this view of infant feeding, which depends upon bottle feeding as a normative model, mirrors the way that obstetrical practice inculcates women into the core technological values of American culture and promotes the idea that babies come from science and not from women's bodies.

But Davis-Floyd would also argue that women's bodies provide the natural origin of babies, and in this move to counter the technological mythology with one about nature we find the major counter-discourse to the formula model of infant feeding. In the fifth chapter I examine La Leche League, the most visible international lay organization that promotes breastfeeding. La Leche League provides a context, both rhetorical and material, to help women breastfeed their babies, and since its inception in the 1950s has promoted a discourse about breastfeeding as the *womanly* and *natural* mode of infant feeding that is also *scientifically* best for one's baby. But before I examine League materials, I take a detour to discuss an increasingly prominent element of breastfeeding advocacy discourses—the use of evolutionary theories to support specific kinds of breastfeeding practices. Evolutionary theory currently provides a set of foundational assumptions in scholarly and lay discussions of breastfeeding advocacy, yet the implications of relying on a specific and narrow understanding of evolution are rarely raised. In the following chapter, I outline and critique the evolutionary support for breastfeeding, and demonstrate why a political perspective on mothering is necessary to temper any strictly biological story about why breastfeeding should be promoted as maternal practice.

CHAPTER 4

Stone Age Mothering

My daughter Rachel was what is known as an easy baby. I didn't know it at the time and even tried various elimination diets to see if she fussed in response to a particular food that I was eating.[1] It turned out that she was fussing, as much as she did fuss, because she was a baby. In general she was an observant, interested infant who loved to nurse, adored her pacifier, and sat quietly or fell asleep in restaurants. When she was two months old, I started leaving her for two to three hours a day five days a week in order to teach; otherwise, she and I were together. Before she was six months old she had been to two professional conferences, an out-of-town lecture, and an on-campus job interview.

Sam similarly went to two professional conferences before he was six months old, but he was not an easy baby. He refused to take a bottle of expressed breast milk. He rejected pacifiers and wanted all sucking to be on me. He didn't sleep more than three hours at a stretch until he was two years old. While Rachel had napped for about two hours each morning while I prepped for my afternoon teaching, Sam napped in twenty-minute stretches and wanted to be held the rest of the time. At some point I figured out that if I strapped him into his car seat and set it on top of a running clothes dryer, he would sleep for over an hour.

I went back to work when Sam was five weeks old. My plan was to be gone two full days per week. He immediately indicated his dislike of the situation. He refused to take any nourishment that was not directly from my breast. We tried different nipples on the bottles, different positions, cup feeding. He wanted nothing of it and would scream for hours at a time. So twice a week he was delivered to me at my office to nurse after my first class and I rushed home to nurse him when I finished teaching the second. Soon we found a sitter who would pick up Sam from my office after my husband brought him in and take him home while I was teaching in the afternoon. During the spring semester, two days a week I came home in the middle of the day for a stretch, bringing Sam back with me in the afternoon to be cared for by a sitter in my office while I taught. On other days we were pretty much together all of the time, as I took him to department and committee meetings, lunches with colleagues, and other professional events.

While I hadn't anticipated needing to be available to Sam at least every two to three hours for almost an entire year, I consistently accommodated myself to what I perceived to be his needs. Throughout his first two years of life I felt I was being stretched to my limits as a human being (I just never got enough sleep and never had enough time to get my work done), but I accepted his demand for close contact and frequent nursing and rearranged my life rather than force him to adhere to the routine I had anticipated before he was born.[2] The feedback that I got from most people outside of my La Leche League group was that I should put my foot down and show him "who's boss." My La Leche League friends encouraged me to think of Sam as the boss, to think that I was doing my best with a "high need" baby, and to soldier on with the challenges that I had been given.[3] That's basically what I did.

Sam's infancy and my responses to his behavior during this period demonstrate some of the difficulties of accommodating motherhood with paid employment, especially when the practices of motherhood include close physical contact with the infant, extended breastfeeding, and limited nonmaternal child care for the first year of the infant's life. Clearly, I could have made other choices that would have differently affected my work life and the amount of time I spent personally on child care. Even many mothers who do not work outside the home would have made different choices than I did, as would many who are employed. But this experience also points out how it is possible to make certain kinds of maternal behaviors cohere with certain kinds of employment. As an English professor at a research university, I had an extremely flexible work schedule (as well as a sympathetic department scheduler). My toddler daughter went to full-time day care at a local commercial center, so I was caring only for an infant during the day. Thus, although I was subject to high expectations for research productivity, I had an accommodating employment situation, as well as a very good child care arrangement, and I took what I considered to be full advantage of both in order to engage in maternal practices that felt right to me.

I know that what felt right to me was (and continues to be) influenced by current trends in child rearing advice available in my social circles and immediate cultural context. Beliefs about and trends in child rearing, infant care, and infant feeding change historically. Petra Büskens argues that we are in a period during which Western infant care experts value a romanticized traditional model of "intensive" or "immersion" mothering in which the mother places more emphasis on the quality of her bonded relationship to her children than on the efficiency of her maternal practice in terms of schedules, hygiene, and child development (75). Büskens suggests that the rational-efficiency model of child care prevalent earlier in the twentieth century always exists in tension with the romantic model of traditional care but has given way (at least in much of the advice literature) to the latter in the contemporary period (75). This description of child care advice as divided into two broad traditions, the rational and the romantic, provides an astute interpretation of the contemporary archive of prescriptive literature about child development and rearing.

It seems to me, however, that Büskens uses sources that represent trends rather than a wholesale transformation in maternal ideals. I would argue that while it is true that some popular advice manuals such as *The Baby Book* (William and Martha Sears) and *Your Baby and Child* (Penelope Leach) promote the kind of "intensive mothering" criticized by Büskens, most contemporary advice to mothers expects *some* aspects of her experience to be immersed in continuous availability to her child but *other* aspects to enforce separation from the child and to enhance the efficiency of her actions as a mother.[4] Indeed, authors like Penelope Leach promote maternal availability at the same time they caution mothers to set limits to the child's access; in other words, intensive mothering exists in tandem with practices like feeding schedules and solitary sleeping that are the hallmark of scientific motherhood as it developed in the early twentieth century.

If general infant care advice books tend to mix ideals of intensive maternal attachment with expectations of efficient and modern maternal practices, La Leche League links successful breastfeeding solely with the ideal of immersion mothering, encouraging mothers to stay at home with infants and small children and to resist efforts at maternal–child separation. My little group of breastfeeding advocate mothers, most of whom met at monthly La Leche League meetings, felt ourselves embattled by the infant-rearing norms promoted by some local pediatricians and what we termed the bottle-feeding culture. We sought out and created narratives to support our practices (such as breastfeeding on demand and sleeping with our infants), which were belittled or simply dismissed by many of our doctors, mothers, and mothers-in-law.[5]

Significantly, at League meetings I attended during Sam's infancy, I heard other mothers talk about specific nursing practices in conjunction with ideas about evolutionary development and adaptation. These stories generally referred to practices of mothers in Africa during the long period of early hominid development, and they suggested that certain patterns of lactation and maternal practice were appropriate to human physiology as a result of species adaptation during this period. The lay version of this is the idea that we should nurse the way that the most primitive humans did, because that is how our bodies adapted to a specific form of nursing as an advantageous practice. The best mothers, in this model, were Stone Age mothers, because they didn't have the distractions and deformations of a highly developed and technologically sophisticated culture to impede natural infant feeding.

This chapter is an attempt to make sense of evolutionary arguments in breastfeeding advocacy, as well as an attempt to understand how such arguments are related to my own experiences of breastfeeding and mothering. Originally, I hadn't thought much of this discourse, even though my own maternal practice replicated many of the requirements of Stone Age mothering—almost continuous availability to my infant, extended nursing on demand, prolonged night nursing, cosleeping, and late weaning. In the summer of 1999, however, I attended my first La Leche League Seminar on Breastfeeding for Physicians; there I heard a lot of medical references to evolutionary ideas about breastfeeding and infant care. At that point I realized that scholarly and medical promotion of breastfeeding through evolutionary arguments deserved extended critical attention, primarily because evolutionary narratives were becoming significant throughout contemporary culture and this was yet another venue for their influence. I also felt compelled by this topic because my own experience suggested the importance of an evolutionary paradigm (Sam's demand for intensive maternal availability) at the same time that I was wary of the prescriptive aspects of its articulation.

Academics like Katherine Dettwyler, an anthropologist who is perhaps the most visible proponent of an evolutionary approach to scholarly breastfeeding advocacy, and James McKenna, an anthropologist who specializes in sleep research, espouse the evolutionary paradigm as a way to understand infant behavior and to promote infant care patterns that deviate from American norms that emphasize scheduled behaviors. Dettwyler's work, in particular, argues that extended breastfeeding is a feeding and psychosocial experience that human infants are "designed to expect"; organizations like La Leche League use her research to connect the paradigm of immersion mothering with evolutionary ideas through the concept of natural mothering. Thus, part of the unstated lure of what Büskens calls the traditional model is the idea that such a model is imitative of infant care practices that follow an ancestral pattern that is biologically appropriate to the human species; in other words, that it is not only traditional, but *adaptive* in a biological sense. The idea that specific, supposedly traditional, mothering practices are really evolutionary adaptations—rather than cultural constructions that emerge at specific historical junctures—is a persuasive rhetoric, delineating natural and unnatural maternal practices within a speculative evolutionary paradigm.

Evolutionary ideas that appear in breastfeeding advocacy discourses touch on the entire gamut of breastfeeding and infant care issues (sleeping, feeding patterns, child spacing, weaning, etc.). The ways that ideas about the biological appropriateness of breastfeeding as part of hominid evolutionary heritage are linked to questions about weaning, in the work of Katherine Dettwyler for example, demonstrate in particular how scientific theories about evolutionary development can be used to support specific practices of infant care in the modern world. La Leche League literature is certainly based on this perspective, as its discussions of weaning demonstrate. *The Womanly Art of Breastfeeding* presents extended nursing as part of attentive mothering and appropriate to a child's need for emotional and nurturant caretaking. The book cites Dettwyler's research on a "hominid blueprint for weaning" to support the League's view that extended nursing is natural for humans and a potential choice for nursing mothers (La Leche League, 6th ed., 249). La Leche League encourages extended nursing and child-led weaning as natural patterns for the breastfeeding relationship, although the organization does not take an official stand on breastfeeding duration, since its general philosophy is simply to support the mother's choice to breastfeed (which includes her choice of when and how to wean). The idea that child-led weaning is natural suggests that mother-led weaning is cultural and thus not appropriately biological.[6]

Studying these discourses reveals how their articulation contributes in no small part to what Sharon Hays has called "the cultural contradictions of motherhood." As Petra Büskens points out, "the ascendancy of childrearing practices which stress primary maternal availability and care ... sit in awkward relation to the (often opposing) bodily experiences and self-identities of most Western people, including, of course, new mothers" (75–76). Indeed, as the specific instance of a modern engagement of a so-called traditional practice, child-led weaning may not itself be a natural practice linked to evolution at all, at least not in all societies where it occurs, but may instead represent a modern adjunct to extended nursing in developed societies that has emerged recently, as breastfeeding itself has enjoyed something of a resurgence in these societies.[7] Some of the groups currently perceived to still follow the ancestral pattern of extended breastfeeding have rather abrupt methods of weaning their offspring (see discussion of the !Kung below).

In this chapter, I analyze the stories about evolution and evolutionary development that are told in the process of supporting a specific view of breastfeeding and its attendant maternal practices. I am interested specifically in the links between advocacy discourses (particularly scholarly advocacy discourses) that use evolutionary ideas and the promotion of particular modes of mothering in the contemporary United States. I consider these evolutionary discourses both as narratives and as rhetorical arguments that are meant to persuade. Evolutionary discourses are all around us in contemporary American culture: evolutionary medicine is a burgeoning field, and books about the evolutionary adaptiveness of a variety of perceived behaviors—rape, divorce, adultery, monogamy, for example—seem to come out regularly.[8] The general sense one gets from such texts is that evolutionary theory can explain how behaviors or diseases in society today can be understood as the outcome of previously successful adaptations, and therefore are hard-wired into our genetic heritage.[9] Understanding the evolutionary situation, it seems, will help us to accept the inevitability of such behaviors or diseases, or to combat them more effectively.

What is missing in the current love-fest with evolutionary ideas—in culture in general and breastfeeding advocacy in particular—is a political analysis of their rhetorical purposes and ideological effects. Evolution is brought into breastfeeding advocacy as a way to argue for and rationalize particular breastfeeding behaviors in the context of *idealized familial arrangements* (the middle-class, nuclear family in which the wife-mother stays at home and the husband-father earns a living in the paid labor force) and *idealized stereotypes of mothering* (mother as sacrificial figure who lovingly negates her personal needs or desires in service to her children). Advocates use evolutionary theory to support specific breastfeeding practices that they feel optimally insure successful lactation, but because they rarely consider the political context of their support for breastfeeding, they often end up delegitimating other breastfeeding experiences. They imply that women who eschew the maternal practices endorsed by the evolutionary paradigm are enculturated dangerously to particular American ideals (such as women's autonomy as individuals), even though other American ideals, such as the nuclear family and the wage-earning husband/stay-at-home mother duo, are promoted by that paradigm. Articulating evolutionary theory in the service of breastfeeding advocacy thus often ignores the political contexts of contemporary motherhood in favor of an essentialist notion of universal, biologically-determined, maternal practice.[10]

That breastfeeding advocacy so consistently utilizes arguments based in science to promote its cause demonstrates the extent to which it continues to be difficult to argue for women's *political* rights when reproduction is at issue. By arguing for breastfeeding through evolutionary theory, breastfeeding advocates subscribe to the view that science should be a significant arbiter of human social experience. This is not to say that the evolutionary perspective on human lactation behaviors is incorrect *scientifically*. I would have to say that in listening to discussions of species-specific nutrition, patterns of mammalian maternal–infant interaction and sleep arrangements, and the evolution of particular behaviors appropriate to the fat/calorie content of human milk and the psychophysiology of lactation, I am convinced that evolutionary ideas are a powerful way both to understand infant feeding behaviors and needs *and* to rethink the paradigm that defines infant feeding and caretaking in the developed world today (i.e., what breastfeeding advocates call a bottle-feeding culture). In this way, I think that scholars and breastfeeding advocates who use evolutionary theory to promote breast-feeding and to identify problems with the formula paradigm are basically right in a scientific sense. But the evolutionary perspectives put in play in the context of breastfeeding advocacy and research also function *rhetorically*, and they operate in predictable ways to focus attention on the infant's needs and experiences, seeming to ignore the mother and her role as an agent of the process. If breastfeeding advocates want to suggest that socially accepted behaviors for American mothers detour from the evolutionary adaptations of the infant to a particular mode of biological caretaking, then I'd also like to see the discussion extended to considerations of how expectations of mothers that are based in evolutionary paradigms can actually be realized— not on an individual basis, concerning the mother's specific commitment to breastfeeding, but on a group basis, concerning all mothers regardless of the kinds of resources they control personally and their specific life situations. Such a consideration is necessarily political, and draws attention away from the scientific discourse that grounds it toward the material circumstances that are the immediate determinants of most mothers' daily practices.

After all, what allowed me to continue to nurse my son and to work at a demanding career was not simply my commitment to breastfeeding but, certainly more significantly, the flexibility of my job situation and the resources available to me in my home life. If one could call my maternal practices evocative of the ancestral pattern, it is only because I was able to marshal significant resources to realize such practices. This is why the use of evolutionary discourses to support breastfeeding in the First World is so modern and so obfuscatory. Evolutionary discourses encourage all of us to "do what comes naturally" and eschew the cultural forms that have encrusted around seemingly simple biological functions. Yet the statistics on rates of breastfeeding initiation and duration, so skewed toward women of means and education—and women of the dominant race—should tell us that there is more at stake in infant feeding as a social practice. Educating women about breastfeeding may augment their personal commitment to it as part of their maternal repertoire, but in the end it is women's diverse material situations that set the context for their decisions as mothers. If "doing what comes naturally" in America is a lifestyle choice available to specific post-traditional women with privilege,[11] then breastfeeding is a political issue concerning maternal rights, and advocacy discourses should recognize that.

Evolutionary Discourses as Rhetoric

I first started to think about evolutionary discourses used to promote breast-feeding as *rhetorically* interesting at La Leche League's 27th Annual Seminar for Physicians in July 1999. At that conference, "Breastfeeding: Protecting the Future," a number of presenters suggested an evolutionary model for understanding the lactating human female (Klaus, "Perinatal Care," 1999; McKenna, "Dance of the Sugar Plum Fairy"). In the context of this model, the idea that contemporary humans have the same body as humans 400,000 years ago is, for some medical breastfeeding advocates, a way to encourage what they call "natural feeding." The reasoning is that our physical makeup is primarily the same as those early humans who hunted and foraged for millions of years, because the time that has passed since their emergence is only a blip in an evolutionary sense. For example, Katherine Dettwyler writes, "It is reasonable to assume that the five to seven million years of evolution as hunting and gathering hominids on the East African Savannah have resulted in an organism that relies on nursing to provide the context for physical, cognitive, and emotional development" ("A Time to Wean" 65). The environmental conditions the early humans endured shaped their physiology and their biosocial practices: danger from other animals (thus the need to have infants close at hand and to stifle immediately any loud cry, usually by nursing), a lack of appropriate weaning foods in the hunter-gatherer period (which meant prolonged breastfeeding and late weaning), and a continuous cycle of pregnancy and lactation for fertile females (during which prolonged lactation helped space childbirth at optimal intervals for infant survival). These are only a few of the implications of this view in terms of lactation, but they suffice to demonstrate the kind of evolutionary narrative constructed to support the view that perceived norms of contemporary infant care, such as scheduled feedings, separate sleep arrangements for baby and mother, and frequent separations of mothers from their infants, are wildly out of sync with the evolutionary physiology of humans. In this view, we haven't had enough time for our bodies to adapt to the life of modern industrial capitalism, and we do a severe disservice to our infants if we ignore the essentially ancient physiology of modern humans.

However, the promulgation of the evolutionary narrative about breast-feeding (and infant sleeping, etc.) as a *rhetorical* support for maternal nursing, in a discourse meant to offer physicians a scientific rationale for encouraging specific infant feeding and child care practices among their patients, may not have the desired result (increased rates of breastfeeding). Indeed, the evolutionary narrative—we have the same bodies as our ancestors 400,000 years ago, thus we should treat our infants as they did theirs—brings up some of the most problematic elements of breastfeeding in modern culture, reasons why women choose not to breastfeed or give up breastfeeding after a short period of time: its association with primitiveness (Kitzinger, *Experience*, 230), its apparent inadaptability to contemporary American lifestyles (where mothers are not connected to infants continuously to age three), its seeming propriety to life in previous historical eras. Dettwyler proposes her argument about hominid weaning patterns—that modern humans should expect to nurse from two to seven years—as a way of suggesting that lengthy breastfeeding is normal, not pathological. I wholeheartedly agree with this goal, but linking the argument to the evolutionary narrative of an essentially primitive human body may, for many people, elicit an opposite response. The very idea that our bodies determine our lives and lifestyles, that we must reorient ourselves to the presumed biology of a hunter-gatherer society, is not accepted as a given for many (if not most) Americans, especially in a culture in which we are urged to transform our bodies in line with cultural ideals, in which bodies are perceived as infinitely plastic and malleable. It may not make sense to many women as a way to consider infant feeding methods.

If the narrative is accepted as a guide, it is accepted only insofar as there is both a perceived need and an ability to adapt such an understanding to contemporary life. For example, a La Leche League leader in my local chapter mentioned to me that she feels the evolutionary narrative can be quite helpful in getting women to understand why their infants are behaving in certain ways, whereupon they can use that information to make changes in their lives to adapt to this behavior.[12] I have no doubt that the evolutionary narrative can be helpful for those individuals who (like me) are susceptible to its rhetorical and scientific persuasiveness. Indeed, the narrative itself assumes a certain self-evident belief in the power of scientific ideas to guide social practices like breastfeeding. But as helpful as it may be, conforming to this evolutionary perspective still means changing one's life in consonance with a speculative ideal of prehistoric infant care practices, and it entails having the resources and agency to make those changes. Resorting to the evolutionary narrative suggests one central dilemma of modern medical breastfeeding advocacy, that is, the dissonance between the lifestyle of our ancestors 400,000 years ago and contemporary American modes of living (which generally, for example, involve the separation of adults from children and babies in the sphere of waged labor). The evolutionary narrative thus represents rhetorically the very contradiction it is meant to solve, a contradiction that mothers then contend with socially.

Indeed, the evolutionary narrative suggests that it is the *female body* that hasn't evolved, that is essentially primitive, maintained in its

400,000-year-old state. For while the male body presumably has also not changed in evolutionary terms, its reproductive role is limited to genetic transfer, and thus the man's body is not implicated in this narrative as the woman's is. The female body is the target of a discourse that suggests it can't be modern because it is stuck in the maternal pattern of the gatherer; the male body just isn't an issue here, and thus doesn't seem to be hampered by its similar evolutionary state. The implication, then, is that women in particular are affected by their 400,000-year-old bodies. The idea of women lagging behind men on the evolutionary ladder is an old one, and although not one intended by the physicians and scholars at the meeting, it creeps into breast-feeding advocacy all the same as a well-known story about women's inherent primitivism, their closeness to nature and an ancient way of doing things (Russett 49–77; Hubbard 87–106; Hrdy 82–83). Thus, the evolutionary narrative about breastfeeding suggests to women that they *should* breastfeed because women have always breastfed, that their bodies are not evolved, that they are, essentially, nonmodern. Such a view essentializes women and makes a complex social practice seem like the singular result of biological forces that occurred long ago but continue to organize human life today.

Discussions of the 400,000-year-old human body and its physiological requirements may only serve to highlight the problems of breastfeeding advocacy in (late) industrial capitalist countries. Yet the physicians and other professionals that I heard espousing this view seemed to think that this kind of argument cemented not only the biological case for breastfeeding but for specific breastfeeding behaviors (night feedings, for example, that may continue throughout the first two years of an infant's life, or longer). In addition to the fact that these evolutionary claims are hotly contested (e.g., the idea that human physiology hasn't evolved appreciably since the hunter-gatherer period, or even since the emergence of homo sapiens[13]), the evolutionary rhetoric may not have the intended impact on the culture and its members. After all, Katherine Dettwyler's view that "human children, like their nonhuman primate relatives, are *designed to expect* all the benefits of breast milk and breastfeeding for a minimum of 2.5 years" ("A Time to Wean" 65; emphasis in original) will not necessarily convince mothers to breastfeed if they feel discomfort (or disgust) in comparing themselves to the great apes. Many women express the sense that breastfeeding makes them feel like cows, and this comparison is not meant favorably.

Optimal Development

Scholarly breastfeeding advocacy that uses evolutionary narratives often links the evolutionary discourse with a medical perspective that emphasizes optimal infant health. In this section, I discuss problems that result from this linkage, specifically in the work of Katherine Dettwyler and James McKenna; the latter promotes co-sleeping as an adaptive mother–infant behavior that is intimately linked with breastfeeding as a maternal practice. While the discussion that follows will seem quite critical of their work, I want to state at the outset that both Dettwyler and McKenna are formidable researchers whose arguments are directed against American cultural norms that do not necessarily serve women and children well. My attention to the rhetorical and ideological effects of their discourses is meant as a constructive correction to what I see as a blind spot in this particular form of breastfeeding advocacy.

Materials published by La Leche League use an evolutionary approach to support their view of natural infant feeding. Their usage produces a rhetoric of evolutionary theory as a description of the natural development of human behavior. Katherine Dettwyler has published two essays that exemplify this view: "A Time to Wean: The Hominid Blueprint for the Natural Age of Weaning in Modern Human Populations" and "Evolutionary Medicine and Breastfeeding: Implications for Research and Pediatric Advice." Both essays present their evolutionary argument in an attempt to normalize breastfeeding behaviors (such as nursing longer than two years) that are currently perceived to be somewhat perverse in the U.S. context. The following quotations offer a fair sampling of Dettwyler's approach and rhetorical style:

> [R]ecent research examining nonhuman primate life history variables that are closely correlated with duration of breastfeeding suggests that the natural duration of breastfeeding for many modern humans is somewhere between 2.5 years and seven years, with many predictors clustering at the five-to-six-year end of the range. For example, among nonhuman primates, isochrony of weaning with the eruption of the first permanent molar predicts 5.5–6.5 years of breastfeeding for humans; the relationship of weaning to reproductive maturity predicts almost five years of breastfeeding for a primate species with first breeding at 16 years; the relationship of weaning to gestation in large-bodied hominoids predicts 4.5 years of breastfeeding for humans. ("Evolutionary Medicine" 1)

> It is reasonable to assume that the five to seven million years of evolution as hunting and gathering hominids on the East African savannah have resulted in an organism that relies on nursing to provide the context for physical, cognitive, and emotional development. ("A Time to Wean" 65)

> [H]uman children, like their nonhuman primate relatives, are *designed to expect* all the benefits of breast milk and breastfeeding for a minimum of 2.5 years. ("A Time to Wean" 65; emphasis in original)

> Life history variables refer to the length and characteristics of vari-
> ous stages of the primate life span. [They include] . . . length of gesta-
> tion, . . . infancy, traditionally defined as lasting from birth until the
> eruption of the first permanent teeth . . . juvenile stage . . . adult pe-
> riod . . . reproductive period in females . . . postreproductive period
> in females. . . . Members of the Order Primates have longer stages of
> the life span, and longer life spans, than members of other Orders of
> placental mammals. . . . Every segment of the life span is elongated
> in primates compared with other placental mammals, and every seg-
> ment of the life span *not subject not cultural manipulation* is elongated
> in humans compared with other primates. ("Evolutionary Medicine"
> 4-5; emphasis in original)

> Age at weaning is the *only* life history variable that is subject to direct
> and substantial cultural intervention, and the only life span segment
> for which shortening the duration or eliminating it entirely has come
> to be viewed as normal and desirable" ("Evolutionary Medicine" 21;
> emphasis in original)

Throughout her work, Dettwyler emphasizes the physiological normalcy
of breastfeeding the older toddler and young child, using medical evidence
interpreted through this evolutionary lens to support her conclusions.

In "Evolutionary Medicine and Breastfeeding," Dettwyler presents a series of challenges to the medical establishment, arguing the health benefits
of nursing and suggesting that more studies need to be done to specify
the precise health outcomes of prolonged breastfeeding (over two years, in
her usage of the phrase, although Euro-American medicine often measures
anything over six months as prolonged nursing). She outlines a set of research areas that she feels should be targeted, including "research on how
to mimic the beneficial effects of extended breastfeeding for those women
who do not experience it," "research on how to mimic the beneficial effects of extended breastfeeding for those children who do not experience it,"
"research on how to best meet the sucking needs of children weaned prematurely," "cultural research on the reasons why extended breastfeeding came
to be viewed as abnormal or unnatural in Western industrialized countries
and how to change such perceptions" (40–42), and she specifically argues
that

> The typical Western pattern of shortening the breastfeeding period
> as much as possible and having children close together in age—and
> then spending most of one's reproductive career artificially prevent-
> ing further pregnancies—*makes little evolutionary, biological, or even
> cultural sense.* In such a context, a more rational strategy would be

to return to a pattern of maximizing the breastfeeding investment in each offspring, thereby maximizing the health outcome and cognitive achievement of each child. This requires having those offspring relatively far apart, or tandem nursing two children of different ages (common among women in the U.S. practicing child-led weaning). (42; emphasis added)

The fact that she claims that shortening the breastfeeding period and having children close together does not make cultural sense is nothing short of astounding; after all, given the constraints of the modern capitalist workforce, most women cannot afford to be out of waged labor for long (and a majority of women with infants are in the waged labor force in some capacity), and it is extremely difficult to accommodate prolonged nursing on an ancestral model to the contemporary workplace, unless, of course, one is a university professor who doesn't have to run a laboratory or teach four (or more) courses a semester (this is not, of course, the only exception; see Williams for a discussion of mothers' risk of marginalization at work or from maternity leave). Many women work into their mid-thirties to establish themselves in their careers; if they then want to have children, they face an age barrier that forces them into closely spaced pregnancies. Even women who don't work outside the home find themselves isolated from many of the main currents of civic culture when they immerse themselves in intensive mothering for years on end (as would be the case in Dettwyler's model). As Petra Büskens writes,

'immersion mothering' [based on an idealization of 'natural mothering'] is synonymous, in the end, with social exile. Following the prescribed parenting practice creates for mothers an ontological and physical condition that cannot be readily accommodated in the structures of modern society. The result is either social exclusion or the exhaustion of trying to combine normative opposites (home and work, public and private, childcare and leisure). This is a contradiction at the heart of modern culture that cannot be ameliorated by spurious returns to nature or by appeals to an already invented tradition. (84)

Dettwyler's position advocates the use of evolutionary knowledge to transform contemporary reproductive and infant rearing practices—startlingly like the arguments of turn-of-the-twentieth-century feminist Charlotte Perkins Gilman, who believed that evolutionary theory offered women a discourse for the reform of women's subordinate social position. Here, however, evolutionary theory becomes an optimizing discourse to sustain a mother's investment in her children. It seems to me particularly significant that after a century of modern feminist development we still see advocates for a specific view of women's roles in relation to reproduction arguing out of a rational choice paradigm in relation to evolutionary theory.

Essentially, Dettwyler relies on medical research to sustain and enhance the evolutionary paradigm. The further embedding of breastfeeding into the discursive web of medical research and practice is especially problematic because over the course of the twentieth century pediatrics as a specialty has been linked to the rise of infant formulas and their ubiquitous use in Euro-American societies. When medicine meddles in infant feeding, it does save some babies' lives, but it also has managed (at least in the breastfeeding advocacy view) to compromise the experience and nutrition of many other babies (the majority) who needed no intervention at all (Rima Apple makes this same point in the conclusion to *Mothers and Medicine*). It is interesting to me that many (if not most) American breastfeeding advocates rely on medicine as an arbiter of infant feeding practices, given this history; it is a testament to the power of medical ideas and evidence in contemporary American culture. Now that the medical profession recognizes and promotes the superior biological attributes of breast milk, it is attempting to right the historical wrong of infant formula promotion. To do so, in the context of evolutionary medicine, medical discourses link the optimizing discourse of health promotion to the evolutionary ideas concerning adaptation to particular environments and the slow evolution of humans in Africa during the Pleistocene.

Thus, Katherine Dettwyler writes, "Evolutionary medicine seeks to understand modern human health and disease in light of the conditions under which humans evolved, and recognizes that modern lifestyles and cultural beliefs may conflict with our underlying mammalian, primate, and hominid evolutionary legacies" ("Evolutionary Medicine" 2), but also suggests that certain physiological and developmental "factors [in humans] support the idea that the first six or seven years of a human child's life represent a time when the child is still dependent on maternal care, including maternal breast milk, *for optimal development*" ("Evolutionary Medicine" 17; emphasis added). She is forced by evidence to admit that "Clearly, it is not necessary for mere *survival* that all children in Western industrialized countries are breastfed until they are six years old, or even three or four years old" ("Evolutionary Medicine" 22–23; emphasis in original), but claims that "it is clear from the medical research that the longer a child is breastfed, *the better the health outcome for the child*, even under the best of First World conditions" ("Evolutionary Medicine" 23; emphasis added). Indeed, "Future research may confirm that breastfeeding for the full length of time normal in our species, in evolutionary and physiological terms, may result in children who *thrive*—in terms of physical health, cognitive development, and emotional stability—compared with children who were weaned before 2.5 years" ("Evolutionary Medicine" 25; emphasis in original).

This optimizing discourse emerges out of medicine's current paradigm of health advocacy, developed recently (in the twentieth century) through the technological capacity to actually cure many life-threatening illnesses. Through advancements in various medical technologies, medical professionals have been able to expand their purview to the promotion of health and, consequently, optimally healthy behaviors in seemingly nonsick people. But evolutionary theory itself does not provide an optimizing discourse about child development, either physiological or psychological. Evolutionary theory doesn't provide an optimizing discourse about anything; evolution describes the process of natural selection as it works on individuals to reward good enough behaviors and traits with succession into the next generation of the species. Natural selection favors better adaptations over those that are less good; there is no guarantee that the adaptation that wins out is the best in an absolute sense. Marc Lappé comments that the "net effect of selection is to give the new holder of a genetic repository that confers a modest survival advantage greater representation in the next generation" (32). Selection merely offers an advantage to the best adaptation that has appeared as a genetic mutation.[14] As Ian Tattersall writes, "[Natural selection] is a blind, mindless mechanism that lacks any intrinsic direction" (81).

The tension between evolution as a random process that rewards better adaptations and a medical perspective bent on promoting optimal health permeates evolutionary discourses in breastfeeding advocacy. This tension occurs in tandem with an increasingly medicalized perspective on breastfeeding as an infant feeding practice. For example, when Katherine Dettwyler writes, "Only a few studies have defined breast milk intake as a dose-response variable," she is explicitly referring to the need to precisely define what breastfeeding in medical research means and to accurately assess how much breast milk a particular infant has ingested, but she implicitly suggests through this terminology a view of nursing in which breast milk intake is perceived in terms of medicinal dosage ("Evolutionary Medicine" 23).[15] This view that breastfeeding itself is medicinal and in need of supervision by medical experts contributes to the view that breastfeeding is an evolutionary adaptation that optimizes infant health and well-being (rather than just insuring survival).[16]

One area in which this conceptual muddle is evident is in recent research on co-sleeping, especially the work of James McKenna. McKenna is interested in changing current paradigms in sleep research to acknowledge co-sleeping as a normal infant sleep arrangement, so that the research will not always consider the isolated baby as the standard for research protocols. McKenna argues that because of the design of infant sleep research studies, we only currently know

> how infants sleep physiologically when they sleep alone. While this arrangement may be culturally appropriate [in the United States], a different question is whether it is biologically appropriate. I do not dismiss as unimportant present socio-cultural values or lifestyles that promote solitary infant sleep both in the home, and as a standard research condition for studing infants in the laboratory. But socio-cultural values underlying infant sleep research and recommended infant sleep arrangements change much faster than does the biology of the infant whose developing nervous system reflects millions of years of successful adaptations to infant-parent co-sleeping. (McKenna, "Dance of the Sugar Plum Fairy")

McKenna sees infant sleep research as integral to the fight against Sudden Infant Death Syndrome (SIDS), since he believes arousal from deep sleep to be a problem for SIDS victims. Some of the discussion of evolutionary adaptation to specific familial sleep arrangements refers to SIDS as a possible outcome of evolutionarily inappropriate infant sleeping, that is, infants sleeping alone. McKenna is careful to qualify any published statement with regard to SIDS: "Given the kinds of subtle and complex co-factors relevant to each SIDS death, it is not appropriate to conclude that co-sleeping is dangerous across all family circumstances and sleeping conditions, across all cultures or that it cannot protect some infants from SIDS. *These findings do not disprove the hypothesis that infant-parent co-sleeping can protect some infants from SIDS*" (McKenna et al., "Infant-Parent Co-Sleeping in an Evolutionary Perspective," 269; emphasis added). Still, at the end of the article, McKenna and his coauthors write in a synopsis,

> Although we enjoy tremendous medical advantages over nonindustrial western people, the link between the infant's biological status and co-evolved patterns of parental care cannot be understood only by examining infancy in its contemporary biological context. Hunting, collecting and foraging and, indeed, parent-infant co-sleeping represents the evolutionary context within which modern humans were sculpted and designed biologically and psychosocially for well over 95% of our existence as a species. Mismatches between recent cultural changes in child care practices and the more slowly changing biological needs of infants that emerged throughout millions of years of human evolution may emerge as the source of many physiological and psychological disorders. (McKenna et al. 280)

This claim is made even though one of the authors, Evelyn Thoman, argues that "evolutionary processes were neither kinder nor gentler than they are today. For example, in contrast to [McKenna's] assumption, it could reasonably be argued that during evolution, co-sleeping served to eliminate some of the 'less fit' infants, say, those with fragilities or deficiencies that made them less able to respond vigorously to smothering and laying-over type experiences, which can occur during co-sleeping. Thus, there is reason to question the assumption that the co-sleeping environment is optimal because it is 'natural' " (McKenna et al. 274). In other words, claims made about the evolution of sleep patterns and their meaning in the Pleistocene are speculative.[17]

The speculations are meant to help doctors and ordinary folk decide where babies should sleep and what kind of sleep arrangements might be healthiest for infants. The hypothetical benefit is both physiological—reduced risk of SIDS, which is the biggest cause of death for infants in the United States, at an incidence of .77 per thousand births in 1997 (American SIDS Institute)—and psychological—the psychological disorders suggested by McKenna and colleagues as a potential result of the ill-fit between culture and the evolved biology of infants. No one wants babies to die, and the situation is even more significant because the cause of death in SIDS is by definition unknown, so the significance of the sleep research in relation to SIDS is self-explanatory (although one could argue perversely that SIDS deaths may represent selection for isolated infant sleep). But the risk of psychological disorders is a far more diffuse and difficult risk to calculate, and much more problematic as a reason to co-sleep. Caring about the psychological well-being of infants is a very new phenomenon even in Euro-American cultures, dating back to the nineteenth-century model of the mother as the emotional and moral center of the family and coming to full fruition with the advent of psychoanalysis in the twentieth century (Dally 85–103). In emphasizing emotional well-being as an outcome of infant sleep arrangements, we are back at the optimizing paradigm that results when evolutionary ideas are utilized to support medical practice and advice: sleeping with your baby is not about mere survival, but about creating babies who are healthier than those maladaptive infants who somehow survive sleeping on their own in cribs.[18]

James McKenna is fighting a sleep research establishment and a culture that believe that co-sleeping is dangerous to infants, either as a specific risk for infant suffocation or the more diffuse risk of harming the child's development of independence and good sleep habits.[19] And it's possible that he is using evolutionary discourses rhetorically. In a talk at the 2001 Seminar on Breastfeeding for Physicians ("Never Sleep with Your Baby?") he suggested that his use of the term *babies designed to expect* was meant to counter, in a rhetorical manner, the Consumer Products Safety Commission's statement on co-sleeping and infants sleeping in cribs, since that statement suggested that cribs were designed for babies and thus the only appropriate venues in which they should sleep. Yet at other times McKenna used the designed to expect discourse to clearly indicate adherence to the evolutionary viewpoint; design in this sense suggesting adaptations that over millennia create a certain design to babies' anatomy and physiology. It's hard to discern whether there is a distinction in his mind between the rhetorical strategy and the truth value of an evolutionary perspective for medicine.

As a mother who has slept with both her babies, I sympathize with McKenna and believe that contemporary American beliefs against bed-sharing are wildly paranoid and, when understood in a global context, ethnocentric to the point of being xenophobic. And, to a certain extent, I am sympathetic to his arguments: "The composition of human milk, which provides fewer calories per feeding, indicates the need for more frequent feedings, requiring infants to remain close to their mothers, where they can nurse often. Ethnographic evidence suggests that co-sleeping at night and the carrying of infants in body shawls during the day were used to satisfy the need to keep infants close for feeding. Today, the majority of human beings continues to exhibit this pattern of child care" (McKenna et al. 266). And, the "established norms of infant sleep/wake patterns were established in the 1950's and early 60's when breast feeding [in the United States and other Western nations] was at an all time low" (McKenna, "Dance of the Suger Plum Fairies"). These positions seem eminently logical; lactation is an evolved behavior, with different mammalian species producing milks with different compositions appropriate to the growth and development patterns of offspring in those species, and appropriate as well to the way adults in the species obtain food. Animals that leave offspring for a lengthy period of time (cache species) secrete milk that is high in fat and proteins, while human milk and the milk of other primates is watery, low in fat and protein. Much research on infants (and even adults) still takes place in artificial environments and does not control for those cultural factors that the researchers don't even realize may have an effect on their results because the researchers themselves are so embedded in the cultural paradigm that they don't notice them, let alone consider them theoretically. While infant formulas represent exemplary attempts to provide breast milk equivalents to human babies, they cannot imitate exactly the immunological aspects of living human milk. In the developing world, babies gain critical health advantages by being breastfed and by helping their mothers inhibit subsequent pregnancies by nursing frequently; in the developed world, infants that are breastfed are able to avoid what are now considered the ordinary annoying illnesses of infancy and toddlerhood, such as chronic ear infections, gastrointestinal illness, and frequent respiratory infections, and they may be protected against some of the most serious health problems of the contemporary period, for example, diabetes, childhood leukemia, and so on.[20]

I am convinced by McKenna's research that our social expectations of infant sleep are skewed by sleep researchers' lack of a cross-cultural perspective in considering how infants sleep across the globe and the relationship between infant sleep and breastfeeding.[21] Nevertheless, that same research promotes an optimizing version of evolutionary ideas in the service of a medicalized view of biosocial behaviors like breastfeeding.

The optimizing view of breastfeeding has begun to bother breastfeeding advocates, including Dettwyler, who seek to return breastfeeding to the status of normal or ordinary infant feeding in order to highlight the deficits conferred to infants through formula feeding. (McKenna also attempts to reorient sleep research to accept co-sleeping as a normal and widely practiced arrangement, rather than as an aberration.) As long as formula feeding remains the standard, breastfeeding will always be perceived as optional, although preferable. Still, because the default of infant feeding in American culture is the bottle (it's the method most people are familiar and comfortable with, and the majority of American infants are bottle fed by the time they are a few months old), education to mothers encouraging breastfeeding continues to focus on the advantages of breastfeeding and its contribution to optimal child development and growth.[22] The evolutionary discourses utilized by breastfeeding advocates continue this trend, harnessing the health optimizing trends in medical practice to suggest that the human body evolved through millions of years to expect breast milk as both its default and optimal infant food.

This contradictory linkage of the evolutionary concept of competitive adaptation and the medical goal of health optimization remains the central tension of these discourses. Attempts to ameliorate this tension occur through claims about culture and the idea of an ancestral pattern, exemplified in these discourses by the !Kung San of southern Africa. That is, cultural differences in relation to perceived evolutionary adaptations regarding infant feeding come to absorb the tensions that derive from contradictions between evolutionary theory and modern health paradigms. In these scenarios, distinct cultural groups that currently feed their infants according to the perceived ancestral pattern of hominids during the Pleistocene represent proper evolutionary adaptation; American cultural paradigms represent dangerous deviations from this adaptation, as evidenced in increased susceptibility of American infants to a variety of diseases.[23] The problem no longer appears to be one of optimization, but of demonstrating the deficits of a particular cultural paradigm in relation to the ancestral pattern as it is lived by particular groups in the present. Thus, contradictions between health optimization (American medicine's paradigm) and evolutionary adaptation through natural selection (a nonoptimizing and random process) dissolve in the context of cultural comparison: surely those practices that represent the evolutionary adaptation that developed over millions of years must be better than newly developed practices, the logic goes, and our health care system can produce statistics to demonstrate the benefits of such adaptive practices.[24] The modern health paradigm is called in to evaluate and prove the health efficacy of the ancestral culture and its infant care practices, thus demonstrating that evolution as a process does result in optimization.

The Pleasures of the Pleistocene and Those Who Represent Them

This section analyzes how evolutionary narratives evoke the hunter-gatherer lifestyle with specific examples from contemporary foraging groups, typically in Africa. As examples of this discourse in anthropological literature, I use two books that refer to the !Kung San, and examine their representation of this foraging peoples' lactation practices. In all, the discussion in this section strongly suggests a complex set of motives and meanings in any reference to hunter-gatherers as the basis for contemporary child care practices in the West. I explore these issues by taking a look at how the !Kung came to represent the ancestral pattern of infant caretaking and by examining one feminist anthropologist's extensive interactions with the !Kung.

Another anthropologist, Elizabeth Whitaker, opens her recently published study, *Measuring Mamma's Milk: Fascism and the Medicalization of Maternity in Italy*, with a discussion of Italian women's breastfeeding practices, which include precisely scheduled feedings that are preceded and followed by infant weight measurements on hospital-grade scales, practices that quickly lead to reduced milk supply and the early cessation of nursing for most Italian women. She then proceeds to "Breast-Feeding in Biocultural Perspective," beginning this section of chapter 1 with a subsection "Evolution and Health." Here we see a narrative very similar to Dettwyler's: "These past several thousand years [of sedentary agricultural society] have not been long enough for our genes to change significantly in line with our life-style, except for a few elegant adaptations" (11–12); "Evidence of many kinds supports the view that baby-led feeding including parent-infant cosleeping has been the norm for almost all of human history. Anthropologists have sketched this ancestral or traditional pattern by observing contemporary foraging populations and studying past populations as well as other primates" (14). Whitaker also adds a discussion of non-Western groups' breastfeeding patterns, a favorite example being the !Kung San. In the comparison, contemporary foraging societies are used as stand-ins for earlier hominid hunter-gatherers, and their vital statistics with reference to breastfeeding (duration of lactation, length of time between pregnancies, for example) demonstrate the ancestral pattern.

A similar discussion appears in anthropologist Meredith Small's *Our Babies, Ourselves*, a scholarly book written for a lay audience. An introduction to the new field of ethnopediatrics, *Our Babies, Ourselves* charts

> the idea that human babies, and not just their adult counterparts, had evolved under particular ecological and physiological constraints millions of years ago. So far, evolutionary biology has primarily focused on adult members of species; these ethnopediatricians were asking us to step back and think about the human species from the earliest months of life. Thousands of years ago human infants were typically carried at their mothers' sides, nursing continuously. Why did this close physical relationship between mother and infant come about? And what, if anything, does that ancient behavior have to do with how we care for infants today? (xii)

While Small provides a short discussion problematizing distinctions between traditional and industrial societies (76–77), she nevertheless provides the cross-cultural comparisons that many U.S. citizens associate with basic anthropology, especially after their first encounters with it in grade school (my curriculum was called "Man: A Course of Study"). In addition, while she cautions against assuming that traditional peoples today have not changed from historical hunter-gatherers, she nevertheless articulates that very idea on the next page, where she writes about smelling an artifact of the !Kung San peoples: "In that small apron lies the history of a people, the feel of a lifestyle that all humans once shared, and it reminds me what makes anthropology such an intriguing field of study" (77). And then she repeats the typical evolutionary argument:

> Since the human line has been around about four million years, agriculture and the settled life that comes with growing one's own food is only a small fraction of our history; an industrialized lifestyle, in which only a tiny fraction of the population is involved in food production, has been the lifestyle of some humans for only about two hundred years. Anthropologists point out that for the vast majority of time our species has been in existence, we have been hunters and gatherers. More important, our bodies and minds evolved to aid us in hunting and gathering—we have shifted from a subsistence pattern but our biological selves have not yet caught up. (78)

In her discussion of breastfeeding patterns across cultures, Small writes

> !Kung San infants, for example, feed every thirteen minutes on average. This pattern of frequent feeding, with the infant soon able to guide the process himself, probably echoes how the first human

infants fed until they were able to walk, sometime during the first year or so. Human infants long ago must have also been carried all the time; they probably slept with their mothers and fed frequently throughout the day and night. In fact, during 99 percent of human history this was surely the pattern of infant eating, sleeping, and contact. The current pattern of some cultures of long intervals between feeding, no night feeding, and supplementation of mother's milk with other species' milk or artificial milk is very recent for the human species. (184)

The use of existing peoples to represent the ancestral patterns of infant feeding and infant care ends up casting contemporary cultures in a competition for evolutionary-friendly versus evolutionary-unfriendly practices. Ethnopediatrics thus uses culture to argue for a particular view of human evolution: "ethnopediatrics combines culture and biology; with this approach it breaks through our traditional accepted notions of child care and presents options for parental strategies that might be more in tune with evolved infant biology" (Small xiii). Those cultures that are most developed and advanced in terms of economy and standard of living end up being worst for babies, and vice-versa (although non-Western developed countries like South Korea can sometimes be anomalous in this respect). There seems an odd nostalgia at work, if Small's reverence for the !Kung apron is to be taken seriously, since many peoples who are part of the cultures that exhibit the ancestral pattern are themselves at risk of cultural extinction.

Primatologist Sarah Blaffer Hrdy, in *Mother Nature*, offers an important, critical account of how evolutionary theory and references to hunter-gatherer peoples became central to contemporary views of infant care and child development. She credits John Bowlby, a British psychoanalyst at midcentury, with initiating interest in evolutionary psychology by coining the term the *Environment of Evolutionary Adaptedness*, or EEA, which refers to "the millions of years during which the 'behavioral equipment which is still man's today' would have evolved" (Hrdy 98). Bowlby is, not coincidentally, the object-relations psychoanalyst whose interest in infant attachment has led to the development of "attachment theory," propounded by child advice gurus William and Martha Sears among others (see *The Baby Book*). As an object relations psychoanalyst, Bowlby believed that infants primarily seek relationship and love (rather than being completely narcissistic and pleasure-seeking from birth and seeking relationship only as an adjunct to receiving nutritional sustenance; see Chodorow 62–67). Thus, Bowlby was interested in "the human infant's emotional attachment to its mother.... Compared to other behaviors that Bowlby might have focused on (such as how mothers care for their infants), the infant's powerful desire to be held close by its caretaker has changed remarkably little over the ten million years since humans, chimpanzees, and gorillas last shared a common ancestor" (Hrdy 98). The emotional attachment was necessary to connect the infant physically to the mother, who represented the relevant environment to the infant. Hrdy argues, "Since 1969, Bowlby's concept of an Environment of Evolutionary Adaptedness has been enormously valuable for explaining infant attachment to a caretaker," but, in the last decade or so, "the EEA had become synonymous with a specific period, the Pleistocene. This more narrowly circumscribed million-and-a-half-year phase in our evolution was then used by evolutionary psychologists to explain the totality of human nature" (98–99). In this more narrow understanding of the EEA, the !Kung of the Kalahari desert become representative of all hunter-gatherer peoples, since "Most people assume that [the anatomically modern humans who emerged from Africa to populate the world] were hunters of the African savannas" (100).

Hrdy goes on to argue that anthropologists are now beginning to understand how varied hunter-gatherer lifestyles could be, suggesting that the repeated reference to the !Kung as particularly representative of the ancestral pattern of extended breastfeeding ignores groups like the Aka and the Efé, in which individuals other than the mother take care of infants for extended periods, or groups such as the Hazda, in which the mother weans after two years (Hrdy 101, 495). Indeed, "[The] extended half-decade of physical closeness between a mother and her infant [supposedly typified by the !Kung] so typical of other apes tells us more about the harshness of local conditions and the mother's lack of safe alternatives than the 'natural state' of *all* Pleistocene mothers. As Emory University anthropologist and nutritionist Daniel Sellen joked recently, the only people in the world who nurse their babies for five years are the !Kung and women anthropologists" (100–1; emphasis in original). Hrdy also suggests that Bowlby's initial interest in groups like the !Kung was the result of personal bias against mothers allocating care to others.[25]

Hrdy points out that in all cases where possible, mothers seek to extend infant and child care to helpers she terms *allomothers* in order to promote their own productivity. As soon as agriculture made soft weaning foods more available, weaning occurred earlier and babies were spaced more closely together (Hrdy 201–2). Her point is simple: human adaptation to local environments moves in a steady direction away from !Kung patterns of infant feeding, child care, and fertility, which are, as noted above, extreme because of the harsh conditions in which the !Kung have historically lived. To argue that human biology is engineered according to the !Kung model seems to ignore human impulses and historical patterns that consistently leave such a model behind. It is also an argument that ignores !Kung cultural

traditions and treats the group as passively representative of human biological patterns—in this sense, the !Kung do not really act to create a culture
of their own, but simply stand for human evolutionary traits, biologically
defined.

Reading about the !Kung reculturizes their practices, making those practices seem integral to a specific culture rather than an effect of biological
conditions and adaptations. (This is the central contradiction of Meredith
Small's *Our Babies, Ourselves*, and perhaps of the whole field of ethnopediatrics. See DeLoache and Gottlieb, *A World of Babies: Imagined Childcare
Guides for Seven Societies*.) In addition, if the selection of the !Kung to represent the ancestral pattern is somewhat biased, so is the selection of !Kung
child-rearing traditions that become part of the alleged ancestral pattern.
For example, the adaptation of the human female pelvis to bipedalism makes
a birthing infant usually emerge from the vagina back side up, essentially
forcing mothers to have others to assist in the delivery of babies (unlike
chimpanzees and apes who can grab the infant and assist its expulsion from
the vagina by pulling it toward them). The !Kung ideal, however, is to de-
liver alone (Shostak, *Nisa*, 180–1). In addition, !Kung babies are not fed the
colostrum from the new mothers' breasts (even though such a practice, given
the nutritional and immunological benefits of colostrum, would certainly
have conferred a benefit on infants that obtained it), and may not be fed at all
for two or three days until the mother's milk comes in (Shostak, *Nisa*, 181).
Infants may nurse long into toddlerhood, but if their mother gets pregnant,
they are not allowed to nurse and may be weaned with bitter herbs pasted on
the mother's nipples. As feminist anthropologist Marjorie Shostak writes,

> Assuming no serious illness, the first real break from the infant's
> idyll of comfort and security comes with weaning, which typically
> begins when the child is around three years of age and the mother is
> pregnant again. Most !Kung believe that it is dangerous for a child to
> continue to nurse once the mother is pregnant with her next child.
> They say the milk in the woman's breasts belongs to the fetus; harm
> could befall either the unborn child or its sibling if the latter were
> to continue to nurse. It is considered essential to wean quickly, but
> weaning meets the child's strong resistance and may in fact take a
> number of months to accomplish. The usual procedure is to apply
> a paste made from a bitter root (or, more recently tobacco resin) to
> the nipple, in the hope that the unpleasant taste will deter the child
> from sucking. Psychological pressure is also employed, as was clear
> from one woman's memories of being weaned: 'People told me that
> if I nursed, my younger sibling would bite me and hit me after she

was born. They said that, of course, just to get me to stop nursing.'
(*Nisa* 46)

Nisa's own story of her weaning is quite dramatic: her mother tells Nisa that she (Nisa) will die if she nurses while the mother is pregnant with her brother; Nisa's father hits Nisa repeatedly for trying to nurse and finally leaves her in the bush alone at night, in an attempt to stop her from seeking her mother's milk (51–52). The story Nisa tells of her brother's birth suggests a complex psychological game played by her mother in order to get her to accept her brother. After her mother gave birth to the infant, Kumsa, she told Nisa to get her digging stick so she could bury the boy, in order that Nisa could nurse again. A worried Nisa hurried to tell her aunt, who then helped the mother with the baby, cutting his umbilical cord, wiping him off, and bringing mother and baby back to camp. After the baby's birth, Nisa still wanted to nurse at her mother's breasts: "when she nursed him, my eyes watched as the milk spilled out. I'd cry all night, cry and cry until dawn broke" (57).[26]

Clearly, weaning in traditional !Kung society is not necessarily a gentle experience for the child except, perhaps, for the last one: "If the mother does not get pregnant again, a child may nurse until the age of five or older, stopping only when social pressure such as mild ridicule from other children makes it difficult to continue" (Shostak, *Nisa*, 47). The !Kung traditions around weaning are much harsher than current American expert advice for child rearing, which stresses the psychological sensitivity of the child. Only contemporary views concerning infant sleep, especially those that recommend variations on the "cry it out" regime to instill "positive sleep habits," rival the !Kung examples presented in *Nisa* in terms of their brusque and, at times, manipulative approach to the child's feelings. All of this goes to show that nursing behaviors in the !Kung society, like beliefs in particular sleep patterns in Western societies, are fully enculturated behaviors, although the !Kung behaviors may also be more in tune with basic biological survival simply because the !Kung people tend to live at their biological limits more than most Americans do.

Nevertheless, the experience of close contact with the !Kung motivated Marjorie Shostak to attempt to imitate their traditions with her own children:

> I found many !Kung customs and beliefs so reasonable that I adopted them for myself.
>
> My first childbirth was modeled on !Kung women's experience. After twenty-two hours of difficult labor, I continued to refuse all medication. How else would I have understood the stories !Kung women

had shared with me? . . . I was determined to meet one of the most important people in my life—my child—for the first time without dulling the experience with medication. Much of what came later was also influenced by the !Kung: nursing on demand, sharing a 'family bed,' aiming for a birth spacing of three and a half years. And interpreting children's behavior as essentially senseless: 'When they get older, they won't act that way anymore,' I would say, echoing the !Kung. (*Return to Nisa* 234)

Return to Nisa, Shostak's posthumously published reflections[27] on a trip back to Africa and the !Kung in 1989, is remarkable for its revelation of Western nostalgia for African traditions. That the narrative presented is permeated by this frank nostalgia and Shostak's desire to reconnect emotionally with the !Kung demonstrates her intellectual bravery in reconceptualizing the typical relationship of the anthropologist to her research subjects. Throughout the text she writes about wanting the !Kung to heal her in a traditional trance dance, about her wish to be treated as a friend of the !Kung rather than as an anthropologist, and about her desire for the old bush traditions, all but lost since the !Kung moved into villages and began working as herders and laborers for the Bantu. The statement above suggests the complex relationship that Westerners can have to traditions that they perceive to be humanly valuable but which are difficult to assimilate to Western norms. Shostak appears to be aware of the ways that American culture allows her a post-traditional lifestyle relationship to !Kung cultural practices, yet she also demonstrates a certain blindness to her own privileges. Shostak chooses unmedicated childbirth, but the very fact that she refuses medications distinguishes her experience irremediably from those of !Kung women. She "aims for" a 3½ year birth spacing, but presumably makes sure that happens by using birth control technologies unavailable to even contemporary !Kung women. Indeed, in *Return to Nisa* she discusses having an amniocentesis with her second child and of her fervent desire to have a third child at age forty-one (suggesting that she can choose not to get pregnant or that assisted reproductive technologies were available to her). Shostak's own reproductive life is one sustained by American technological medicine and, in her presentation, enhanced by !Kung practices—it is a perfect post-traditional combination. Writing of weaning her last child, which occurred in one night when she learned she had to have a breast biopsy (and perhaps a mastectomy) the next day, Shostak writes, it "broke my heart. What conversation could we ever invent that would match our practiced duet? And how could I give up the vision of myself, a Bushman woman, nursing her last child until the child herself chose to stop, perhaps at the age of five?" (*Return to Nisa* 121). The personal pain of this event is palpable, yet how could Shostak ever imagine herself, about to embark on aggressive anticancer therapies, as a Bushman woman?

Shostak's represented desires to replicate aspects of the traditional !Kung lifestyle suggest that the !Kung operate in complex, symbolic ways for Western theorists (and mothers). The appeal of the !Kung seems to be their more direct experience of physical life, but it is precisely the real consequences of such experience that most educated American mothers (the ones likely to read books advocating !Kung traditions) try to avoid: for example, unplanned pregnancies or abrupt weaning due to a subsequent pregnancy. Indeed, anthropologists believe that !Kung women sustain such long interbirth intervals because of a confluence of environmental factors: lack of adequate weaning foods for infants and young toddlers, round-the-clock nursing, and mothers who, while not necessarily malnourished, are constantly on the move and working to the extent of their physical ability (Shostak, *Nisa*, 66–68). Few Western women really want the lifestyle of the hunter-gatherer period, because it entails many risks that we no longer consider threats to our survival, or our children's, but the appeal of specific aspects of that lifestyle is clear, since it appears consistently in the references to the ancestral pattern of infant feeding in breastfeeding advocacy.

The appeal relies on the idea of a culture without the overlay of negative cultural traditions, a culture that seems to be determined by children's intense physiological need for their mothers. The !Kung are represented as natural human beings. Not only is the representation demeaning (because what else defines being human than that we are so impressively unnatural?), but it denies—by leaving out—!Kung traditions that don't concur with Western sensibilities. Indeed, as Petra Büskens writes, "Numerous histories of 'the family' show that intensive, romanticized caregiving carried out by biological mothers in the private sphere is an 'invention' of modern economic and political arrangements" (76). Idealizing the !Kung is part of a Western romantic view of maternity that oscillates historically with a perspective that mothering should be rational and maternal practices mediated by scientific experts. In our current climate of immersion mothering supplemented by scientific motherhood, mothers are directed by experts to be natural in their maternal practices: hence the significance of the !Kung as exemplars of the ancestral pattern of breastfeeding and infant care. But as Büskens points out,

> isolated caregiving [by mothers] is a product of the modern gendered split between public and private spheres. *There is nothing "traditional" about this.* . . . Mothers are thus attempting to carry out rigorous schedules of attached mothering in an increasingly fragmented and unsupportive social context. And while *some aspects* of the

> attachment style may be derived from non-industrialized cultures,
> the fact that this style of care is first encountered through the purchase
> and consumption of books themselves written by experts and then
> carried out by privatized mothers in isolated nuclear families, means
> "natural" or "attachment" parenting cannot claim in any truthful
> sense to be outside of modern practice. . . . The expectation for "tra-
> ditional" styles of care in a context that lacks traditional systems
> of integration and social support is thus to force a "cultural con-
> tradiction" on women; it is to force them to be against the social
> structuration of *their own* culture. (81–82; emphases in original)

The !Kung represent for Westerners a specific relation between mother and
child (continuous, close contact for the first three to five years of an infant's life) that is currently less and less common in American practice,
as more and more mothers return to waged labor during their children's
infancy or are otherwise involved in public contexts that do not welcome
infants or children. They serve a symbolic function in discourses meant
to support the so-called traditional nuclear family (in which the mother is
available to her children in specific ways), to ground that family form in
the natural history of the human species. Thus, as symbols, they serve an
ideological function in American breastfeeding advocacy—to promote not
only a form of infant feeding practice, but also to provide a template for maternal adequacy that is fundamentally at odds with *her* dominant cultural
context.

Thus, it is not surprising that most U.S. mothers who nurse their babies for
an extended period (longer than six months) are white, educated, middle-
class women.[28] These are the women most likely to have the resources, both
personal and financial, to mimic the ancestral pattern of breastfeeding. This
is the paradox of the evolutionary perspective on breastfeeding, exemplified
in Katherine Dettwyler's comment that it would make more "cultural sense"
for mothers to space out births and nurse their children for years. Her view
is that women should choose what is determined by evolutionary theorists
to be the best adaptation. What is really at stake in her view is women's
choices as mothers; evolutionary discourses privilege certain choices over
others. Expert advice concerning infant care, infant feeding, and other maternal practices always has as its goal the control of women's actions as
mothers. The evolutionary narratives articulated in breastfeeding advocacy
discourses operate to promote specific behaviors on the part of privileged,
white, American women, on the basis of an interpretation of the practices of
primitive, non-Western others. American culture loses because its cultural
practices are deemed nonadaptive for infants; but it also wins because it
can incorporate the evolutionarily appropriate practices of other cultural

traditions through scientific rationalism. American (white) women can be both primitive and modern and, thus, always in their proper place.

Displaced from this relationship are those American women who are neither economically privileged nor white, whose lack of access to medical care and support ironically jeopardizes their ability to re-create the "ancestral pattern" of infant feeding and care. While in the 1990s many of the gains in breastfeeding initiation and duration occurred in mothers involved with WIC (Women, Infants, and Children, a government program providing supplemental foods for poor women and children), class and race remain substantial demographic indicators for breastfeeding. Unlike the black African women who are revered through their continued practice of what are perceived as ancient maternal behaviors, black African-American women are represented as neglectful and dangerous mothers in U.S. public culture (Roberts, *Killing the Black Body*). I discussed this issue at length in chapter 1. Similar issues emerge in relationship to the American nostalgia for primitive maternal norms. The !Kung women's specific nursing behaviors that have been inscripted as the ancestral pattern are represented as being linked to their harsh ecological context of foraging; such behaviors change once they have settled in a village and have more options open to them. Many American women, of course, enjoy some choices with regard to infant feeding and care. It is more than ironic that poor American women are among the least likely to breastfeed their infants, especially since such a practice would offer their children health advantages not likely to be made up through excellent medical care (as occurs for middle-class bottle-fed infants). Poor American women (white or black) cannot afford to be "primitive" in the same way that better resourced women can, even though such behavior might be economically beneficial in terms of health care costs for their infants. It is one thing for a black woman in Africa to nurse her baby for years in a context where that is not unusual; it is another to consider how black women in America might negotiate this highly charged field of symbolic meanings and material consequences.

In an evolutionary sense, breastfeeding evolved in specific ways because there were no other safe choices for infant feeding. Now there are some choices that in specific sorts of contexts—safe water supplies, adequate resources to purchase formula, access to medical care for the acute and chronic illnesses that may result from bottle feeding—seem to offer women an alternative. Evolutionary theory is now used to try to convince women to make the right choices—to choose to be natural as that concept is defined biologically. As appealing as it might be for educated and well-off white women to imitate the infant feeding practices of African foragers, it is far more complex for poor and/or black American women to do the same. In a country where older toddlers are taken away from their mothers because they are still nursing, mothers whose practices are not supported by social and material resources may not choose to risk behaviors that are perceived as exotic. Thus the appeal to an evolutionary paradigm for infant feeding ignores the racialized norms of mothering in the United States (and elsewhere), and makes it seem as if all mothers make their choices outside of particular historical and cultural circumstances that include chronic racism. Incorporating the "other" into one's own lifestyle helps to define racialized, post-Enlightenment, whiteness in America; the evocation of !Kung infant feeding practices participates in this algorithm.

Evolutionary Maternalism, or the Possibility of Feminist Evolutionism

Not all evolutionary theorists, or even sociobiologists, believe that the Pleistocene defines the totality of conditions through which humans evolved. One of the main points of Sarah Blaffer Hrdy's book, *Mother Nature*, is to reorient sociobiological thinking about mothers by demonstrating that mothers throughout the animal kingdom, but especially primate and hominid mothers, make conscious and unconscious decisions about their investment in offspring, based on ecological circumstances, maternal condition, the existence and age of prior offspring, and perceived infant viability. Mothers are not indiscriminate, and their actions have consequences for reproductive outcomes. In a book that focuses on the variation in maternal commitment, it thus makes sense to elucidate the variety of foraging contexts that contributed to human evolution. In addition, Hrdy links contemporary mothers to Stone Age mothers through their decision-making practices, conscious or unconscious processes of attending to the complexities of infant care:

> As birth intervals grew shorter through the course of human evolution and recent human history, pressure on mothers to delegate caretaking to others became even more intense. Whenever they safely could, or when they had little choice, mothers handed babies over to fathers or alloparents, weaned them early, or swaddled them and hung them from doors. At the psychological level, these decisions differ little from those a contemporary mother makes every day when she asks her neighbor to babysit or contracts for more or less adequate daycare. She is playing the odds, and evaluating her priorities. (Hrdy 379)

When newborns seem less than likely to survive, when their survival might endanger that of an older sibling, or when the mother feels investing in the infant would be dangerous to her own survival, infanticide or abandonment have been the historical responses (Hrdy 288–317). The chapter on infanticide and infant abandonment, "Unnatural Mothers," is the bravest in *Mother Nature*, because here Hrdy argues that those mothers most likely perceived by Americans as unnatural are in fact only responding appropriately to difficult situations: "It was not the response of mothers in ancient Rome, or eighteenth-century France, or twentieth-century Brazil that was unnatural. In fact, what was unnatural was the unusually high proportion of very young females, or females under dismal circumstances, who, in the absence of other forms of birth control, conceived and carried to term babies unlikely to prosper" (317). In other words, it is in this depressing discussion devoted to infants dying, killed, or left for dead that Hrdy most effectively demonstrates that to be historically accurate we cannot present mother love as innate, instinctual, or a foolproof guarantee of maternal attentiveness. If mothers are willing to kill their offspring in order to assure their own survival or the survival of other offspring, then clearly mothers make determined decisions—weighing cost and benefit to themselves and others—about their caretaking practices.

Hrdy shows that this can be demonstrated within the context of evolutionary theory itself. Thus, evolutionary theory does not simply suggest what food or behaviors might be biologically appropriate for human infants, given millions of years of adaptations during hominid development in hunter-gatherer groups, but can account for maternal agency as a factor as well. Mothers need to be the subjects of evolutionary theory, in addition to the infants whose adaptation so interests certain scholars, and the infants' adaptations (and adaptability) to maternal interests must be considered as well.

One idea that breastfeeding advocates seem unwilling to accommodate is that babies seem to be quite adaptable, although medical syndromes such as SIDS may suggest that there is a cost, spread over the entire population, of infants' adaptability to American norms of separation from mothers, especially at night (this is McKenna's hypothesis). Hrdy would respond that mothers constantly weigh their decisions in a cost-benefit analysis. Feeding with formula, especially when mothers know (as most American mothers do) that breast milk is better for their infants, is one way of reducing the cost to one's own body, and, in some ways (as Hrdy might also argue) of reducing one's investment in offspring. Reducing maternal investment in offspring, if even by a little bit, can provide breathing space for mothers expected to be sacrificial, attentive, and ever-patient. In addition, breastfeeding advocates are often not willing to acknowledge infant adaptability, arguing that not breastfeeding is the cause of many infant deaths and illnesses, even in the First World, where formula feeding can proceed relatively safely because of sanitary water supplies and programs such as WIC that provide supplemental formula to needy children.[29] In the context of Hrdy's analysis, the representation of the costs of bottle feeding across the population can be seen as a hyperbolic political argument—it's merely one effect of mothers' decision making in an economic and ecological context that makes formula feeding an acceptable option, which provides necessary autonomy for many mothers, especially when the support of the all-important allomothers seems to depend on it.

One option for feminist breastfeeding advocates, then, is to acknowledge infant adaptability and to remain skeptical of medical arguments for breastfeeding that utilize evolutionary narratives to suggest that recent history is insignificant, at the same time that we not give up on the significance of breastfeeding as a biosocial practice. Breastfeeding advocacy, while resting partially on the idea of maternal nursing as natural mothering, most often looks to science to verify its value and promote its interests. Such advocacy is problematic, I think, when it relies increasingly on the scientific case in its favor, because that reliance simply knits a complex biosocial practice ever more firmly into science as the final arbiter of what we, as humans, should eat, how we should sleep, what kind of relationship we should develop with our children, and so on. When Dettwyler says that lactation is the only primate life-span variable that humans have manipulated (and shortened), she is correct: humans manipulate infant feeding because we can.[30] She acknowledges this when she suggests that we can make rational choices now to prolong breastfeeding and space births for optimal nursing behaviors. But to suggest that breastfeeding is biologically beneficial to babies and that this fact should determine all women's maternal feeding behaviors leaves aside all of the other constraints and material aspects of women's lives that contribute to what Hrdy calls "Hamilton's equation," which defines altruistic behavior in relation to cost to the giver and genetic relatedness.[31] Humans have discovered how to manipulate infant feeding (although the jury is still out on some of the biological and social effects of not nursing at all) through thousands, perhaps hundreds of thousands, of years of trial and error with a variety of substances and care arrangements.[32]

If the idea that medical advocacy for breastfeeding is just using science in the service of ideology seems a predictable argument, then the idea that science should be the arbiter of human feeding practices is no less problematic; indeed, what's interesting about this issue is that it allows the problem of infant feeding, the breast–bottle controversy, to be played out entirely on the terrain of science. The scientists get to decide, in the end, what the implications of breastfeeding or not breastfeeding are, whether it's good for women and babies, and what kinds of accommodations should be made for nursing mothers (in the workplace, for example, if it's decided that nursing is indispensable). The dependence on science (or evidence-based medicine, which is medicine's way of saying, "Hey, we're scientific!") as the rational support for breastfeeding promotion is a way of obscuring the political dimensions of breastfeeding advocacy, for women. Most physicians are not women, although the seminars for physicians run by La Leche League tend to be attended by many more women than men. The dependence on scientific discourses to promote breastfeeding, even when such discourses are obscured by references to natural mothering, serves to subordinate women's practices to the paradigm of scientific motherhood, in which mothers' own views and experiences take second place to the advice of (male) experts.

What if a benefit of breastfeeding is the specific way it makes sexual difference a political difference? Breastfeeding divides humans into two groups as kinds of persons who can care for children in specific ways, it allocates to women a much larger reproductive burden than that of men, and it makes it politically easier to group women with children (that is, away from power) in male-dominated societies. Recognizing women's right to breastfeed, as well as what it costs her (physically and economically) to do so, would begin to transform the expectation that she must or should do so on account of her baby. A country with breastfeeding-friendly workplace policies would, of course, be a better place for everyone to work, but it also would force men to acknowledge that their positions of power occur by virtue of women's exclusion from the public sphere. By relegating maternal nursing entirely to the domain of science, through its evocation of evolutionary narratives, breastfeeding advocacy misses a crucial opportunity to position itself positively in relation to women's rights. This is precisely what Sarah Blaffer Hrdy does in *Mother Nature*, a text that demonstrates what a progressive feminist view can do with evolutionary theory—that is, make it argue for women by paying attention to the mindful and material ways that mothers assess their options in constrained social circumstances.

In the next chapter, I examine how La Leche League, an organization initiated by seven middle-class, midwestern Catholic mothers in the 1950s, addresses the constrained social circumstances that continue to confront mothers in the twenty-first century. In attempting to make breastfeeding an ordinary or typical practice of motherhood, at a time when it was nearly a lost art, the founding mothers of La Leche League espoused (and continue to espouse) a traditionalist maternalism that prizes a child-centered domesticity at the expense of women's autonomous independence. Yet to understand League as only a retrograde organization is to miss their continuous interaction with developing trends in women's experiences through the last half of the twentieth century, and to too easily dismiss their reliance on domesticity as a cause of rather than a response to mothers' circumstances.

CHAPTER 5

Womanly Arts

When my children were infants and toddlers, La Leche League meetings were the primary place I went to get support for being a breastfeeding mother. As a member of La Leche League, I was understood to be an expert based on my experiences with my own children. At the beginning of each meeting, we would all introduce ourselves, our children (whether they were present or not), and something about our nursing experiences. Because I nursed each of my children past one year of age, I embody the League ideal of a mother who allows the child's need to nurse, rather than social perceptions encouraging early weaning, to structure the breastfeeding relationship.[1] (The fact that I work full time and put my children in day care when they were a year old was less than ideal from a League perspective.) A classic overachiever, I like being good at things; nursing was something I was good at (although not at the start), and at League meetings I could share my success with mothers still trying to figure things out.

I stopped attending La Leche League meetings when I felt I was treating the meetings like graduate seminars. I felt argumentative; I talked too much. Since I was already working on this book at the time, much of my knowledge about breastfeeding extended beyond my own personal experience; League explicitly encourages women to share information from their own experiences *as mothers*, rather than from other sources. My contributions tended toward the academic, and I sometimes felt awkward because I took such an intellectual interest in breastfeeding. At that point, I rarely took my kids to meetings; my interest in League had become the other mothers, although I continued to need advice about and support for breastfeeding with my second child. Yet I was always welcomed, regardless of the nature of my contributions, by local League leaders who helped me through nursing difficulties and have taken a profound interest in my academic work.

La Leche League is an international, volunteer organization of mothers who provide "mother-to-mother support" for breastfeeding. At League meetings mothers share experiences and knowledge about breastfeeding and parenting. The emphasis on mothers' own expertise in relation to their own children is purposeful; it is meant to challenge the idea that physicians are the only authoritative experts concerning infant feeding and care. La Leche League began when seven middle-class white women in suburban Chicago in the 1950s created an international organization that, over forty years later, has been influential in reversing the dismal midcentury rates of maternal nursing, has brought the American medical profession around to its views concerning the duration of lactation and the introduction of solid foods to a baby's diet, and helped to develop the certification requirements for the new profession of lactation consultant with the International Board of Certified Lactation Consultant Examiners (IBCLE).[2] La Leche League has, of course, done much more, from developing peer counselor programs for poor women to working with government agencies to establish a breastfeeding support system in Latin America. The Founding Mothers, as they are called, in a gloriously ironic commentary on the Founding Fathers of American democracy, are, in many ways, emblematic of the changes in the lives of American women in the second half of the twentieth century—housewives who stayed home to care for their children, they volunteered their time to an organization that grew with such speed that their managerial skills were consistently challenged and thus quickly developed. As their children grew up, some of the founding mothers became salaried employees of La Leche League International. They educated themselves about the medical aspects of infant feeding, and they are now internationally recognized authorities on breastfeeding.

According to Rima Apple, the founding of La Leche League in 1956 initiated the expansion of scientific motherhood to include those women who wanted to breastfeed their infants. "Scientific motherhood is the insistence that women require the expert scientific and medical advice to raise their children healthfully" (Apple, "Constructing Mothers," 90), and as an ideology it developed concurrently with the creation and commercialization of infant formulas in the first half of the twentieth century. "However," Apple writes, "though the league accepted medical involvement, its primary goal was to reach out, woman to woman, to provide a network of female sharing to counteract the sense of isolation faced by many mothers and to teach new mothers [how to breastfeed] by example in an informal atmosphere" (*Mothers and Medicine* 177–78). In the past few decades, La Leche League has heralded the increasing scientific evidence for the health benefits of human milk for human babies, and its leaders are expected to be well-versed in *both* medical literature on lactation and League-approved mothering through breastfeeding.[3] Scientific knowledge about the benefits of breastfeeding exerts a certain tension on the League philosophy of the mother as knowledgeable expert in her own domain.

La Leche League's ideas about mothering, developed in the 1950s and seeming to change little in subsequent decades, make it an interesting organization in the context of second wave feminism and women's wholesale entry into the labor market since the 1960s. Historian Lynn Weiner provides an incisive analysis of the League's maternalism: "Like maternalist ideologies of past centuries, La Leche League motherhood gave public purpose to the private activities of domestic life; like advocates of those past ideologies, too, the league urged that women subsume their individualism for the greater good of the family and society." Significantly, Weiner explores "the paradox embedded in the league's maternalist ideology—the way in which it simultaneously promoted women's autonomy and restricted women's roles" (364), concluding that "The La Leche League reconstructed mothering in a way that was both liberating and constricting and so ironically offered both prologue and counterpoint to the emerging movement for women's liberation" (383). Putting the matter more concretely, Karen and Gale Pryor write that "The league leader of the '60s and '70s was a path-finder, an innovator: she had to be, to teach breastfeeding in a bottle-feeding world. The leader of today is often a family-oriented traditionalist. She may oppose the women's movement and reject some of the ongoing changes in society. While her work and counseling are still sorely needed, they are not directed toward the women whose lives reflect those societal changes" (180).

One ideological problem of the La Leche League's maternalism is, essentially, the tension highlighted when I introduced the chapter with a discussion of my experiences in La Leche League, identifying myself as an authority based on my experiences as a breastfeeding mother. Responses from feminist colleagues and friends that I was doing research on La Leche League are telling: consistently, I was told two things—often by the same person— "those La Leche League women are fanatics," and "I couldn't have done it [breastfeeding] without them." Together, these responses demonstrate criticism of a certain form of maternal practice that nevertheless provides an essential service for many women.

In examining differences between maternalist and feminist political groups, feminist scholar Ann Snitow writes, "Feminism has raised the questions [about women's work that maternalist groups don't raise], and claimed an individual destiny for each woman, but remains ambivalent toward older traditions of female solidarity" (22). Maternalism, in this analysis, is suspect because it doesn't adequately question the sexual division of labor, but works within that division for mothers and children. Thus, maternalist groups usually remain inside the ideological boundaries of traditional social formations, although their effects can be quite radical given the individual empowerment that political organizing can facilitate.[4] Addressing *The Womanly Art of Breastfeeding,* the League's breastfeeding manual, as a feminist, I am uncomfortable with the idealized view of motherhood presented in it, but as a breastfeeding mother, I know that I also couldn't have done it without League. Moreover, I know that the model of breastfeeding offered in *The Womanly Art* empowered me as a mother and deepened my feminism.

In a sense, in this chapter I try to work out that apparent contradiction. Representations of mothering and breastfeeding in the six editions of *The Womanly Art of Breastfeeding* promote a traditional version of heterosexual mothering at the same time that they promote mothers' individual authority as experts, which leads to women's self-empowerment and enhanced autonomy in the face of male authorities such as doctors.[5] In addition, LLL's support for domestic mothering is an effect, at least in part, of the fact that over the course of its forty-plus-year history, work life in the United States has not accommodated the needs of working mothers (let alone those who nurse). *Both* the espousal of traditional mothering *and* feminists' excoriation of LLL as a conservative organization mired in 1950s domesticity emerge from a social context that does not recognize women as having a biological relation to their offspring that is different from men's (that is, physiological rather than genetic).

The apparent impasse between feminist and maternalist approaches to infant feeding and mothering is revealed in the National Organization for Women's initial response to the American Academy of Pediatrics' 1997 guidelines for infant feeding. This set of guidelines, offering advice promoted by La Leche League for forty years, includes recommendations for exclusive breastfeeding for six months, followed by the introduction of solid foods and continued breastfeeding for at least six more months, with breastfeeding continuing as long as is mutually desired by both mother and child. The guidelines also suggest that "companies can help working mothers" by providing breast pumps and lactating rooms with refrigerators. In response, a spokesperson for the National Organization for Women publicly stated that "these guidelines will present a problem for new mothers who have no choice but to go back into the workforce quickly. . . . They might already feel guilty about working, and this might add even more to that" (Elias; see also Galtry, "Extending the 'Bright Line,'" for a lengthier discussion of NOW's evolving response to the AAP's 1997 guidelines). I try to understand the entanglement of representations of breastfeeding with public meanings of La Leche League in order to elucidate why League continues to attract many contemporary mothers, even though it seems to be, to some feminists, a "backward-looking group" (Blum and Vandewater 286).

This exploration of La Leche League is largely the result of close reading, both of the texts that the organization publishes and of the discourses articulated at local meetings of mothers and their larger international conferences. Scholars have already examined La Leche League through the lens of ethnographic analysis, both sociological and anthropological, or through historical study. In each instance, La Leche League written materials were part of the research but largely secondary to the primary impressions and interpretations of ethnography. Attending to rhetoric and discursive strategies allows me to consider how La Leche League functions as a representative symbol of motherhood in relation to breastfeeding, apart from the specific individuals involved and their particular views and involvement.

Ultimately, I am interested in understanding how a consideration of breastfeeding as a practice of embodied motherhood could change feminist approaches to maternity, as well as to philosophical considerations of sexual difference. In the final chapter of *Mother's Milk* I look at feminist critiques of breastfeeding advocacy and examine how feminist inattention to lactation as a biological process has made it difficult to approach breastfeeding as a public health issue with significant racial implications. In this chapter I use La Leche League's attention to breastfeeding within maternal domesticity to stage a more general discussion about the problem of domesticity within feminist scholarship. While feminists criticize LLL for its adherence to a traditional and domestic maternity, it remains the case that the structure of waged employment also privileges traditional domesticity on the part of mothers in order to insure that male employees continue as ideal workers with a flow of family work supporting them (see discussion of Williams below). I argue here that greater attention to breastfeeding as a biological aspect of maternity would enrich feminist considerations of domesticity, and complicate these discussions. More attention to breastfeeding also demonstrates the extent to which LLL, rather than simply toeing a traditional line, contributes to and develops contemporary debates about women's roles as mothers and workers, in the context of a society generally hostile to women's equality.

Thus feminist approaches to La Leche League provide both a background and an interpretive field for my analysis in this chapter. I begin with a consideration of feminist scholarship on LLL, as a way of introducing how the ideological problem of maternalism is represented by feminists through criticism of League values and practices.

Feminists on, and in, La Leche League

In her anti-breastfeeding diatribe, *When Breastfeeding Is Not an Option: A Reassuring Guide for Loving Parents,*[6] Peggy Robin represents La Leche League as an antifeminist, traditionalist cult. If it wasn't so deadly serious, the chapter "More than a Simple Feeding Choice," which details the "Lifestyle of the Breastfeeding Cultist," would be a marvelous send-up of the purportedly extremist views of some breastfeeding advocates, who, according to Robin, never circumcise their sons or vaccinate their children, treat their nursing babies like lovers and never have sex with their husbands, sleep together as families, "wear" their babies and eschew strollers, don't use artificial birth control, refuse all medications during childbirth, home school their children, and only wear cotton clothes. To anyone who has read the history of La Leche League, this representation of League mothers is comical, since from the very beginning the organization has stressed that ordinary mothers can breastfeed discreetly, without drawing attention to themselves in public or in the company of squeamish family members. The League's founders were all respectable, middle-class, Catholic women who, in the 1950s, sought greater control over their reproductive lives and more information and support for breastfeeding. They saw breastfeeding as a way to be better mothers within the predominant middle-class, midcentury paradigm of separate spheres and beliefs in innate gender differences. As feminist scholars are quick to point out, La Leche League is a conventional, middle-class organization that promotes class-specific ideals of mothering through breastfeeding, even though League itself has sometimes called attention to its "radical" support for wholesome natural foods and nonregimented forms of child rearing.

Yet Robin's overblown critique of League as a cult is not without precedent. Feminist scholarship on La Leche League has emphasized, to a lesser extent, similar views, generally targeting League as an organization that mandates specific behaviors and ideas from its members. For example, Florence Kellner Andrews, in an article entitled "Controlling Motherhood: Observations on the Culture of La Leche League," has written,

> The League has a cohesive philosophy which has tremendous influence over the lives of its active members. This philosophy has been amended and extended during the three decades of the League's existence.... Prescriptions and proscriptions regarding a variety of activities have been generated over time as responses to the increased devaluation of the mother/homemaker role since the League began. These constructs have two results: the first is a control function. It is primarily through their handling of the extensions and their control of unconventional behaviour that League members communicate ideal standards and permissible deviations from these standards. (86)

In the conclusion to a recent article in *Gender and Society,* Christina Bobel asks "Are women so desperate for a community of like-minded women that they are vulnerable to League philosophy, even if it jeopardizes their own sense of self? Do members adapt to this particular ideology because the alternative—isolation—is unbearable and the human need to 'fit in' looms large?" (148). Elizabeth Bryant Merrill's 1987 contribution to this literature, "Learning How to Mother: An Ethnographic Investigation of an Urban Breastfeeding Group," concentrates much of its methodologically-oriented discussion on the way in which League leaders "repair" the broken structure of meetings that are "damaged" by mothers who are not fully integrated into the League way of sharing knowledge (in this example, only presenting opinions from one's own personal experience, rather than knowledge based on research or other forms of expertise). In "'Mother to Mother': A Maternalist Organization in Late Capitalist America," Linda Blum and Elizabeth Vandewater compare La Leche League to Alcoholics Anonymous (in terms of size, LLL is second to AA "among U.S. self-help groups" [286]), suggest that League's promotion of traditional maternalism is "backward" and "nostalgic," and argue that League views create an "alternative morality": "the League offers both a strong moral rationale for their [mothers'] efforts, affirming the value of women's caregiving. . . . La Leche League thus offers an especially vivid case [of conservative groups' nostalgia for modern patriarchy]: where other groups have religion and God's design as their moral core, La Leche League directly places mothers' nurturance and children's needs at its moral core" (297). These statements suggest that recent and contemporary feminist scholars warily approach League as an ideologically suspect organization with rigorous social controls over the women who become involved with it—much like a cult.

How refreshing to read Julia DeJager Ward's less judgmental and yet equally incisive book, *La Leche League: At the Crossroads of Medicine, Feminism, and Religion,* where she writes in her introduction,

> [T]here are strong indications that the League is evolving. It is, however, evolving in its own way. The manner in which League mothers make choices about motherhood duplicates neither the approach of strict traditionalists nor that of liberal feminists. They are forging a singular path, one that can appeal to a broad spectrum of mothers both in the United States and across the world. Its uniqueness assures us that League will continue to play a positive role in the "politics of the family" in which the world is now engaged. It is just as true that many mothers will find League policies unappealing. This invalidates neither their views nor those of League mothers. It simply means that the La Leche League is one of many good approaches to parenting. (6)

Even Linda Blum's *At the Breast: Ideologies of Breastfeeding and Motherhood in the Contemporary United States,* the larger project of which her earlier coauthored article is only a part, contains a more measured account of La Leche League, which instead of emphasizing its focus on "backward" visions of mothering argues that "the group's practices ... combat the excessive commodification of the breast as objects for the marketing gaze" (106). Her interest in the "unfixed" body of the mother allows Blum, at this point, to see League as having made a "radical contribution" to contemporary discourses of motherhood.

Feminist scholars are rightly concerned with La Leche League's emphasis on "good mothering through breastfeeding," since, as Molly Ladd-Taylor and Lauri Umansky point out, "the definition of a 'bad' mother intertwines with that of the 'good' mother, itself a relatively recent invention" (6). In *Seven Voices, One Dream*, an interview book with the La Leche League Founding Mothers compiled and written by cofounder Mary Ann Cahill, Mary Ann Kerwin states that the original motto of the organization was "Better Mothering through Breastfeeding," which they quickly ditched in favor of "Good Mothering through Breastfeeding." According to Kerwin, "Now our motto is simply, 'Mothering through Breastfeeding' with no reference to 'good' or 'better.' Because in the end, that is our goal—to help women mother their babies by helping them to breastfeed their babies" (56). Feminist scholars resist the implication that certain types of mothering are better than other types, or even good as compared to bad, because such distinctions are almost always used to control mothers' actions as mothers and define their mothering according to external, and usually unattainable, standards. The Good Mother/Bad Mother dichotomy also serves a larger social function. As Ladd-Taylor and Umansky write, "Fundamentally, the 'bad' mother serves as a scapegoat, a repository for social or physical ills that resist easy explanation or solution" (22). Blum notes that the La Leche League mothers she interviewed had constructed the "bad yuppie mother" as one who ignored her children and was personally selfish in the face of their evident need for her (Blum, *At the Breast*, 85–90); here, the "good mothering" of League mothers is bolstered by their ability to point a collective finger at mothers who act according to a different set of values.

Yet the feminist critique of La Leche League consistently points out that the League itself would be a better maternalist organization if it would pay attention to all mothers and all children, and not just those of the white middle classes who seem to make up the majority of its membership. (LLL does not keep demographic figures of its membership.) Essentially, feminists argue that the League itself is a bad mother: it only pays attention to its own children, and promotes the individual mothering of well-off women. As Linda Blum writes, "Although La Leche League is an organization dedicated to maternal nurturance, it demonstrates a lack of political action for low-income mothers and enhanced medical, welfare, and anti-workfare policies needed by increasing numbers of mothers" (Blum and Vandewater 296). La Leche League responds, in a way, with an understated antipathy toward feminism (Blum, *At the Breast*, 91–92). The organization also follows a strict policy of not mixing causes, since to align itself to a specific political cause might alienate women who would otherwise seek breastfeeding advice from LLL. Thus, although LLL has been involved in developing peer counseling programs to support breastfeeding among poor mothers, it has not taken any specific stand on welfare reform or governmental provisions for universal maternity leave.[7] This lack of broad support for maternalist policies beyond breastfeeding means that LLL is perceived to care only about those women who already have the resources available to stay home with their children or manage their workplace experience to accommodate nursing or breast pumping.

If LLL represents for feminism mothers who are too individualistic to be the kind of good public mothers it can support politically, for LLL feminism represents women's retreat from mothering. Indeed, at least one of the founding mothers still thinks that women (feminist or not) who yearn to return to work after the birth of their babies, when economic pressure is not great to do so, "are not developing their potential as wives and mothers, or as women" (Cahill 160).[8] As Lynn Weiner demonstrates in "Reconstructing Motherhood," in the 1950s La Leche League "anticipated a strand of the feminist movement that was concerned with women's control over health care issues centered on childbirth and child rearing. On the other hand, by the early 1970s the league also challenged the emerging feminist ideology by questioning the consequences for children of the movement of women away from the home and into the workplace" (382). In her analysis, League is both proto-feminist and problematically antifeminist; indeed, the general contemporary feminist consensus is that LLL is still caught back in its 1950s nostalgia for domesticity. The ideal League mother stays in the home to be available to her children, and this domestic ideal remains the sticking point for a feminist appreciation of League's understanding of "mothering through breastfeeding."

Yet the problem of domesticity, and the issue of women's relationship to domestic labor, continues to be a sticking point for feminism in general. The conflict between La Leche League and feminist scholars, as each group essentially points to the other and says "bad mothers," is set up by the economic and social structure of the United States itself, in which mothers really have little true choice about how to practice their mothering. Women without means, especially since the 1996 Personal Responsibility and Work Opportunity Act (welfare reform), are expected to work outside the home for wages. Women linked to male providers are encouraged socially to stay home with young children and often have a difficult time making careers mesh with family expectations and needs. Women who stay home say that feminists think they have given up their individuality and their independence. This conflict defines the Mommy Wars that are the subject of so many popular books, and it is this external context that influences the individual situations within which women make their choices about infant feeding and make those choices a reality (or not). If we step back from the fray and see how mothers' hands are tied regardless of which position (employed or staying at home) they find themselves in, we might see how ridiculous the whole conflict is. No one wins the Mommy Wars if we accept the positions staked out for us by the social status quo. It is also this situation that leads all mothers to seek affirmation that we are good mothers.[9]

In calling for a truce, then, I want to place more emphasis than might be warranted on the ironic feminist effects of League literature and League practice. Reading through League materials is always, for me, an ambivalent experience. But one thing I have learned as a feminist mother is that no social practice is uncontested, or unambiguous in its meaning, if it involves mothers and children. In the next section of the chapter, I offer an interpretation of *The Womanly Art of Breastfeeding*, the League's premier breastfeeding manual, that highlights all of the ways in which maternal practices and authority are enhanced through encouragement and a steady supply of information. I also suggest how League's changing views of "womanliness" and "manliness" occur in accordance with developments in theories of gender during the 1960s and 1970s. In my view, La Leche League isn't an organization that looks back, but one that at each step in its development engages with its changing social and cultural context.[10] It may not, as an organization, be changing fast enough for feminists, but neither is the society at large.

The Womanly Art of Breastfeeding, 1958–1997

Part I: Nature, Science, and Working Women

The Womanly Art of Breastfeeding was first published in 1958 as a mimeographed collection of $8^1/_2$ by 11 inch sheets of papers bound in loose leaf folders. It was written as a group effort, with three women doing most of the composing and the other founding mothers contributing comments and editorial suggestions.[11] Subsequent editions, in 1963, 1981, 1987, 1991, and 1997, were published professionally as bound volumes. Originally conceived as a "Course by Mail," *The Womanly Art* has become what some League members call the "breastfeeding bible." Because it has gone through so many editions since its inception, and because it is meant to help women breastfeed and introduce them to League concepts and practices, the various editions of *The Womanly Art* provide an exceptionally rich archive with which to explore La Leche League discourse and representation.[12]

In addition to providing basic information about breastfeeding, all the editions of *The Womanly Art of Breastfeeding* encourage the mother to eschew housekeeping and her former homemaking routines in order to make a place for the breastfeeding infant in her life, implying an American norm of a housewife whose primary responsibility is the house and children. The early editions assume a woman at home and a husband at work; this does change with later versions, which argue for this norm rather than presume it. The texts work to get the reader accustomed to the way in which breastfeeding a baby transforms the life of the mother and the whole family. In a sense, the purpose of these manuals is to shake up the mother's expectations that are based on bottle-feeding routines (which free the mother to tend to the house, for example) and to provide an alternative set of expectations about life with a breastfed baby.

It may seem odd that a simple change in infant feeding method would have such a profound impact on women's daily practices at home, but League argues, in the second edition of *The Womanly Art*, that "bottle feeding led gradually to a whole new way of bringing up babies. So many new decisions had to be made; which formula to use, how to prepare it, how much, whether you should hold the baby or not, and if so, how long—a mother could easily begin to regard her baby as a most complex digestive system instead of a dependent person with feelings of his own. Bogged down in scales and charts and schedules, mothers began to lose confidence in their own abilities, and often missed the easy, natural enjoyment of a new baby" (2nd edition, 5–6). The retreat into a discourse of naturalness represents a counterattack against the norms of "scales and charts and schedules." Bottle feeding thus appears to burden the mother with demands for scientific measurement, at the same time that it seems to (falsely) free her to do unneeded housework. Both upset the natural relation between mother and baby thought to develop in the first weeks after birth.

In the first edition, the discourse of naturalness is linked to religious views concerning "God's plan": for example, in a discussion of natural child spacing, the text reads "Probably there would not be the issue today of 'family planning' if parents would follow through with God's way of doing things and breastfeed their babies" (1st edition, 5). While this particular language is largely absent from subsequent editions, the emphasis on lactation amenorrhea as a form of natural birth control remains.[13] In both the first and second editions, the religious overtones are continued with a short discussion of "Eve," who "had no choice to confuse her" and who "had it easy. Her baby came; the milk came; she nursed her baby" (2nd edition, 5; see figure 5.1). The line drawings in the second edition are particularly interesting, given this emphasis on the natural, since they are so purposefully stylized and idealizing. Representing Eve is important not only because she is a biblical

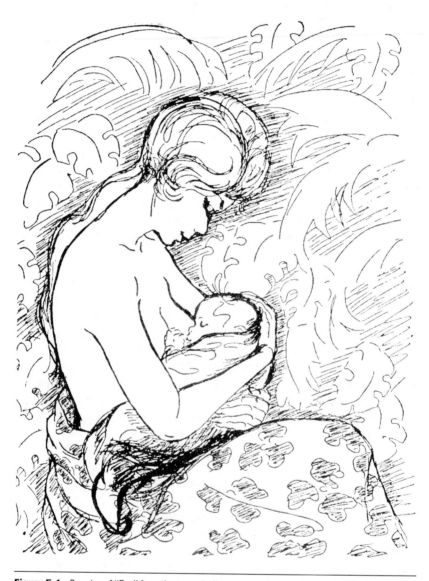

Figure 5.1. Drawing of "Eve" from the second edition of *The Womanly Art of Breastfeeding*. Drawing by Joy Sidor; courtesy of La Leche League International.

figure, and therefore another example of "God's plan," but also because she didn't need help. Successive editions of *The Womanly Art of Breastfeeding* continue to emphasize the naturalness of breastfeeding, but couple this with the understanding that in contemporary society such naturalness must be taught and learned.

La Leche League's position on the value of scientific knowledge for the breastfeeding mother fits into this paradigm: science should support and enhance nature. Any other kind of science interferes with a mother's attempts to establish and maintain biologically appropriate (that is, natural) infant feeding. Thus, in the view of *The Womanly Art's* authors, all information needs the mediating presence of the breastfeeding mother, the League member. For example, the title page of the first edition (1958) proclaims, "This booklet is written by mothers for mothers. It is not intended as a substitute for the writings of the various members of the medical profession who have done valuable research in this field. The mothers of La Leche League are familiar with many books, pamphlets and articles written by doctors and nurses. We quote these sources in many instances and recommend many of them to the mothers for reading." Mother-to-mother support means that any scientific information is distilled and processed through the experience of a mother.

The second edition emphasizes that medical information supports the advice offered in the text itself, but the crucial link in the exchange of information is another nursing mother. In the section "About La Leche League," the text reads,

> Breastfeeding is a part of a womanly heritage, and it would naturally follow, in fact it seems almost inevitable, that mothers should initiate the revival in breastfeeding. Not that professional [medical and scientific] work and interest are not important. Repeatedly, new evidence of the superiority of breastfeeding is brought to light through medical research. The facts are substantial and impressive, although scientific and lengthy. But someone is needed to emphasize and interpret the facts; someone with an understanding of just what a new mother needs to know. Someone must be handy to reassure and encourage her. Why not another nursing mother? She would have understanding, and enthusiasm and, let us hope, a simple touch. (2nd edition, 151)

Doctors are necessary when medical problems arise, "But most of the time, the problems aren't medical, and all that is needed is the practical advice and encouragement of another mother" (2nd edition, 154). In assuring the reader that the organization isn't impersonal or highly organized, the authors write, "You can think of La Leche League if you like as a woman with a baby in her arms and a smile on her face, proud of herself, and eager to share with you the wealth of all she has experienced and learned" (2nd edition, 154).

Dr. Herbert Ratner's foreword to the third edition, published in 1981, links nature with the mother's mediation of scientific knowledge:

> The founding mothers and their legion of followers opted, not for science and technology, but for nature as the repository of wisdom. They did not entrust the development of the mother-infant relationship to the vagaries of scientific advance, but rather, they placed their faith in nature and the promptings of the heart, a mode by which nature communicates many teachings.... How wise LLL mothers were. Their faith, which led them to accept nature's obvious norms, kept them ahead of the scientists. As one LLL Leader wittily stated, "A fanatic is a breastfeeding mother who for twenty years and against great odds has been doing and believing what physicians have only now discovered is a scientific truth." (x)

In this scenario, the mother's faithfulness to nature leads to her vindication by science; this is also a defense of traditionalism, the lifestyle that allows the mother to follow, in their words the "promptings of her heart."

The League's representation of the mother who must learn to be natural and who uses science as the ideological and evidentiary support for her natural mothering practices appears consistently throughout the six editions of *The Womanly Art of Breastfeeding*. One thing that changes, however, is the representation of the mother's relation to the physicians that care for her and her baby. An early advocate of unmedicated childbirth ("Childbirth is a woman's natural function" [1st edition, 8]), the League recommends that breastfeeding mothers be assertive in their dealings with medical professionals.[14] For example, in the first edition, the text reads, "By all means tell your doctor of your plans to breastfeed and enlist his support. (You may have to be a bit firm about it)" (1st edition, 7). The text also advises the new mother to "expect a few raised eyebrows from the hospital personnel" and to go home as soon as possible (1st edition, 8).[15] The doctor is understood to be supervising the mother's feeding practices, but the League encourages mothers to enlist doctors to help them, rather than to direct them. Sometimes this is stated explicitly, as in the following discussion of weaning: "It is not our purpose to set down or even suggest a feeding schedule for your baby. This can be worked out with the help of your doctor, relying heavily on your own special brand of knowledge about your baby. Here, as in all phases of caring for your baby, you can rely on your own motherly instincts. You've gotten to know him pretty well by now, and you do love him so much" (1st edition, 27). On the preceding page, however, the doctor seems to be in more control: "[A]t six months your baby is ready to start the solid foods. In certain, specific cases, a doctor might have a reason for starting solids earlier. As with most of these things, check with your doctor first and find out how he wants you to begin" (1st edition, 26). With their strong ties to medical advocates and advisors, League founders could not resist all facets of scientific motherhood, yet their palpable ambivalence about the doctor's role in making decisions about infant feeding means that the implication of the last quotation is unclear: do the authors mean that the mother should follow the doctor's advice, or simply know how he wants to proceed, regardless of her plans?

In the second edition, there are big changes in the section about "Talking to the Doctor": "Different doctors will react differently to this announcement [the mother's plan to breastfeed], so from here on you will more or less have to play it by ear. ... If the doctor feels very negative about it, try to find out why. In this case you definitely need to be in touch with some mother who knows the ins and outs of breastfeeding because of her own personal experience. Of course, it will be better all around if your doctor does approve of breastfeeding, and this is one of the things to keep in mind when you choose him. Remember, your right and privilege as a patient is the choice of a doctor sympathetic to your needs and desires" (2nd edition, 20). The mother is advised again to take charge of her hospital experience, but "nicely": "Take the attitude that you are being quite progressive. (A recent Harvard study indicates a trend back to breastfeeding headed up by the better-educated women)" (2nd edition, 53); "It won't hurt to mention casually to the nurse that you're glad your baby isn't getting any formula—since you'll be completely breastfeeding him, any formula given now could lead to his developing an allergy to cow's milk when that is reintroduced into his diet several months later. The nursing staff may not know this fact about allergies, and through busy forgetfulness, or simply out of the goodness of their hearts, they may think they are doing your baby a kindness by giving him a bottle or two during those first days before your milk comes in. Knowing this allergy fact may help them remember the doctor's orders [for no bottles]" (2nd edition, 53–54). This last suggestion is particularly interesting in that the mother is advised to educate the nurses in order to elicit their compliance with an order already given by the doctor.[16] In a later passage, the text suggests "If you do run into considerable opposition, don't antagonize the hospital personnel by throwing your weight around and telling them how to run their hospital. You can't win. Be firm about breastfeeding, but otherwise go slow on trying to buck established routines; smile and smile, and get out of there as fast as your doctor will let you" (2nd edition, 58). The League also advises writing a letter to the hospital administration and leaving a League pamphlet for nurses along with the customary gift of chocolates.

In the third edition, there are more changes in the section advising mothers to talk to their doctors about their interest in breastfeeding. In the section now entitled "You and the Medical Community," there are four consistent messages: be a good consumer of medical care, find out your available options, educate your doctor, and be organized in your advocacy of breastfeeding by writing petitions, letters, and memos. While each of these issues was presented in an earlier edition, only this third edition encourages the mother to change doctors if she is not satisfied with the responses she receives in an interview (3rd edition, 28). In advising nursing mothers to speak up about their desires and expectations, the League tells women to be direct in their opposition to advice to terminate or curtail breastfeeding. Women are also told to cry, if necessary, in order to get their point across: "Occasionally parents and the doctor find themselves at cross-purposes, perhaps over the treatment of a sick child, and the situation is enough to make the doctor throw up his hands and a mother dissolve into tears. Some emotion can be good, really—it relieves the tension and expresses more forcefully than words (which can be hard to find at such a time), how strongly a mother feels her baby's need for her" (3rd edition, 28). This is an example of how the book, in advising women to be experts about their own children, encourages women to be active in achieving their desires at the same time that it reinforces certain stereotypical gender behaviors.

The sections on the mother's relation to the doctor in the fourth, fifth, and sixth editions of *The Womanly Art of Breastfeeding* are all consistent with the positions put forth in the third edition, emphasizing the medical consumer's rights, finding the right doctor, and resisting inappropriate medical advice concerning breastfeeding. No longer is the mother working completely under the supervision of her doctor; instead, she is working with him and/or choosing her doctor based on her own beliefs.

Scientization enhances the mother's authority. The more recent editions of *The Womanly Art of Breastfeeding* include an increasing amount of medical information concerning problems that might be faced by a nursing mother and baby, as well as advice on how to manage those problems with or without a physician. For example, the first and second editions do not mention jaundice. The third edition, however, provides extensive descriptions of normal, pathological, and breast milk jaundices, along with a discussion of various treatment options and the information that it is never necessary to wean because of jaundice. Subsequent editions are updated, offering the mother information about what causes the different forms of jaundice and the appropriate treatments. Mothers are advised, in the sixth edition, that "Parents have input into treatment decisions, and you should let your doctor know how important it is to you to continue breastfeeding and not be separated from your baby.... While some physicians may still recommend a day or two without human milk to bring down the bilirubin level, many have come to recognize that this advice is not in the best interest of either a breastfeeding mother or her baby. Instead they may suggest the use of phototherapy along with continued breastfeeding, if the jaundice needs to be treated at all" (6th edition, 281). The advice in this section is obviously meant to give the mother information to consider the options before consulting the physician, as well as while the physician is making treatment decisions. In this way, the mother's experience of breastfeeding and monitoring her baby's health becomes scientized and her authority is extended and enhanced by the medical knowledge presented in the text.

The illustrations that accompany the text also contribute to the sense that the succeeding editions of the manual are more scientific, but that the science is filtered through the mother. We have already seen Eve nursing one of her children; other line drawings from the second edition continue this romanticized version of nursing. For example, one illustration from the second edition shows idyllic family members asleep together in one bed (figure 5.2). Illustrations like this one seem humorous and manage to make this edition seem cute and accessible—not like a medical text at all. Beginning with the

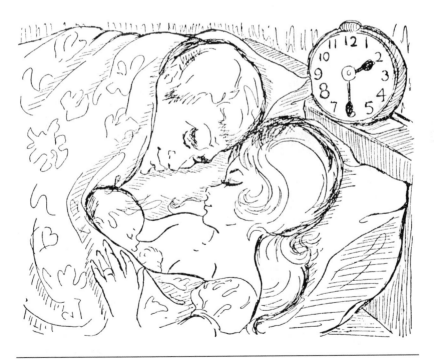

Figure 5.2. The family bed, from the second edition of *The Womanly Art of Breastfeeding*. Drawing by Joy Sidor; courtesy of La Leche League International.

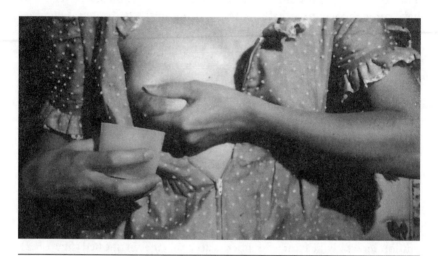

Figure 5.3. Manual expression of breast milk demonstrates some of the less romanticized aspects of breastfeeding. From *The Womanly Art of Breastfeeding,* 6th edition. Courtesy of La Leche League International.

third edition (1981), *The Womanly Art* includes photographs instead of line drawings. While continuing the romanticization of motherhood to a certain degree, these photographs more successfully represent the material exigencies of nursing (see figure 5.3, a woman expressing milk). Illustrations and photographs in the fourth, fifth, and sixth editions are all very similar; the photos demonstrate the scientific advance back to the natural and provide detailed advice about positioning the baby properly to address the problem of slow weight gain, for example, or how to position premature babies for "kangaroo care" (figure 5.4).[17]

Unlike the drawings, the photographs represent real mothers nursing their babies.[18] Because of this, they emphasize the mother-infant relationship as crucial to successful breastfeeding, and they also show mothers successfully breastfeeding in a variety of circumstances (pictures of babies with cleft lips and palates, for example, might be particularly helpful in convincing women that their babies with the same anomalies can nurse). There's a big difference from the first edition, which tells mothers to hold the baby in a comfortable position and that a pillow on the lap might help support the baby (1st edition, 14), to the sixth edition, which includes a section entitled "Breastfeeding in Slow Motion" that details the mother's position, the baby's position, the correct way to offer the breast to the baby, and the proper physical encouragement for the baby to latch on properly and suck effectively, all of

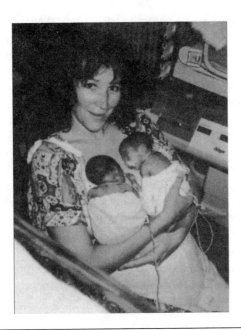

Figure 5.4. "Kangaroo care" is an amalgam of low- and high-tech care for premature babies, borrowed from contexts where advanced technological procedures and machines are not available. In kangaroo care, the mother's body is engaged to help warm and stabilize babies whose bodies will not do this without support. This kind of care demonstrates the scientific return to the natural exemplified in La Leche League discourses. From *The Womanly Art of Breastfeeding*, 6th edition. Photograph by Mühlmann, Austria; courtesy of La Leche League International.

which are accompanied by realistic drawings and photographs of the entire procedure (6th edition, 48–51). Through the illustrations and the extended discussions of positioning, avoiding plugged ducts and breast infections, and even how to handle what they call a "nursing strike," *The Womanly Art of Breastfeeding* provides the necessary technical information to initiate and sustain breastfeeding in contemporary Western society. Rather than an art, the breastfeeding practices presented in this text are really a craft, utilizing science and motherly know-how to pass on the practice from mother to mother.[19]

Because the League founders felt that successful nursing depends on "information and support" (Lowman 11), League practice mandates that mothers be offered the best information available in an encouraging manner so that they may make informed decisions about infant feeding. The *Leader's Handbook* states flat out that a "Leader's goal . . . is to *empower each mother*. She does this by giving the mother the facts she needs to make an informed choice and by supporting her as the expert on caring for her own baby" (Sachetti 12; emphasis added). The text emphasizes supporting the mother first, advising her about breastfeeding second. Thus, promoting positive relationships between women as they "share information rather than give advice" (Sachetti 23; paraphrase) structures League's approach to breastfeeding advocacy on the individual level.

This sort of woman-centered practice, in which the emphasis is on helping mothers make choices (often in the face of opposition from physicians; see Sachetti 27–28), has always seemed profoundly feminist to me. Julia DeJager Ward agrees, arguing that "La Leche League mothers are not some group apart from women with feminist concerns" (110), and "La Leche League's faith that women can change the direction of culture has extended beyond the help offered to individual mothers. League leaders work unceasingly to bring their concepts to the attention of the wider community" (100). League leaders are entrusted to help the mothers who come to them succeed in their own self-articulated goals. In addition, League has developed an informal critique of consumerism that, although it is often directed against women in the workforce, represents its philosophical bias of "people before things." Such a critique aligns the League with some forms of feminism and other radical groups.

Throughout the tumultuous years since its founding, La Leche League has also dealt with political conflicts concerning key issues in the women's movement. For example, in *Seven Voices, One Dream*, it is made clear that the legalization of abortion threatened the cohesion of the organization. The founding mothers are all Catholic. Some felt that League should take a public stand against abortion, in keeping with their focus on babies and mothering. Other founders argued that to take such a stand would unnecessarily alienate existing League leaders and future League members who believed in a woman's right to abortion. The latter position won the day with the Board of Directors, but not without intense, public friction: at the 1971 International Conference in Chicago, Mary White (a founding mother) "made a plea for La Leche League to take a stand in support of all mothers and their unborn babies. She received a standing ovation, though not everyone was pleased. The Board of Directors again met, and this time passed a motion stating that any LLL member who brought up the subject of abortion at an LLL function would summarily be dismissed from La Leche League" (Cahill 134). League has since developed a statement against mixing causes, and has generally refused involvement with other organizations so as not to compromise its ability to help all mothers, regardless of their beliefs and political activities, to breastfeed.

Nevertheless, League beliefs and practices end up sending a political message about women's place in contemporary society, although that message has changed over the decades and continues to develop. Because the practice of breastfeeding promoted by League is so all-consuming, the authors of *The Womanly Art of Breastfeeding* have a difficult time incorporating a positive assessment of working mothers within its purview. The third edition of the book includes a chapter called "Are You Thinking of Going Back to Work?" This chapter was not present in earlier editions, which simply assumed a stay-at-home mother. While the chapter begins with representations of women in a variety of experiences, it quickly devolves into a discussion of why women should stay home. Thus, while exhibiting some support for the idea that working women can breastfeed, the text moves immediately to problems attendant to the mother's absence from the house and her separation from the children. There is an extensive argument in favor of the rewards of at-home mothering. Much of the discourse involves rethinking staying at home as an intellectual challenge rather than a place of boredom and routine. The discussion involves two overriding assumptions: first, that a woman's income is secondary to her husband's, and second, that mothering is a career valuable in and of itself.[20] The chapter ends with the following statement: "We hope that these suggestions are helpful to you and that you will be able to stay home with your baby. But if you can't be an at-home nursing mother, we hope we can help you to breastfeed your baby as a working mother" (3rd edition, 71). The information about working and nursing comes in a completely separate chapter, entitled "Special Circumstances." The message is very clear: working mothers should be considered special and not the norm.

In subsequent editions, there is a complete chapter with information on breastfeeding and working, which is followed by a chapter on "making a choice" to stay at home. Both appear in a separate section of the book entitled "Going Back to Work." While the League remains committed to full-time mothering, it recognizes that many nursing mothers work outside the home and that they need reliable information about how to manage breastfeeding while being employed. Sections on pumping, manual expression of breast milk, and storage of breast milk have become more detailed in the recent editions. At the 2001 La Leche League convention, sessions on breastfeeding and working, and on corporate lactation programs, drew standing-room-only crowds, and many women in attendance expressed the view that helping working mothers breastfeed successfully was going to be crucial to La Leche League's success and growth in the coming years. In other words, accommodating itself to the working mother is now one of La Leche League's biggest challenges.

Part II: The Manly Art of Fathering

Concomitant to League's change in attitude about working women are changes in attitudes about gender roles in the home and what League now calls "the manly art of fathering." The first printing of the first edition contains a chapter, "The Father's Role," which, in a nutshell, is a peroration against women's rights and suggests that fathers are "most useful to their children" as authority figures, protectors, and moral influences (1st edition, 18–20). Much of this section is an extended quotation from University of Chicago psychoanalytic psychologist Bruno Bettelheim. In his view, the time a father spends with his children matters less than if he has "inner convictions" about his relationship to them and "answers all of his child's questions and handles emergencies well" (1st edition, 20). This edition exhibits distaste at the notion that a husband and father might perform a household chore, and suggests that if his wife asks him to do so it demeans her womanhood as well as his manhood.

Apparently, the founding mothers very quickly changed their minds about the wisdom of this presentation of "The Father's Role," because, according to Kaye Lowman in *The LLLove Story*, "This section as originally written... didn't seem quite to suit, though, and by the time of the second printing six months later, it had been re-written by a League mother, Dorothy Vining, on the basis of the ideas about fathers expounded by Dr. Ratner. Interestingly, search has so far failed to turn up any copies of that first printing with the Father's Role à la Bruno Bettelheim" (24n). I must have found the only existing "Bettelheim edition," through interlibrary loan, and Lowman's commentary cleared up the confusion I experienced after reading Julia Ward's discussion: "The earliest edition of the manual urged a rethinking of the traditional division of roles within family life. It argued against the prevailing ideology, which ruled that certain actions such as child care or household chores were 'woman's work' and that any man who valued his masculinity should avoid them at all costs. It was far more important, from a League viewpoint, to consider who a father *is* within the family than what he *does* when at home" (103–4; emphasis in original). Clearly, Ward read a different printing of the 1958 edition than I did.

The second edition includes a similar chapter on "The Father's Role" that plays up the father as protector of the mother; he shields her from unwanted advice that would inhibit her breastfeeding. A short discussion of the father's protective role appeared in the first edition as well. While in the Bettelheim edition the blurring of the family's sex roles was seen as dangerous, the second edition supports "manly men" and "womanly women" without worrying so much that blurring these roles will be a problem: "We are all in favor of manly men. And La Leche League was formed for no other purpose than to help women be more womanly. As you might guess, we're going to urge breastfeeding in order to help keep these father and mother images clear! ... As long as women continue to bear babies and to nurse, there is not much danger that the roles of mothers and fathers will be badly confused" (2nd edition, 115). The emphasis here is on the biological differences that allow women to breastfeed. But biological differences (as in men's strength) also suggest a natural division of labor: women cook and clean while men do carpentry and paint the house. However, "The fact that certain duties are ordinarily performed by father or mother does not mean under some circumstances they cannot be performed by the other. . . . If a wife has been up much of the night, a husband grows in stature as a man when he has the thoughtfulness and foresightedness to let her nap with the baby while he takes the older children out for a walk"; and "The authoritative, masculine man knows his dignity and stature are not in jeopardy when he performs a kitchen chore" (2nd edition, 116).

It is clear that, at least in terms of the Bettelheim edition as a reference point, there has been a shift from a role-centered view of gender differences to an identity-centered view, commensurate with the shift in psychological literature of the time.[21] Thus, if the initial position is that the sexual division of labor is essential to normal parenting, the second position (and the more enduring League view) is that transgressions of sex role stereotyping aren't much of a problem if one's essential gender identity remains intact. Indeed, certain kinds of transgressions—on the part of men—are valued because they demonstrate his "manly" concern for his family.

The third edition includes a chapter entitled "The Manly Art of Fathering," which emphasizes biological sexual differences in reproductive behaviors. This chapter seems intent on countering the seeming advance of the father wanting to be involved with the feeding of the baby. The authors offer instead a scenario of complementary parental attributes and responsibilities: "Beginning with the conception of their child, the roles of father and mother complement each other. It has never ceased to impress and reassure us to see how the unique abilities of one parent balance out and complete those of the other. . . . Mothers and fathers both nurture their children, but they do not provide the same kind of nurturing" (3rd edition, 145). Fathers can't count on the mothering hormones (prolactin for example) that help mothers develop nurturing behaviors, but they do have special qualities to soothe a fussy baby: "daddy lifts the little one out of her arms, hoists him onto his shoulder, and promptly puts the baby to sleep! It is a trade secret known only to fathers, whether it is the broad shoulders, the large strong hands, or the deep baritone voice that does the trick" (3rd edition, 150). Indeed, mothers feed and cuddle while dads bounce and tickle.

This edition, then, while stressing the father's active role with the children, and promoting the husband and wife as a team, continues to assume a sexual division of labor and an interpretation of biological sex differences that give sense to that division of labor. However, men are certainly expected to help out without feeling that their manliness is endangered (or enhanced): "Most men today are willing to help with work around the house. If they have any misgivings about the subject, it's usually because they don't know what's expected of them" (3rd edition, 153). This more enlightened attitude about the father's experience of parenting a breastfed baby continues throughout the subsequent editions of the manual, which include testimonials from fathers waxing eloquent about their relationship to breastfed offspring.

It is interesting to consider why, of all the activities an engaged father can become involved in, feeding the infant takes on such significance. At my Bradley childbirth education class in Chicago, a mother from a previous class told us that she chose to bottle feed so that the father could participate in feeding. At many of the League meetings I attended where a new mother or expectant mother introduced herself, the issue of the father's wanting to help feed the baby was brought up. Even if the mother was breastfeeding, it was often thought to be important to provide an opportunity for the father to feed the baby from a bottle. Certainly, feeding a baby is much more pleasurable than changing a diaper, although the diapers of exclusively breastfed babies are mild and generally inoffensive. I think that feeding is privileged over other parent-baby interactions as a way to get dad involved because of the hype about bonding that has been linked to feeding. In *The Complete Idiot's Guide to Bringing Up Baby,* one stated advantage of bottle feeding is that "[b]oth parents can participate equally in feeding and take advantage of this opportunity to bond with their child" (Larson and Osborn 30); *What to Expect When You're Expecting* makes a similar claim ("Bottle-feeding allows the father to share the feeding responsibilities and its bonding benefits more easily" [Eisenberg et al. 253]).

Men's responsibility for their children has both real and symbolic value. Nancy Scheper-Hughes notes that in poor communities in Brazil, fathers indicate their acknowledgment of paternity by providing the first few weeks of formula for their babies (323–25). Other anthropologists do not see this practice negatively, given that this kind of practice shifts the burden of infant nutrition from an overtaxed female body to the father's cash resources (Maher, "Maternal Depletion"; Martha Ward 79–81). Breastfeeding advocates worry about the material effects of such a symbolic system: mothers whose babies die of malnutrition or gastrointestinal diseases, or who lose their milk because they don't nurse their infants enough to stimulate adequate production. In the United States, the majority of infants are unlikely to die because they are fed formula, yet the idea that infant feeding decisions are made in order to enhance equal parenting is problematic from a biologically informed perspective. After all, most feminists don't promote extra-uterine gestation as a way to make becoming a parent a more egalitarian process. It is the fact that infant feeding is no longer perceived as an inextricable part of biological reproduction that causes it to become so successfully accommodated to norms of social equality in many people's minds.

Of course, League materials espouse the bonding hypothesis about breastfeeding—that as a mode of infant feeding it is better at promoting bonding than formula feeding, which makes it easy to leave the infant alone with a propped bottle. (All infant care guide books warn against bottle propping, and advise mothers and fathers to bottle feed infants with the kind of close attention that breastfeeding necessitates. The practice is clearly widespread, since all the experts feel a need to address its negative effects.) It is clear, however, that while La Leche League promotes active and engaged fathering, it accepts as necessary the father's absence from the home in order to make possible the continuous presence of the mother, whose bonded relationship with the child is far more significant than the father's. The League member magazine, *New Beginnings,* is often a site for member testimonials about involved fathers who support breastfeeding through active caring, but the emphasis on mother–infant bonding generally assumes that fathers work to support mothers at home (the column "Staying Home Instead" often discusses financial issues and conflicts resulting from one-income families). League accepts, in other words, a biologically-based understanding of the mother's primary significance to the infant, and accepts the sexual division of labor that such an understanding mandates in the current economic structure of American society. In contrast, feminists start from the presumption that the sexual division of labor is wrong and argue that it is bolstered by ideological rhetoric about the biological significance of the mother to the baby. Shared parenting, as a way to end the sexual division of labor, is valued over biological views of maternal nurturance.

Yet many feminist scholars also acknowledge that the grand experiment of shared parenting to end the oppression of mothers has largely failed. Women still do more child care than men, do far more housework than fathers, and often find themselves marginalized in the workforce (or from the workforce) after they have become mothers. While mothers of young children are clearly in market work to stay (in 1998, 55.2 percent of women with kids under age one were employed [Cohn]), those women are not getting much relief from their traditional duties as mothers and wives. Breastfeeding does confer substantial burdens on women: it takes time, it can be physically challenging, and it binds the mother to the baby in a demanding physiological relationship. It can also be tremendously rewarding, but, as Sarah Blaffer Hrdy argues, all women make decisions as mothers that balance perceived rewards with actual costs (288–317).

La Leche League's reliance on maternal domesticity can be understood as pragmatic—to feed a baby in what she perceives to be a biologically appropriate manner, a mother needs to be available to her child—and the ideological bias, the promotion of *good* mothering through intensive maternal–infant contact through toddlerhood, follows from that pragmatism. Their overall approach throughout the editions of *The Womanly Art* suggests such a reading: they counsel mothers to be reasonable in the face of opposition, to stand firm in their beliefs but not upset others, and to be discreet about their own practices in public. In fact, the encouragement offered to women to stay home if they possibly can is probably as strenuously ideological as *The Womanly Art* gets, but as a strategy to support breastfeeding it makes sense, given the structure of work and family in the United States. The problems that feminists have with La Leche League's domesticity concern how domesticity has continued to cause problems for feminism. The ideological problem of domesticity continues to haunt feminism itself, and not just La Leche League.

In the next section of the chapter, I explore La Leche League's representation of maternal domesticity, as well as a recent feminist consideration of how domesticity structures gendered experiences for most working women. Joan Williams's *Unbending Gender* provides important insights into the ideological problem of domesticity, but I argue that her discussion would be improved by a consideration of breastfeeding. In examining the problem of domesticity within LLL breastfeeding advocacy and feminist theory, I try to show that feminist criticism of La Leche League is somewhat misplaced and thus misses what is interesting about the organization's representation of motherhood as embodied experience.

The Ideological Problem of Domesticity

La Leche League's approach to domesticity is ambiguous: on the one hand, *The Womanly Art* cautions mothers to "always put people before things" and suggests that "Meeting the needs of family members should always come before immaculate housekeeping or caring for material possessions," but on the other hand, the chapter entitled "Meeting Family Needs" spends five pages discussing methods of more efficient housekeeping (6th edition, 199). Mothers are encouraged to put baby first, but the text also assumes that mothers at home are responsible for domestic chores like cooking, cleaning, and laundry. This echoes the traditional division of labor common in the United States since at least the nineteenth century: mothers at home in charge of the domestic space and the children within it; men elsewhere in the public sphere making money. In actual practice, the ostensible reason for mothers being at home—care of children—often recedes in significance to the material necessity of taking care of the domestic realm itself, but even La Leche League's earliest publications challenged the rigorous household standards of the 1950s middle classes, which League founders associated with the advent of bottle feeding.

Of course, if mothers are at home with infants and small children, some-one else has to be in the workforce to make the money to allow them to be home—at least in the two-parent, heterosexual family that League imag-ines. That someone else is referred to by Joan Williams as the "ideal worker," who, in order to command top dollar in market work, must be freed from the family work performed in the home (24). As Williams shows in her excellent study *Unbending Gender: Why Family and Work Conflict and What to Do About It*, early feminist calls to liberate women from the isolation of domestic life assumed that full participation in market work was es-sential for women's emancipation. Domestic labor, including child care, was thought to be fully commodifiable—that is, cleaning, cooking, laun-dry, and child care were to be outsourced to the market in order to allow women equal access to waged employment (40–45). Yet "the drawbacks of the full-commodification model became evident as early as the 1970s," as women began to realize that "entering the workforce without changing the conditions of work resulted in longer working hours for women" (456). Significantly, "feminists' dream that day care facilities would be as common as public libraries [and as free] never came true" (49).

Thus, while European women largely enjoy generous and lengthy paid maternity leaves, government subsidies for child care, and even cash bene-fits on the birth of children, U.S. women who become mothers experience marginalization in the workforce and sharply stratified opportunities for nonmaternal child care. Only the most well-off women can afford the best care, either in well-staffed centers or at home with nannies; most mothers send their children to relatives or unlicensed caregivers in family homes. Of course, some of this care is quite good due to the commitment of the caregivers, but child care in the United States is among the lowest-paid pro-fessions and mothers often get what they pay for. Williams argues that "the time has come to abandon the fiction that both mothers and fathers can perform as ideal workers in a system designed for men supported by a flow of family work from women" and concludes that "it is time to acknowledge the *norm of parental care*" (51–52; emphasis in original).

Joan Williams sees many women's choice to stay home with their children as less a free decision than a result of the structure of work in contempo-rary U.S. society. While acknowledging many women's preference for the domestic realm, she argues that such preference is produced in an envi-ronment in which both women and men are penalized if they cannot live up to the ideal worker norm. The choice to stay home is not made freely, since "the decision to work part time generally means restricted prospects for advancement and lower pay, despite comparable qualifications" (72). Many mothers would opt to "keep their hand in" through part-time work while their children were small—indeed, many women do, which is why women are segregated to professions where overtime work is low and part-time work often an established possibility (82). Yet while most women with small children continue in market work, they are either marginalized from well-paying jobs or forced to work longer hours than they would like—or they choose to leave the market in favor of family work that will allow them to help husbands be ideal workers. Women and children are also severely disadvantaged by mothers' inability to work to their capabilities, Williams argues, because in the event of divorce women's family work goes unrecognized and they do not retain a high enough share of the erstwhile family wage of the male provider through alimony or child support.

Williams argues that domesticity operates as a force field pulling women back into traditional gender arrangements because of the lack of change in the labor market and structure of work. Many of the women quoted in Williams's book express relief at the end of family tensions caused by trying to balance family life with the needs of two working parents. La Leche League provides a practical paradigm for those families that, in Williams's words, express "commodification anxiety over the intrusion of the market into family life" (150); that is, for League, breastfeeding is a mode of maternal care that eschews the market not only in terms of the infant's food, but also in terms of the presence of the mother in the home. (Of course, League presumes a father fully engaged with the market and bringing its benefits home in the form of a family wage.) And, as Williams also argues, a belief in innate gender differences (such as League espouses) justifies women's choice to stay home as a result of their "priorities as women" (191–92).

To Williams's analysis of domesticity as a force field that enforces traditional gender arrangements I want to add a consideration of the material exigencies of breastfeeding, since her notion of women's orientation toward domesticity is based on the idea that gender is a social construct without biological significance. For example, Williams uses Sweden as an example of how women continue to refuse the full-commodification model of child care even when it's made available as high quality care and subsidized by the government. She notes that "As of 1986, 43 percent of working women were employed part time. Women continued to do a disproportionate share of family work and took fifty-two days of leave for every day taken by a man" (51); to Williams these data clearly represent women's lack of social equality. Yet according to international breastfeeding advocate Ted Greiner, Sweden has extremely generous maternity leave policies, and has implemented social policies to promote women's independence from men so that their ability to take maternity leave is not dependent on their ties to a male provider. In 1997, 98 percent of Swedish mothers breastfed their infants, and three-quarters of Swedish babies were breastfed for six months, most of them at home (Greiner, "Return"). Swedish women do not rely on breast pumping at work to continue breastfeeding while working, which is the American norm for employed breastfeeding mothers, because they take paid maternity leaves. Williams's figures on Swedish women's work experience and repudiation of the commodification model of child care need to take this into account.

The Swedish example raises a number of questions in relation to issues of domesticity and shared parenting: To what extent do extended maternity leave and prolonged breastfeeding lead to women permanently taking on increased domestic responsibility and seeking part-time work to accommodate that responsibility? Patterns of domestic labor set up during a child's infancy often persist even after the child begins schooling, especially when they are supported by other social structures. Do Swedish women work part-time in large numbers because they become accustomed to being the primary parent while they are on maternity leave? If we support women's right to breastfeed, the goal of establishing a norm of parental care cannot, in an infant's early months and/or years, involve the expectation of equal parental care, unless provisions would be available to support equal leaves for both parents (for those families with two parents).[22] Greiner argues that to support breastfeeding, pumping at work should not be a goal or the norm, and that what is necessary is "a policy environment and a legal environment [that] make it possible for women to be at home for six months" (Greiner, "Return").[23] He believes that putting too much emphasis on pumping, and not enough on the experience of breastfeeding itself, makes breastfeeding as a practice vulnerable to increasingly sophisticated attempts to technologically duplicate human milk. His statements also imply that given the option to work and pump or to be home with a baby, most breastfeeding mothers would choose to stay home for a six-month maternity leave (given the evidence of the Swedish example).

The latest edition of *The Womanly Art of Breastfeeding* encourages mothers who will go back to work after the birth of a baby to "bargain for as long a maternity leave as you can possibly manage," the implication being that such a leave will be unpaid (what you can manage) and specific to each employment situation (156). The U.S. context (lack of social and governmental support) is assumed. While the section on breast pumps is in another chapter, much of the chapter "Breastfeeding and Working" is taken up with methods of collecting and storing milk and feeding it to the baby; thus the work environment is understood to exclude nursing babies. (Examples of working *with* a baby appear in the next chapter, "Making a Choice," which concerns choosing to stay home with the baby.) Expressing milk at work to feed a baby cared for by others assumes, in Joan Williams's terms, a masculine norm of the worker and an individualistic response to the lack of universal maternity leave policy in the United States.

In *At the Breast*, feminist sociologist Linda Blum argues that the focus on providing breast milk through pumping leads to a "kind of disembodiment . . . in which the maternal body and embodied experience are devalued and all but erased" (59). Blum criticizes the American emphasis on breast pumping as the solution to maternal employment, and demonstrates how maternal disembodiment can occur even in contexts promoting breastfeeding. Along the lines of her analysis, LLL's emphasis on choosing home over work is not just a way to put people before things, but is a resistance to what Blum terms the "Supermom" disavowal of biological maternity and the physiological relation of mother and infant through breastfeeding. Thus, La Leche League promotes stay-at-home mothering to succeed at breastfeeding, but imagines working mothers to have to resort to pumping in order to maintain their milk supplies and provide milk for their babies during their absences. To a large extent, this is a pragmatic approach to the exigencies of the U.S. labor market, although most women in the workforce lack access to jobs that would allow pumping or have the private space to do it. But it's clear that League values the domestic model of breastfeeding over the pumping model; such a valuation is not only based on a preference for domesticity but a belief in a specific form of physiological proximity between mother and child.

What domesticity means is influenced by the mother's body and how it operates in domestic space. As Williams notes, "in the important early weeks, when family patterns change to adjust to the new baby, the baby's demands will be tied to the mother alone rather than to the father as well" under current pregnancy disability rules that link maternity leave with the mother's recovery from childbirth (225). She goes on to argue that "the best design for [workplace leave] policies would offer, from the beginning of a child's life, leaves for both recovery from childbirth (available to postpartum women) and for caregiving (available to all parents), with the provision that such leaves could be taken either simultaneously or sequentially" (225–26). But this proposition assumes that childbirth is the *only* compelling biological experience linking the mother to the baby—caregiving can be offered either by mother or father. Breastfeeding as a norm of infant feeding disrupts this easy distinction between the biological experience of childbirth and the social organization of infant care. This is an issue I explore further in the final chapter; here I just want to point out that while breastfeeding does not encompass other sorts of caregiving, when practiced as a continuous close physiological relation between mother and infant, it usually means that the mother is the primary caregiver for the infant. In U.S. society, in two-parent families, both parents rarely stay home with an infant; either one parent stays at home or the child receives nonparental care. Gender-neutral parental leave policies like the Family Medical Leave Act deny the specificity of maternal embodiment by treating caregiving by either parent as equally desirable, given that most families cannot afford to have both parents absent from work without pay (indeed, most families can't afford to have one parent absent from work without pay).

If infant feeding is understood as domestic labor, then some forms of domestic labor cannot be shared equally between men and women without practices which disembody mothers by denying breastfeeding as a particular, and important, form of maternal embodiment. Breastfeeding is simply a difficult practice to continue in the context of women's paid work as it is structured in the United States. Although bottle feeding became the norm in American society before mothers returned wholesale to the labor market, integrating waged employment with maternal nursing continues to be a major challenge to increasing the duration of breastfeeding, a stated U.S. public health goal (employed women are just as likely to initiate breastfeeding as other women, but are more likely to wean early [Riordan and Auerbach 578]; for public health goals, see Department of Health and Human Services, *HHS Blueprint for Action on Breastfeeding*). As Nancy Scheper-Hughes points out in her study of impoverished Brazilian women (who have given up breastfeeding almost completely), "they must often work as temporary wage laborers and rear their infants as best they can and with whatever is at hand. In the desperate situation in which many Alto women find themselves, bottle-feeding is really the only possible 'choice' " (323).[24] As described above, Joan Williams compellingly demonstrates that mothers' choice to leave market work for family work is overdetermined by the U.S. economic structure; infant feeding choice is similarly constrained by economic forces.[25]

Conclusion

Challenging domesticity from within, which is Joan Williams's strategy of "domesticity in drag," may "use domesticity's momentum to bend it into new configurations . . . [such as] using domesticity's norm of parental care to deconstruct the ideal-worker norm in market work" (260), but any theory which purports to make new feminist overtures to stay-at-home mothers must confront the mother's sex as well as her gender. Including breastfeeding in the paradigm of domesticity means rethinking the meanings of the reproductive female body in relation to the social roles that women play—specifically, not assuming that pregnancy is the only significant way in which female bodies are engaged in biological reproduction. In the years since its founding, La Leche League has attempted to bring infant feeding back to a biological paradigm of pregnancy, childbirth, and lactation, yet in sociological terms it has been most successful in creating breastfeeding as a lifestyle choice available to well-resourced women. League has challenged domesticity from within, by promoting mothering, rather than housewifery, as the primary activity of women at home, but such a strategy also plays into the intensifying expectations of all mothers (see Hays, Büskens). League has also challenged some of the traditional presumptions about men's domestic labor, yet by maintaining rigid ideas about essential differences between men and women the organization continues to support the sexual division of labor, a position that makes public politics concerning the right to breastfeed at work difficult. Finally, LLL has empowered mothers with explicitly medical information about breastfeeding to use in augmenting their authority in relation to physicians, but in so doing has also contributed to the contradictions of scientific motherhood.

Thus, feminist scholars continue to decry La Leche League's lack of involvement in public politics (for example, Bobel; Blum, *At the Breast;* and Blum and Vandewater), and they also criticize the implicit class bias of League's breastfeeding advocacy. In a class- and race-stratified health care system, scientific motherhood is less disempowering for white middle-class women, whose loss of authority as mothers can be partially made up for by other status categories, than for those women who lack other discourses of social power to rely on. Yet feminism has neglected breastfeeding as women's right, or only paid attention to its demise in situations like that described by Nancy Scheper-Hughes, where the decline in breastfeeding, in the context of other complex social and economic developments, has led to astronomical rates of infant mortality. But the real problem *both for feminism and for La Leche League* is the lack of change in the relationship of market work to family work, as Joan Williams has so aptly pointed out. I am not blaming organized feminism or La Leche League for this failure, but marking the intransigence of U.S. social and economic structures concerning women's place; organized labor has not made much headway on these issues either. Within the context of this failure, La Leche League continues to promote full-time mothering to accomplish biological breastfeeding, just as feminist groups have largely supported full-time market work for women who are then expected to outsource child care and housekeeping: both positions, it seems to me, need adjustment. LLL is not ignorant of the feminist critique; the organization sees its promotion of full-time mothering as the best option for women and children in the current context.[26]

Julia DeJager Ward points out that "there exists in the League's ideology a tendency to overestimate women's ability to overcome biases against the 'mommy track'" and to "underestimate the actual economic desperation of many employed mothers" (158), pointing toward economic structures as the culprits in mothers' dilemmas concerning market work. Such over- and underestimation are, however, part of the League strategy of encouragement. Its founders believed that successful breastfeeding was in large part a confidence trick; they perceived many of the problems new mothers encountered to be caused by discouragement, coming from both friends and professionals. The cheery tone of all League publications is another aspect of this strategy, and it grates on feminist sensibilities because the cloying optimism about the wonders of mothering through breastfeeding seems to fly in the face of many women's realities: poverty, single motherhood, sex and race discrimination. But surely we can interpret this optimism about women's capabilities as a rhetorical strategy; in the least, it reflects the overachievement of the founders' own experiences, based as they are in solid middle-class resources and educational attainments. I wonder what La Leche League's position on working mothers would be if our economic structure had undergone significant feminist changes since 1956, if mothers' choices were not so constrained by the ideal worker norm, and if the ideal worker norm was not dependent on the norm of the male body. It's my hope that LLL would be far more in the vanguard of social change, because mothers would have more power generally and would not need to rely on traditional discourses of gendered domesticity in order to retain social status and authority, but ultimately, it's impossible to tell.

The question of whether La Leche League supports maternity leave legislation in an enthusiastic enough manner, or whether it has argued (or will argue) against workfare on the grounds that it keeps new mothers away from their infants, is an interesting one. The League's web site suggests that some members and leaders see a need for greater attention to the U.S. situation and specific U.S. governmental policies. There is a new movement afoot to organize a LLLUSA, which would focus on the United States, at least partially to pay more attention to WIC and developing legal issues.[27] Most feminists see League's apparent lack of sustained attention to political contexts and the material circumstances of most women's lives as a reflection of privileged bias. Yet La Leche League is, in a real sense, a very young organization: as of fall 2002, the Founding Mothers are all still alive, and some are very much involved in the organization still. When League began, fewer than one-quarter of American mothers breastfed (La Leche League, "A Brief History"); most of its attention has been on helping women breastfeed, and trying to keep up with an organizational structure that is always already outdated because of League's constantly expanding membership.[28] LLL's studied emphasis on breastfeeding as a maternal practice has helped it to develop a specific expertise that an organization with a broader agenda might have lost.[29] La Leche League is the world's foremost authority on breastfeeding, and it is, for the most part, a voluntary organization of mothers.

Yet until La Leche League addresses how its optimistic focus on individual women excludes the experiences of many or most poor women, women of color, and working women in the United States, it will not succeed in promoting a cultural climate in which all women can really choose to breast-feed. Similarly, until feminist scholars address breastfeeding as a biosocial practice, one that is both cultural and embodied, they will not adequately address the needs or experiences of mothers, employed or not. Feminist scholarship hasn't yet provided the theoretical terms with which to address breastfeeding as a reproductive practice of the female body, with the result that it is consistently subsumed within the notion of domestic labor or family work. As a result, feminist scholarship has neglected to appreciate how its lack of attention to breastfeeding has impoverished its overall approaches to motherhood, to embodied sexual difference, and to racial disparities in maternal/child health. It is to these topics that I now turn.

CHAPTER 6

Breastfeeding, Feminism, Activism

I ran into one of my son's former day care teachers the other day, and got a chance to meet her two-and-a-half-month old son. He's a big, happy baby, obviously well fed and healthy. In the course of our short conversation, and because she knows I'm interested in childbirth and breastfeeding (before her baby's birth I plied her with books about birthing and nursing), she told me some things about her birth and subsequent nursing experiences.

A week before her due date her doctors told her that they would have to induce labor because they were convinced the fetus was measuring 10 pounds 14 ounces. After 16 hours of pitocin-induced labor, she hadn't dilated at all, so they performed a cesarean section. The baby was a bit over nine pounds. A difficult (and probably unnecessarily interventionist) start to life with baby, but she had no trouble breastfeeding. The baby did, however, develop late-onset jaundice. Her pediatrician's office suggested supplementing with formula, since there was "probably a hormone in her milk that the baby's immature liver couldn't metabolize."[1] More recently the nurses at the pediatrician's office have suggested supplementing with formula because the baby has stopped having a bowel movement every day.[2] The mother told me that she and her husband are thinking of changing their pediatrician, since all they hear from the office is "supplement with formula."

It's the kind of story that breastfeeding advocates hear often, and, depending on the outcome (whether the mother resists such advice or not), agonize over. The contemporary American medical management of childbirth and infant feeding never cease to amaze me, especially because so many women allow themselves to be guided by scientifically erroneous beliefs that are nevertheless promoted by medical personnel.[3] Most of these beliefs teach women to distrust their own experience and their interpretation of their bodies. Women are not merely pawns in this process either; many seek out physicians who will actively manage labor and delivery with pain relief medications, labor stimulating hormones, and other technological interventions. It is not the specific medical practices that bother me, but the overall context of medical intervention that is accepted as the proper way to experience childbirth and manage infant feeding. Robbie Davis-Floyd interprets the current medicalized birth scenario as a cultural ritual whose purpose it is to accommodate birthing (a function of physical embodiment) to the core technological values of American society. A corollary purpose is to make it seem as if babies are the products of doctors and hospitals rather than women's bodies; in Davis-Floyd's analysis, this purpose validates the patriarchal nature of the core technological values.

While the medical management of childbirth has received a lot of attention from feminist scholars, until very recently the medical management of infant feeding has received relatively little (aside from early works discussed by Lauri Umansky in *Motherhood Reconceived*). As Pam Carter remarks, "no feminist practice has evolved around infant feeding," as opposed to feminist attention to childbirth (19). Even though Rima Apple demonstrated the process through which infant feeding came to be supervised by experts in the context of the development of scientific mothering in the twentieth century, most feminist scholars interested in reproductive issues do not see the decline of breastfeeding to be as important as (for example) the rising rate of cesarean section or (in another example) the social implications of the new reproductive technologies. The fact that infant feeding is supervised by physicians as a routine aspect of the medical care of infants (known colloquially and in terms of insurance coverage as well-baby care) is, in fact, a relatively recent historical phenomenon (Apple, *Mothers and Medicine;* Golden), as recent as the shift of childbirth from home to hospital and the subsequent increase in technological management of birth in the West.

Why hasn't infant feeding drawn more attention from feminist scholars? In years of research on this book, I have wondered about this question. In the introduction to the book I discussed historical approaches to breastfeeding and breastfeeding advocacy; clearly women's historians have been interested in these issues. But until quite recently, other feminist scholars have only infrequently approached what is often called "the breast–bottle controversy." Penny Van Esterik, an anthropologist and breastfeeding advocate I discuss later in this chapter, writes, "lactation seems to have moved out of the consciousness of western women. It is not a central concern of women's health clinics or reproductive rights groups, nor is it something likely to be brought up in meetings on women's pay equity. It is surprisingly absent from contemporary feminist thought—much as if women no longer had breasts, or considered them merely as optional equipment" (*Beyond* 67). Linda Blum, a sociologist whose work I also discuss in this chapter, concurs, writing that "Breastfeeding . . . has attracted little attention, perhaps because it seems a more optional aspect of motherhood" (7). A catalog from any hip cultural studies publishing house will always offer a feminist take or two (or three) about reproductive technologies (including medicalized childbirth, infertility treatments, and routine technological interventions practiced during gestation and labor/delivery), but few (if any) texts about breastfeeding are available. It is clear that the pregnant body takes pride of place as the subject of feminist inquiry into reproduction.

A similar focus on pregnancy occurs in feminist discussions of embodiment and its relation to sexual difference, maternity legislation, and the more generalized "equality versus difference" debates. For example, in Zillah Eisenstein's fascinating *The Female Body and the Law,* which argues for perceiving women as equal through (and not in spite of) embodied differences, it is the pregnant female body that stands for the generic sexual difference that matters:

> [M]y focus reintroduces the pregnant body in order to decenter the privileged position of the male body. This approach contrasts markedly with the dominant discourses, which use pregnancy to differentiate women and subordinate them to men.
>
> I do not mean to imply, of course, that equality requires that everyone is, or should be, pregnant. . . . The ultimate significance, then, of the pregnant body for developing a theory of sex equality is that it *reminds* us of at least a *potential* difference between females and males that makes sameness, as the standard for equality, inadequate. (1–2; emphasis in original)

In her argument, Eisenstein uses pregnancy as an example of the continuing state of motherhood, as a signal of the duration of caring and relationship; as such, she argues that pregnancy cannot be considered a temporary disability, as it is in the law:

> [P]regnancy marks the beginning of a state that lasts as long as motherhood does. Pregnancy leave recognizes only the fact that women bear children. The model of pregnancy as generic temporary disability does not meet the complex needs of women in an engendered society. Pregnant women are usually not just pregnant; they most often are also or will become mothers. (100)

Yet if she were to consider lactation as an embodied maternal practice, Eisenstein's argument would be even more powerful.[4] After all, pregnancy, while inaugurating motherhood for most women, is not really like the rest of motherhood, given that during pregnancy the offspring is contained within the mother's body as a fetus. Breastfeeding models maternity (in the sense that Eisenstein highlights) in that it establishes a specific kind of relation between the mother and the infant through the mother's body, thus demonstrating a radical embodiment in which two individuals share a physiological relation. It is true that pregnancy is becoming, in medical and popular opinion, more like lactation (in that the fetus is increasingly perceived to be an individual separate from the mother), but this new social phenomenon only suggests that the specific maternal embodiment of lactation should be getting more attention.

In the example of my son's former caregiver, the mother might spend more time negotiating with her doctor(s) over infant feeding issues than she ever did negotiating with her OB/GYN or birth attendant about birthing issues or prenatal care. Indeed, if mothers breastfeed for the length of time recommended by the American Academy of Pediatrics (one year or longer), their infant feeding experiences would last longer than their prenatal care, labor and delivery, and routine postpartum obstetrical care combined (except in cases of treatment for infertility). Most women who breastfeed in American society experience numerous medical interventions, as well as the imposition of medical views about the female body and about a woman's ability to manage her body and that of her child. Certainly a maternal practice of such duration deserves the kind of attention paid to methods of getting pregnant, technological methods of monitoring pregnancy, and medical practices for labor and delivery. Most of the academic women I know have breastfed their children, and this is precisely the cohort producing feminist theories about the body and critiques of the medical management of childbirth.

For most American women, "breast or bottle?" defines a question about feeding in the social world, rather than a reproductive decision. Infant feeding is perceived as a nutritional issue for the child, as well as an issue within the domestic division of labor. And for most women in the United States, breastfeeding lasts for a brief period, far shorter than the time spent gestating. In addition, it is difficult to locate the proper subject of lactation—is it the mother or the infant/child? Medical discussions of breastfeeding tend to focus on the health benefits of breastfeeding for the infant and child; only recently has there been concerted and public attention paid to the effect of breastfeeding on the mother's health (see Blum, *At the Breast*, 50–52 and passim, for a discussion of this issue). At one medical conference on breastfeeding that I attended, an OB/GYN told a pediatrician that "the breasts are your responsibility."[5] Yet insofar as breastfeeding is a condition or function of the maternal body that provides direct nutrition to offspring, there is no one subject—lactation describes a relation.

There are a few reasons why feminist scholars have stayed away from breastfeeding as a research topic. They may be confounded by the problem of the mother's apparent lack of autonomy in breastfeeding literature and public perceptions of nursing mothers. This is only a problem, however, if autonomy is understood to reside in or adhere to a body without encumbrances. Current conceptions of female embodiment typically assimilate women's embodied experiences to the norms of male embodiment. Focusing on pregnancy allows us to do that; focusing on lactation makes that assimilation more difficult. Furthermore, feminist scholars may feel that breastfeeding as an issue works against a general feminist interest in sexuality as a defining factor in female embodied difference. Since breastfeeding is perceived socially as a nonsexual function of human breasts, to suggest lactation as a maternal embodiment that is threatened through the manipulations of technological medicine seems to challenge the core feminist definition of female difference as sexual.[6] (How maternity became separate from sexuality is another question.) Finally, feminist scholars tend to be critical of what they perceive to be the conservativism of breastfeeding advocates.

The relative inattention to breastfeeding in feminist scholarship means that lactating women lack a feminist discourse to frame their experience, both as embodied mothers and as social beings who interact with others in a society that discourages their use of their bodies to feed their infants.[7] If feminists have no theory that takes account of breastfeeding as an ordinary practice of maternity, lactating women will continue to be ignored as significant subjects of feminism. This goes along with the lack of maternity rights in the United States, which has a tradition of pressing equality as sameness. Some breastfeeding advocates are trying to bridge the gap between feminist theorizing and women's experiences of maternity, but have trouble because they are seen as avowing a problematic relation to scientific data and the idea of women as good mothers. Breastfeeding advocates may place too much emphasis on child welfare for many feminist theorists, who perceive such emphasis to promote maternal sacrifice and the dissolution of a mother's autonomy into the bodies of her children. This antagonism delineates a set of dilemmas we need to explore and resolve.

I want to understand more clearly why feminist scholars don't seem perturbed by the situation faced by my son's former day care teacher, who consistently contacted her infant's doctor for information concerning the child's feeding and elimination patterns and who was given incorrect information about managing lactation as it related to other conditions experienced by her son. I remember distinctly my anger at my own OB/GYN, when he told me that nursing beyond eighteen months offered no health advantages to the child (thus implying that it wasn't necessary to continue), even though I hadn't asked him for any advice on the matter. (I had asked how long I should wait for surgical anesthesia to wear off before I nursed my two-year-old son.) Even more startling was the advice—given to me when my son was eight days old and recovering from a fever of unknown origin—that I could begin to schedule his feedings, a practice which, at the time, would have led to nursing difficulties (because I was engorged since he wasn't nursing well). Physicians' lack of education concerning breastfeeding is an accepted commonplace at medical conferences concerning breastfeeding and its promotion within the profession, yet in feminist considerations of breastfeeding, the effect of this lack on women almost never comes up.[8]

Feminist scholars are more concerned with the pressure placed on women to breastfeed (what Linda Blum calls the "exhortation to breastfeed"); the notion that there is a culture of misinformation about breastfeeding, a belief of most breastfeeding advocates, does not emerge as significant in feminist work. Feminists disregard physicians' misinformation concerning breastfeeding, in my view, for the same reason that they think of arguments in favor of maternal nursing as political: they distrust science as a repository of information concerning how women should lead their lives, since science has for so long promoted essentialist and deterministic approaches to women. Medical misinformation concerning the management of breastfeeding doesn't matter that much, in this paradigm, since the medical arguments for breastfeeding are themselves problematical and not trustworthy.

As I demonstrated in the introduction to the book, the medicalization of infant feeding, which occurred through physicians' increasing promotion of artificial infant foods, has provided a complex legacy for breastfeeding advocates. Physicians and other health care professionals mediate the meanings of scientific evidence concerning human health, and yet many (if not most) medical personnel do not know how to practically assist women with breastfeeding, nor do they seem to be aware of misinformation about lactation that they provide. The paradigm of scientific motherhood demands that women seek expert medical advice in order to act as good mothers, yet the general admonition "breast is best" often conflicts with the actual advice for a specific infant feeding issue. Breastfeeding advocates use biomedical evidence of the health benefits of breastfeeding, yet criticize medical professionals for their lack of knowledge about the science and practice of lactation. Thus, advocates both depend on and criticize the medical establishment for its equivocal support for breastfeeding. Given this scenario, it is easy to understand how breastfeeding advocacy comes to represent, for many feminist scholars, just another political discourse to regulate mothers.

Women, however, are not simply caught in competing political ideologies, but must make concrete decisions on a daily basis concerning how to feed their infants. In chapter 4 I cautioned against the reliance of breastfeeding advocacy on scientific narratives of evolution, because attention to politics must be a part of such advocacy. In what might seem to be an about face, in this chapter I argue for increased attention to bodies from within the biological accounts of breastfeeding's health advantages, as well as more attention to lactation as a form of embodied motherhood. If I claimed earlier that we should not allow scientific research to be the arbiter of maternal feeding practices, here I demonstrate what happens when science is thrown out of the window altogether: breastfeeding advocacy is perceived to be a completely political enterprise, only about controlling women through putative, but not reliable, claims about health. Breastfeeding itself, in a metonymical relation, comes to be defined as a political practice (defined by ideological commitments) without biological consequences for women or children. This last point represents a significant trend in recent feminist scholarship on breastfeeding and breastfeeding advocacy.

I believe in the scientific evidence for breastfeeding as a maternal practice that confers substantial health benefits both on nursing infants and children and on lactating mothers. This premise informs the interpretations that I offer throughout this book; it is also a belief that divides those few feminist scholars who examine breastfeeding. In the main argumentative sections of this chapter, I examine three discourses that frame feminist approaches to breastfeeding. First I look at feminist critiques that refute the scientific evidence for the biological advantages of breastfeeding in order to argue for completely political interpretations of both advocacy and breastfeeding itself. I call the authors of these critiques the "feminist critics," and I argue that their refutation of the scientific evidence is a rhetorical move that allows for an emphasis on political meanings. Next I examine two feminist anthropological treatments of breastfeeding that are cited, alternately, by the feminist critics and by breastfeeding advocates. The approaches differ according to the value placed on biological arguments about lactation. In other words, the same opposition between science and the political structures both the feminist critique and the anthropological discourses that critics and advocates rely on. Finally, I provide an example of a feminist breastfeeding advocate, also an anthropologist, whose work offers a synthesis of biological and political arguments. Cited sparingly or not at all by the feminist critics, Penny Van Esterik's work merits greater attention in feminist scholarship, because it demonstrates how to work with both biological and political discourses concerning breastfeeding. In addition, Van Esterik refuses to separate First and Third World contexts, as the feminist critics tend to do in order to argue against the health advantages of breastfeeding in the developed world. An ecologically astute theorist, Van Esterik provides a significant response to recent feminist critiques of breastfeeding and breastfeeding advocacy, even though her book was published over ten years ago.

In the final section of this chapter, I consider the disparities in rates of breastfeeding among women of different races and classes in the United States. In comparing this analysis to that of the feminist critics, I argue that approaching breastfeeding as an issue of health activism for women and children is really about approaching breastfeeding as an aspect of women's rights. Instead of finding that women are compelled to breastfeed by health promotions that make them feel guilty about alternative choices, I find that the system consistently works the other way around, especially for poor women and women of color. The irony, of course, is that breastfeeding advocacy continues to work to educate women and health care professionals, as individuals and as groups, while a political movement for breastfeeding as woman's right would target a different audience entirely.[9]

The Feminist Critics

Feminist scholarly approaches to breastfeeding generally follow disciplinary lines. Historians, such as Rima Apple, Janet Golden, Ruth Perry, and Adrienne Berney, have approached changes in breastfeeding as a maternal practice in relation to other social transformations in the United States and Europe. Anthropologists, among them Vanessa Maher, Katherine Dettwyler, Elizabeth Whittaker, and Penny Van Esterik, have studied the effect of cultural ideals, material practices, and economic structures on breastfeeding initiation and duration. Other anthropologists, like Nancy Scheper-Hughes, address breastfeeding as part of a larger project about women's experiences in changing Third World economies. Literary critics, like Mary Jacobus and Marilyn Yalom, have provided interpretations of breastfeeding in representations; these scholars have also offered historical analyses of lactational symbolism. Breastfeeding advocates have produced a literature defining and criticizing the "breast–bottle controversy," especially in developing countries; these authors include Gabrielle Palmer, whose influential *The Politics of Breastfeeding* is based on the premise that capitalistic enterprise is robbing women of their natural capacity to nourish their infants, and Naomi Baumslag and Dia Michels, authors of *Milk, Money, and Madness*. Economist Judith Galtry focuses on the implications of ignoring breastfeeding in examining women's position in the labor market and in assessing economic development.[10]

In the mid to late 1990s a new genre of feminist scholarship on breastfeeding emerged. While continuing to be defined, at least in part, by disciplinary paradigms, this literature seeks to understand the meanings of breastfeeding for women in contemporary Western contexts, as well as to address feminist concerns about how the culturally dominant meanings of motherhood are mediated through breastfeeding advocacy and ideas about maternal nursing. Thus, this emerging genre does not directly address how women experience breastfeeding, as Cindy Stearns does in her recent article, "Breastfeeding and the Good Maternal Body," but seeks to use information about women's experiences to develop theories about how breastfeeding is part of contemporary ideologies of motherhood (to borrow from the subtitle of Linda Blum's book).[11] Breastfeeding, then, serves to focus an analysis that addresses, in a more general sense, the politics of motherhood, domesticity, and sexual (in)equality. In addition, these new works, while remaining disciplinary in some senses, identify themselves as explicitly feminist works of scholarship; that is, their stated purpose is to enhance feminist understandings of breastfeeding and mothering, rather than to contribute primarily to the scholarship of their own disciplines.[12]

Pam Carter's *Feminism, Breasts, and Breast-Feeding* (1995), Linda Blum's *At the Breast: Ideologies of Breastfeeding and Motherhood in the Contemporary United States* (1999), and Jules Law's "The Politics of Breastfeeding: Assessing Risk, Dividing Labor" (2000) represent this new trend in feminist scholarship on breastfeeding in the United States and the United Kingdom. These works share a crucial rhetorical strategy: refute scientific claims to the health benefits of breastfeeding, at least in the developed world, so as to argue that breastfeeding promotion is largely political, having to do with the promotion of certain kinds of mothering.[13] This strategy is most evident in the work of Blum and Law, but appears subtly in Carter's book as well. *Feminism, Breasts, and Breast-Feeding* looks at working-class women's experiences of infant feeding in northern England from the 1920s through the 1980s. In it, Carter emphasizes a science studies critique of the ideological (or discursive) enmeshment of scientific facts. Consider the following statements from *Feminism, Breasts, and Breast-Feeding*:

> Rather than examining the case "for" breast-feeding it is more useful to chart the way in which "facts" about the virtues of breast-feeding have been connected with certain ideas, images, beliefs, and favoured subject positions for women. (34)

> This is not however to argue that breast-feeding is unnatural, rather to try to explore the discourses of which it is a part, and to disrupt the scientifically endorsed culture versus nature dichotomy which has become fundamental to gender divisions. (70)

> For example, it is not simply a "fact" that breast-feeding is better for babies. Rather, this needs to be explored, evaluated and its meaning deconstructed in relation to particular contexts. (237)

All three scholars hold in common the view that infant feeding practices are best understood in the context of an analysis that emphasizes political concerns by repudiating scientific ones. While they all acknowledge, at some level, the biological superiority of human milk as an infant's nutritional mainstay, they argue against the use of this information as the primary determinant of maternal feeding practices, given social and political constraints on women's lives. They ask, in short, that biological considerations of infant feeding be subordinated to political ones.

I agree that infant feeding practices must be analyzed through a perspective that takes account of politics and the social construction of the body. In this sense, I support the second statement from Carter cited above. As Judith Galtry writes, "privileging biomedical knowledge is ... problematic [because] such 'knowledge' has come to represent the only legitimate understanding of the body and its processes, supporting, in many instances, prescriptions and practices that have adversely impacted women" (" 'Sameness' and Suckling" 78). But in the context of the other two statements by Carter, both of which question scientific evidence on the basis of contextual analyses of ideology and discourse, I find myself resistant to the cumulative meanings conveyed in all three. In constructing arguments against medical breastfeeding advocacy on the basis that the scientific evidence is faulty or misleading (Law and Blum) or on the basis that the scientific evidence is itself culturally mediated (Carter), these authors refuse the idea that biological approaches to breastfeeding can have anything meaningful to offer feminist considerations of the practice. The effect of such arguments is to remove breastfeeding from the realm of biological reproduction and to place it into what Jules Law calls "social reproduction," the sphere apparently amenable to negotiation and social change. This definition of breastfeeding as part of social reproduction allows feminist critics to critique the sexual division of labor that breastfeeding is enmeshed in, but the definition also provides a convenient method of denying the biological specificity of female lactation. Feminist critics, while arguing that they are not really against breastfeeding, offer up more reasons why nursing isn't really all it's cracked up to be, may not confer any significant biological benefits on infants and toddlers, and may really be more of a drag than mothers currently admit.[14] It is unclear why any woman would want to breastfeed, given the constraints articulated by these theorists.

In the rest of this section, I examine these three scholars' discussions in detail, demonstrating how their arguments concerning the overemphasis of the health benefits of breastfeeding coincide with a general cultural view that underemphasizes those same benefits. The feminist critics of breastfeeding and breastfeeding advocacy offer some very compelling insights concerning the difficulty of managing lactation in the context of Western women's familial and economic roles, and their insistence on approaching the topic through attention to women's social subordination provides a necessary corrective to the overoptimism of La Leche League. Indeed, the feminist critics' preoccupation with the political meanings of scientific information have struck me as crucially significant, ever since I attended my first La Leche League Seminar on Breastfeeding for Physicians and realized that the interesting talk on postnatal maternal-infant bonding had been refuted in the scientific literature decades previously. Yet the feminist critics' move to set aside scientific support for breastfeeding is essentially rhetorical: it allows them to sidestep a significant engagement with science and its findings in order to focus on political meanings. Childbearing continues to carry biological significance, but infant feeding becomes, in this scenario, a practice defined completely by hegemonic social discourses. In the discussion that follows I try to show why that doesn't make sense—why, in other words, accepting the scientific evidence doesn't have to mean giving up on politics.

Law argues, in general, that the scientific arguments for breastfeeding incorporate assumptions about the traditional sexual division of labor and present erroneous ideas about the health risks of formula feeding. What is presented as scientific support for the benefits of breastfeeding really isn't scientific, but "misleading at best and false at worst" (412). In this same vein, Carter remarks that there is a "concern that the benefits of breastfeeding have been overplayed," even "with regard to developing countries" (64). Law's particular formulation of the problem is presented with some significant insights, as he points out that formula use in the developed world may be a health risk for infants, but that most people don't really understand what the level of that risk is compared to other risks of bringing up baby: living in polluted areas, extensive use of potentially dangerous car seats, and so on. In an argument similar to Sarah Blaffer Hrdy's treatment of maternal agency, Law sees parents consistently making decisions in the context of relative risk, "balanc[ing] health risks (relative to finances, likelihood, and seriousness) all the time" (415). This balancing act occurs each time we weigh the potential effects of taking our children to McDonald's (in order to save money or time, for example, or simply to please them) as opposed to more healthful alternatives.[15]

Yet in his attempt to demonstrate that "the relative 'risks' of formula feeding are far from clear" (415), Law makes some problematic claims: for example, "City air is clearly more toxic than infant formula" (415). "In what way?", I want to ask; surely some statistics would be helpful here in sorting out what Law has already claimed is a context of relative risk. He also argues that if breastfeeding confers immunological protection, this may lead to a "lack of immunological experience" so that the breastfed child is more susceptible to illness in the preschool years, but he neglects to mention that the child's own immune system will be somewhat stronger in the preschool years than it was during infancy, so that the same illness later on may be milder than one contracted earlier (416).[16] While he later argues that "common sense suggests . . . that breast-fed infants and home-cared toddlers will survive their early 'lack of immunological experience' without serious health consequence," he also states that "common sense also suggests that the vaunted health advantages of breastfeeding are equally marginal and relative" (422). Why common sense is less fallible than scientific research is unclear.

Law wants to use certain kinds of scientific evidence against scientific claims for the benefits of breastfeeding, but not other kinds. He claims that "A formula-fed baby may have an incrementally greater risk of developing an ear infection, *but more than half of all infants develop ear infections sometime in their first year anyway*" (416; emphasis added). Yet he finds this figure in Jane Heinig and Kathryn Dewey's "Health Advantages of Breast Feeding for Infants: A Critical Review," an article providing evidence that breastfeeding *is* protective against otitis media (ear infection) (97–98). In one study reviewed, "the effect of breast feeding on otitis media and recurrent otitis media remained significant after controlling for parental history of allergy, presence of one or more siblings, use of day care, maternal smoking, and gender" (97). The DARLING study (Davis Area Research on Lactation, Infant Nutrition, and Growth), reported in part by Dewey, Heinig, and Nommsen-Rivers in the *Journal of Pediatrics* in 1995, suggests that even in affluent populations, breastfeeding has a protective effect against common childhood illnesses. The incidence of diarrhea in breastfed infants was half that in formula fed infants; the percentage of breastfed infants who suffered any otitis media was 19 percent less than the formula-fed group, but even more significant is the fact that the percentage of breastfed infants with prolonged otitis media (longer than 10 days) was *80 percent lower* than in the formula-fed group. The authors conclude that "the protective effect of breast-feeding against illness is of public health significance *even in relatively affluent populations*" (701; emphasis added). In less than affluent circumstances, what Law calls the "incremental" risk of infantile illness adds up, especially if one doesn't have health insurance or has difficulty taking off from work to go to the doctor, or if one is in a demographic group likely to experience other health risks like poor living environment or lack of medical care generally.

The fact that more than half of all infants get an ear infection before their first birthday doesn't mean that the protective effect of breastfeeding is insignificant; this fact may only mean that most infants (even infants initially fed by breast) spend most of that first year feeding by a bottle. In the study mentioned above by Heinig and Dewey, "infants who exclusively breast fed for 4 or more months had half as many episodes of acute otitis media as those not breast fed at all and 40 percent less than those who were partly breast fed" (97). Those do not seem to me to be insignificant statistics, but in Law's critique they are set aside since ear infections are an expected aspect of infancy anyway.

Law's critique of the research supporting the health benefits of breast-feeding is meant to cast doubt on scientists' ability to separate their views of proper mothering from what should be an ideologically neutral investigation. It is also meant to shore up feminist ideas about infant feeding as an activity that should be part of equity negotiations between parents and within communities (422). He is particularly against the idea of the maternal/infant dyad that is common in breastfeeding advocacy discourses—"how can risks be openly weighed when breastfeeding advocates regard women and children as a single biological unit?" (421)—arguing that mothers and infants have different interests that must be "disaggregated" in order to assess the different types of risk involved in different feeding scenarios. Clearly, it is on the premise that mothers and infants are separable entities that he makes his argument concerning "imaginative, fully deliberated, ethical, and responsible caregiving" (423). Carter also criticizes the "assumption that the mother and baby pair can be seen as a unit" (69). But what if "dyad" is the most appropriate biological way to approach the relation between mother and infant? Law begins his article claiming that "one of the most intractable problems facing feminist analyses of domestic ideology is the seemingly inevitable slippage—in cultural discourse as well as cultural practice—between reproductive and social-reproductive issues: between childbearing and child raising" (408). Childbearing is biological for Law, but breastfeeding is not, because it's always already child raising, presumably because once the fetus exists outside the woman's body as an infant, her relation to it must be understood in social terms.[17] And that, for Law, proscribes a biological conceptualization of the relation.

This refusal to acknowledge the biological continuum of pregnancy, childbirth, lactation, and weaning suggests Law's unstated presumption that the modern paradigm of maternity has transformed the sequence of embodied maternal experience that prevailed throughout most of human history. Indeed, Law eventually separates *lactation* as an aspect of biological reproduction from *infant feeding* as an aspect of social reproduction: "Lactation is a reproductive phenomenon that takes place in a woman's body; infant feeding is a social activity in which the bodies, prerogatives, obligations, and interests of multiple citizens converge" (442). He continues: "Infant feeding ... should be regarded as a practice that engages the entire social body and not just the bodies of women and infants, as a form of social labor whose division is open for negotiation, not as an extension of biological reproduction" (442). This position is necessary in order to designate breastfeeding, and discourses about it, as ideological, by which he means based on myths that obfuscate real material conditions (443). While he rightly points out that breastfeeding advocates often pay less than adequate attention to the domestic division of labor assumed in their promotion of maternal nursing, there is no reason to argue so vociferously against breastfeeding, especially when his argument refuses to address a crucial dimension of breastfeeding advocacy—the biological continuity between birth and breastfeeding. He simply pronounces such a view as incorrect. Law *is* correct that "the very real obstacles that breastfeeding and career pose to one another in our culture tend to be obscured by the myriad subtle ways in which a traditional domestic division of labor is built into the very assumptions and study-parameters of social-science researchers" (432), but since he is only willing to consider "currently imaginable conditions" (410n), he targets breastfeeding advocacy and breastfeeding itself, rather than the structure of market work and women's continued marginalization in the workforce, for extended critique.

Astute as he is to the problematic assumptions of breastfeeding advocates, Law cannot escape his own assumption that infant feeding cannot be conceptualized, primarily, as a physiological relation between mother and infant. His view is based on a formula feeding model, because it assumes in the first place a conceptual separation between mother and infant. He argues that breastfeeding advocacy presumes a traditional domestic division of labor, but only because he understands breastfeeding as child raising, that is, as domestic work. Conceptualizing breastfeeding as a physiological relation holds the potential to free infant feeding from its ties to domesticity precisely because identifying the biological dyad of mother and infant is not the same as marking the woman as domestic servant. Other constraints of contemporary developed societies, including, in the United States, the lack of governmentally-supported paid maternity leave and a gendered wage gap, enforce that latter role. Recognizing and affirming the biological relation between a nursing mother and her infant, if articulated in the terminology of women's rights, represents a political argument for all mothers to have what is now only available for the privileged few—time to experience biological nurturance that began in pregnancy and continues through lactation and weaning.[18]

Linda Blum's analysis, presented in *At the Breast: Ideologies of Breastfeeding and Motherhood in the Contemporary United States*, follows a similar pattern, although she ends up with a more positive assessment of breastfeeding than does Law. Blum enters her discussion against the medical case for breastfeeding by first looking at the developing world, arguing that even there "infant health and its relation to infant-feeding is a contested field of 'facts'" (45), and that "in the contemporary Third World, though breastfeeding *is* optimal, the causes of infant death and disease are embedded in larger social problems" (46; emphasis in original). She faults Nancy Scheper-Hughes for ignoring her own evidence that even when breastfeeding was the norm in northeastern Brazil, "many babies simply died later" (46). Following anthropologist Vanessa Maher (discussed at greater length below), Blum points out that concern for the health of Third World mothers rarely finds its way into standard breastfeeding advocacy. Through this series of claims, Blum minimizes support for breastfeeding in the developing world by making it seem only marginally connected to infant health and welfare, and her argument overall suggests that breastfeeding advocates seem to think that breastfeeding is the most important aspect of health care in the Third World: "On balance, it *is* safer for poor Third World mothers to feed their babies at the breast—but it is problematic to single out breastfeeding if this ultimately only targets mothers" (46; emphasis in original).

Blum, like Law, believes breastfeeding should always be understood as a maternal practice that takes place within a web of interconnected social, cultural, and economic circumstances; it can never be understood as a panacea for poverty or inadequate medical attention. Fair enough. Yet, some hyperbolic discourse to the contrary, most breastfeeding advocates *do* understand that breastfeeding won't compensate for the many ecological and economic disadvantages faced by Third World babies. On the other hand, breastfeeding may offer individual infants the possibility of survival in circumstances no one would wish on any child.[19] In de-emphasizing the health benefits of breastfeeding, First World feminists do a disservice to the most disadvantaged women in the world. For example, Linda Blum misconstrues Nancy Scheper-Hughes's findings. Scheper-Hughes argues that development in Brazil led to what she calls the "modernization of child mortality": "the standardizing of child death within the first twelve months of life and its containment to the poorest and marginalized social classes" (296). Most older children are now protected by immunization campaigns; middle- and upper-class infants are protected further by access to medical professionals and safe water supplies. Scheper-Hughes's point is that breastfeeding *in combination with* aggressive immunization campaigns and other public health efforts would enhance the survivability of the dying infants of the lowest classes in Brazil. Clearly, women themselves are not responsible for the modernization of child mortality through their abandonment of breastfeeding, which Scheper-Hughes acknowledges has many social and economic causes. But it is fair to say that in adverse ecological circumstances women themselves might act to increase the health prospects of their children by breastfeeding. Promoting breastfeeding as a panacea for poverty is ethically questionable; educating women about what they can do in the face of state neglect is not.

The logic of Blum's (and Law's) argument is that if we can question the extent to which breastfeeding matters in the Third World, certainly it confers only minimal advantage in the First.[20] Linda Blum states clearly that "most of the problems [breastfeeding] prevents no longer pose serious health risks in this country and . . . most formula-fed babies thrive" (49). She goes on to argue that "dramatic claims for infant-health benefits" that result from breastfeeding are not really understood well, even by scientists, and that "the exhortation that 'breast is best,' . . . may represent new kinds of middle-class anxieties about children as much as rational health-enhancing advice" (49–50). As I have argued earlier, the linkage of medicine's health optimizing discourses with evolutionary theory represents a problematic trend in breastfeeding advocacy. Blum is correct to point out how the "new cultural imperative" to breastfeed is linked to contemporary perceptions of the good mother that are raced and classed in their conception. Yet it is troubling to see the scientific evidence for the health benefits of breastfeeding so easily set aside.[21]

It is easy to demonstrate that scientific research on breastfeeding is sometimes less than unified in its results, just as it is easy to claim that a certain amount of infant and childhood illness is normal. It is much more difficult to determine, definitively, the benefit or advantage of a specific health-related practice.[22] Yet, as one speaker at a La Leche League Seminar on Breastfeeding for Physicians commented, all the research points in the same direction: perhaps incrementally, perhaps more "dramatically" (to use Blum's term), breastfeeding seems to confer some advantage on human infants, as compared to formula feeding. As Blum herself points out, much of the research on infant feeding tends to "underestimate the benefits of breastfeeding . . . [because] the 'breastfed' measure . . . includes many children fed some, or even lots of, formula" (49).

Then why is breastfeeding advocacy itself felt to be such a problem? The key complaint, for Blum, Law, and Carter, seems to be that breastfeeding is singled out by breastfeeding advocates as something individual women should do to maximize their reproductive effort; it is a burden, another responsibility foisted on women who are already overburdened. The implication is that women can or should resist such social prescription, which is part of a historical pattern of controlling women through ideological regulation of their reproductive activities.[23] Law argues further that breastfeeding advocacy wants women to make up for resources not provided to them and their children by the state or by male relatives: "Breast milk and motherhood have become the symbolic vehicles for a shift in the burden of resources and responsibilities back onto women" (441). Blum ends up arguing that breastfeeding may work, for some women who are opportunely positioned in social and economic terms, as an antidote to late-industrial expectations about disembodied motherhood, but her argument depends upon separating breastfeeding from any biological understanding of its practice. In other words, for Blum breastfeeding as an embodied practice can serve a resistant function to late-industrial capitalist ideology, but only when the embodiment of breastfeeding is understood as primarily ideological in its effect. In her analysis, bottle feeding can *also* serve a resistant function, especially for black mothers; I discuss this issue at length in the last section of this chapter.[24] For Law, breastfeeding advocates' representations of breastfeeding function ideologically to mask women's real relation to the state's organization of gender (441). To make such arguments, the biological argument for breastfeeding has to be discounted as a justifiable reason for engaging in it as a maternal practice.

Within Pam Carter's Foucaultian framework, the scientific evidence never exists outside the other discourses—on maternal duty and the maternal body, for example—within which it is articulated. Overall, she tries to demonstrate that addressing health inequality in general is more important than specific breastfeeding campaigns, especially when the latter are targeted at disadvantaged women as a requirement for proper motherhood (235). Carter takes as her starting point the "point of view of the kinds of women who have long been seen as a problem with regard to low rates of breast-feeding" (189–90), using ethnography as her basic research technique. This enables her to present the experiences of her informants from their perspective. Clearly, any breastfeeding advocacy program that does not seek to understand the experiences and perspectives of those people it hopes to engage will be a failure; Carter is adept at demonstrating the women's relationships to infant feeding prescriptions and their thoughts about their own practices. She concludes that it isn't clear that breastfeeding itself is always in women's best interests (213); she also argues that bottle feeding "did not liberate [women] to become like men; bottle feeding is not a route to gender neutrality" (233).

Carter does not take a clear position here, as she believes that any practice is necessarily contextual; she does, however, argue against breastfeeding advocacy, although she implies that working for women's autonomy may improve rates of breastfeeding (240). Yet in the absence of a discussion of the benefits of breastfeeding, there is no clear rationale to choose breastfeeding over bottle feeding, no reason to believe that given more autonomy and control women would choose breastfeeding. Ted Greiner argues that breastfeeding rates in Sweden are high because women's autonomy from men has been enhanced through governmental supports (extended maternity leaves and job security, for example), but Sweden is also a country with a tradition of advocacy to promote the practice of maternal nursing (Greiner; Riordan and Auerbach 49). The choice to breastfeed would seem to necessitate some sort of advocacy, especially given the negative portrayal of its burdens in the work of Carter and Law. Yet Carter's conclusion (that breastfeeding may follow attention to women's autonomy and control) does support her position

206 · Breastfeeding, Feminism, Activism

that feminism is about creating real choice for women, choice that does not divide women into good and bad mothers. She states that "attention to differences between women and to women's wish to have control over their bodies and their lives, has alerted us to the need to expand women's choices about how they engage with reproduction and sexuality ... neither form of feeding can in itself represent a goal for feminism" (240).

I agree with these authors that breastfeeding advocacy, especially in the developed world, can be somewhat blind to the material circumstances of many women's lives, circumstances that make breastfeeding not only bur-densome as a reproductive practice, but unattainable as a social accomplish-ment of maternity. The strategy of optimistic encouragement employed by La Leche League, for example, can make it seem as if a mother just hasn't tried hard enough when, for a variety of reasons outside her control, breast-feeding doesn't work out. Blum's discussion of working-class white women demonstrates the difficulty of trying to breastfeed without adequate social and financial resources, especially when medical professionals don't offer support. The particular books that Jules Law focuses on, Jellife and Jellife's *Human Milk in the Modern World* and Baumslag and Michels's *Milk, Money, and Madness,* are particularly guilty of this oversight, the first because it is so focused on demonstrating the biological superiority of breast milk and the second because it is written in the hyperbolic discourse of journalistic ex-posé. Many breastfeeding advocacy materials tend to overestimate women's abilities to control their environments; Pam Carter aptly demonstrates that many working-class women live with other relatives and thus are not even in charge of domestic space.[25] Breastfeeding advocacy also, as Law insightfully demonstrates, can distort the scientific record on bonding and incorporate evolutionary discourses to bolster current idealized familial arrangements. But just because these advocacy discourses problematically collude with antifeminist ideologies does not mean that the practice of maternal nurs-ing is itself a purely political experience, determined by conservative social discourses and solely defined by their meanings. Just because scientific re-search seems less than unified on the health benefits of breastfeeding (and not just of human milk) does not mean that the evidence that does ex-ist isn't compelling. Judith Galtry comments that "denunciations of 'best practice' recommendations for infant feeding as merely another example of patriarchal prescription tends to ... trivialize the influence of this advice on women's lives" (" 'Sameness' and Suckling" 78).

The main problem, it seems to me, is that the discourses of breastfeeding advocacy and feminist critique are incommensurable: the first advocating a straightforward use of scientific evidence to press its promotion of a biosocial practice; the second questioning any nondiscursive understanding of the same evidence and casting doubt on even the possibility of arguing for lactation using scientific research. To use scientific evidence in support of the biological benefits of breastfeeding is only engaging in a rhetorical debate the very structure of which divides feminist critics and breastfeeding advocates into two opposing camps who refuse to speak each other's language and to accept the other's evidentiary claims.

This rhetorical impasse is evident in the anthropological literature used by both sides as evidence. Anthropology itself is split between sociocultural and physical perspectives. Blum, Law, and Carter rely on Vanessa Maher's 1992 edited volume, *The Anthropology of Breast-Feeding: Natural Law or Social Construct* (Law very heavily). Breastfeeding advocates, on the other hand, are more likely to cite Katherine Dettwyler's work, principally the two essays published in *Breastfeeding: Biocultural Perspectives.*[26] Comparing these sources demonstrates profound disagreements in how to consider breastfeeding as a maternal practice, and reasons why feminist scholars tend to criticize breastfeeding advocacy.

Biological Function or Cultural Practice, or Both?

In *The Anthropology of Breast-Feeding: Natural Law or Social Construct*, Vanessa Maher, the volume's editor, contributes two individually authored chapters and one coauthored chapter. In these essays, Maher presents a persuasive and interesting account of breastfeeding as a culturally embedded activity that depends on numerous factors: the specific organization of society, role of the father in caring for his children, significance of family formation on the sexualization of girls and women, social expectations concerning male sexual privilege, the impact of industrialization on family structure and mothers' work, and the economic status of the family, among other factors. In her chapter "Breast-Feeding and Maternal Depletion: Natural Law or Cultural Arrangements?" Maher argues that "infant mortality has probably less to do with women's 'failure' to breast-feed than with poverty and inequitable gender relations," and states unequivocally, "It is important to stress that none of the essays in this volume, and this one is no exception, is intended to make a case for or against breast-feeding or bottle-feeding. In bracketing breast-feeding with maternal depletion, my quarrel is not with breast-feeding itself, far from it, but with a simplistic approach to its practice which neglects the multiple roles of women in regimes of gender inequality" (153, 154). She consistently argues against the "medical model," suggesting that poverty and lack of resources, not lack of breastfeeding, lead to infant death, and she forcefully maintains women's right to shift the burden of infant feeding costs from their overburdened bodies to the pockets (and cash) of men (who buy formula). But in order to make these claims, Maher must throughout the essay contest the specific biomedical claims that breastfeeding significantly benefits infants' health without endangering the mother's health in compromised situations in the developing world.[27]

Discussing the evidence that malnourished women seem to make perfectly adequate breast milk ("The idea that the nursing woman's body manages somehow to compensate for a net loss of vital resources is an optimistic one" [160]), Maher indicates the cultural contexts of women's decreasing share of nutritional and economic resources in the Third World, and argues that women should not be asked to provide, with their bodies, "more resources while their own share continues to diminish" (174). Yet despite her stated emphasis on breastfeeding *advocacy*, and not breastfeeding *per se*, the chapter, in making a case for women's rational decision making concerning infant feeding in the Third World, seems to argue that because there is no biological basis to claims of breastfeeding's intrinsic advantages, infant feeding methods should be analyzed in terms of their cultural meanings and economic effects. The strategy of raising questions about medical evidence in order to assert the primacy of cultural meanings of breastfeeding is the one articulated by both Blum and Law and alluded to by Carter. Maher, of course, is not only concerned with cultural meanings; she is concerned with women's material welfare and wants more respect accorded to their decisions. She is clearly angry with assumptions that women must be educated to make the right choices concerning infant feeding, believing that most women make such decisions in ways that appropriately respond to their economic and social circumstances. For Maher, culture creates the necessary meanings for breastfeeding, and culture itself is influenced by the meanings breastfeeding takes on (9).

But Maher also notes that (Western) medicine creates a context in which it is difficult to sustain breastfeeding, because the medical model involves a mechanistic and regulatory view of the female body that many women may unconsciously resist (32); this analysis alludes to the bottle-feeding culture that breastfeeding advocates work against. Breastfeeding in the medical model still follows the rationalized practices initiated in the early part of this century in the United States (Berney). These practices, including scheduling and adherence to dietary guidelines, encourage bottle feeding by making the requirements for breastfeeding seem onerous while also making the actual practice of breastfeeding difficult. In addition, while I agree that as feminist scholars we must approach women's decision making as rational and responsive to their specific circumstances, we must also take account of decisions that are made based on systematically erroneous information provided to mothers. In an analysis that continues the outlines sketched by Maher, Linda Blum offers examples of working-class mothers given advice to wean because of a baby's jaundice or "allergy to the mother's milk," and states that La Leche League offers alternate information to counter such "common misconception[s]" (*At the Breast* 118–23). Yet Blum consistently focuses on the women's sense of failure that attended their cessation of breastfeeding, and thus pays inadequate attention to the culture of misinformation that surrounds infant feeding. This may seem to present a woman-centered interpretation of their experiences, but does little to address the fact that women routinely make decisions based on these common misconceptions. At the end of her chapter on working-class mothers, Blum expresses concern about state promotion of breastfeeding and the effects of enhanced breastfeeding promotion campaigns on these mothers; concern for the adequacy of the information and support that they receive is completely absent from the discussion.

Katherine Dettwyler, whose work on evolution and breastfeeding I discussed in chapter 4, also believes breastfeeding to be a culturally embedded activity, but she understands the relation between culture and biology a bit differently than Vanessa Maher. For Dettwyler, lactation is first and foremost a biological function of the female breast; this function is influenced by culture insofar as culture can distort, denigrate, or enhance the meanings of breastfeeding. Other cultural practices and beliefs can help or hinder the practice of maternal nursing in a given society. Thus, different cultures interact with the biology of breastfeeding, aiding or abetting, in particular ways. Because she understands breastfeeding to have an intrinsic value that is universal for all humans, Dettwyler focuses more insistently on cultural practices and beliefs that inhibit women's ability to nurse their babies. In the United States, she identifies four "fundamental assumptions that underlie beliefs about breasts [and that inhibit breastfeeding]: (1) the primary purpose of women's breasts is for sex (i.e., for adult men), not for feeding children, (2) breastfeeding serves only a nutritional function, (3) breastfeeding should be limited to very young infants, and (4) breastfeeding, like sex, is appropriate only when done in private" ("Beauty and the Breast" 174). These beliefs permeate the culture, and have far-reaching effects on women's behaviors; for example, the emphasis on breasts as sexual for men has created, in Dettwyler's view, the widespread phenomenon of breast augmentation, what she calls "female mammary mutilation." She compares breast augmentation with foot-binding and female circumcision (201–2). These practices distort, in a basic way, any realistic perception of what breasts are for; Dettwyler is insistent that the primary function of female breasts is lactation, an argument she promotes by showing that only in a very few cultures are women's breasts included as part of sexual activity between adults. Finally, she believes emphatically in using scientific discourses and evidence to promote breastfeeding. Indeed, in her conclusion to "Beauty and the Breast," she presents an optimistic view of changes in U.S. culture and public policy that would support maternal nursing, and she specifically uses the example of changing attitudes toward tobacco smoke as a model for how a society can alter both its views and its practices concerning activities that risk optimal health.

At first glance, it would seem that Dettwyler's view is problematic from a cultural studies perspective: she enforces a universalizing conception of the female body and its functions, and her model for the interaction of culture and biology emphasizes the primacy of biology in the context of its distortion by cultural practices and beliefs. Yet all of the scholars discussed in this chapter acknowledge the biological superiority of human milk as compared to infant formulas—they just differ concerning how much of an advantage it really confers, given social arrangements and the constraints on women's lives. The real difference between these anthropologists concerns their attitudes toward women's relationship to society and culture. Dettwyler believes that cultural representations and ideas about female bodies and breasts negatively influence women's choices and practices around infant feeding. Culture here is a force that, in addition to simply offering women incorrect information about breastfeeding, encourages in women ideas about their own bodies that work against successful breastfeeding once those women become mothers. The emphasis is on what keeps women from breastfeeding. The choice not to breastfeed, or to breastfeed only briefly, is not considered irrational, but is based on culturally embedded ideas that are themselves not rational. In Foucaultian terms, Dettwyler's view of the negative impact of cultural ideas concerning breasts and infant feeding is both repressive *and* productive. But, like other breastfeeding advocates, Dettwyler is more likely to focus on a culture of misinformation, that is, the repressive function of ideology.

Maher, on the other hand, pays more attention to the material exigencies of women's lives that make breastfeeding difficult, and not breastfeeding a viable option and rational choice for many women. The emphasis here is on the productive aspect of power—how women use whatever agency is available to craft opportunities for themselves and their children. Like Dettwyler, Maher believes that breastfeeding is made difficult by a variety of social and cultural practices, but rather than concentrate on how society and culture should change, she focuses on women's abilities and choices in a constrained context. In her view, breastfeeding advocacy should not focus so much on the biological properties of human milk that it neglects attention to the circumstances of the women who provide the milk, as well as other forms of child nurture.

Understood in this manner, the differences between these two kinds of anthropological approach seem more a matter of emphasis than of substantive disagreement. Yet neither Law nor Blum cites Dettwyler as a source, even though her chapter, "Beauty and the Breast: The Cultural Context of Breastfeeding in the United States," draws on feminist approaches to women's experiences in a misogynistic culture.[28] The real issue, it seems to me, is precisely this matter of emphasis. Feminist scholars in general want to see more positive emphasis on women's experiences as they occur now, with due attention to women's rational decision making in the context of the constrained circumstance of misogynistic and capitalistic societies, while breastfeeding advocates are more likely to see women as the unknowing dupes of formula companies and uninformed medical personnel. Feminist scholars also want some acknowledgment of infant formula as a healthful option for feeding babies; in their view, to put so much emphasis on the biological properties of human milk is to risk reifying it and making it possible to enforce regulations on the bodies of women that produce it. But breastfeeding advocates will insist that we must pay attention to biology; moreover, to them human milk represents the specificity of the maternal body and its evolved practice of infant nurture. For them, to ignore breastfeeding as a crucial aspect of maternal practice, in all but a few cases, is to miss what is significant about women in the first place—their unique reproductive function. Feminist scholars, however, are likely to criticize these descriptions of maternity and infant care as essentialized perceptions of femininity (see Carter's critique of Van Esterik, 189–90).

Clearly, breastfeeding advocacy calls on and reinforces certain views that are prevalent in some strands of feminist theory. In the next section, I discuss the work of one breastfeeding advocate/scholar who makes explicit claims about breastfeeding as a feminist practice, addressing feminism's lack of attention to lactation and assessing the implications for thinking of breastfeeding as a feminist issue. Penny Van Esterik's work challenges the pieties of both traditional breastfeeding advocates and the feminist critics, providing a model for thinking about infant feeding practices in a global context. Her work, I believe, deserves more attention from feminist scholars interested in breastfeeding (she's already well known within advocacy circles), as well as feminist scholars seeking global approaches to maternity and feminist body politics. I offer an extended reading of her research here, as a way to set up the final section of this chapter, which considers breastfeeding as an issue of women's rights within the perspective of health activism.

"Thank You, Breasts"

Penny Van Esterik, anthropologist and author of *Beyond the Breast-Bottle Controversy* and a number of articles linking breastfeeding and feminism, tells a funny story in a number of her published works: At the completion of her doctoral exams, her committee suggested that they all go out for a beer. Van Esterik writes that "the milk for my three-month-old daughter let down and ejected forcefully across the seminar table." During preparation for the exams, she came to associate drinking beer with nursing her infant daughter because, upon returning home after an afternoon of study, she breastfed the baby while imbibing. Reflecting on the meaning of the experience, she writes, "I think the memory was directing me to include bodily experience and maternal praxis in what otherwise might have been a review of why feminists ignore breastfeeding and the pros and cons of various feminist approaches to motherhood. Thank you, breasts" ("Thank You, Breasts!" 76).

Like most breastfeeding advocates, Van Esterik staunchly supports breast-feeding as the optimally healthful method of infant feeding, although she acknowledges that she supplemented with formula because "I doubt that I could have combined the demands of breastfeeding and graduate school had I not used occasional substitute bottles of infant formula" (*Beyond* 22).[29] Her main object in *Beyond the Breast-Bottle Controversy*, however, is not to focus on breast milk as the definitive infant food, but to examine how debates about infant feeding should be framed. She argues that "breastfeeding is a feminist issue because it encourages women's self-reliance, confirms a woman's power to control her own body, challenges models of women as consumers and sex objects, requires a new interpretation of women's work, and encourages solidarity among women" (*Beyond* 69). She is careful to qualify her discussion to large-scale issues rather than simply the choices of individual women:

> By framing the breast-bottle controversy around the issues of poverty environments, empowerment of women, medicalization of infant feeding, and the commoditization of food, attention is shifted away from the infant feeding decisions of individual mothers and on to the conditions affecting their decisions and lives.
>
> The trajectory goal becomes not to have every woman breastfeed her infant, but to create conditions in individuals, households, communities, and nations so that every woman could. The first step is to create conditions that make breastfeeding possible, successful, and valued in a given society. (*Beyond* 211)

We can see the concerns of Maher, Law, Blum, and Carter reflected in the first paragraph, but the second paragraph shifts the discussion back to an advocacy paradigm in which promoting breastfeeding as a practice is a goal. In addition, Van Esterik sees breastfeeding as having widespread significance for "rethinking basic [feminist] issues such as the sexual division of labor, the fit between women's productive and reproductive lives, and the role of physiological processes in defining gender ideology" ("Breastfeeding and Feminism" 542). Unlike Jules Law, then, Penny Van Esterik believes that feminist attention to breastfeeding in the context of advocacy research can make important linkages between problems that continue to haunt feminist theory (difficulties in making shared domestic labor a reality, for example) and the practice of maternal nursing.[30]

For feminists, a major problem with promoting breastfeeding is that "lactation as a process smacks of essentialism and biological determinism" (Van Esterik, "Thank You, Breasts," 80). Unlike pregnancy and childbearing, however, for which there are no substitute disembodied practices,[31] breast-feeding seems to have become an optional physical practice of maternity. Van Esterik argues,

> [T]he physiological process of lactation must be included in any analysis of the relation between production and reproduction. This is not biological determinism but common sense. The biological facts of pregnancy, birth and lactation are not readily compatible with capitalist production unless profits are expended on maternity leaves, nursing facilities and childcare. Thus when mothers enter the workforce, they are forced to seek marginal, low paying kinds of work. ("Thank You, Breasts" 81)

Here we can see the advocacy truism that locates breastfeeding with other aspects of biological reproduction, a grouping strenuously repudiated by Jules Law, who wants to see infant feeding count in social reproduction as an aspect of domestic labor. Yet even when Van Esterik addresses infant feeding in the context of infant care, as opposed to reproduction, she argues that regardless of feminists' desires to more equitably divide the work, "the fact remains that it is women who have the capacity to provide food for their infants, ensuring women's self-reliance and their infants' survival for the first few months of life" (*Beyond* 75).

Thus, a major opposition between feminist arguments critical of breast-feeding advocacy and breastfeeding advocates who claim feminist goals is the question of whether women can be empowered through biological practices of reproduction and how such practices affect (or support) the traditional sexual division of labor. Van Esterik contends that supporting breastfeeding can encourage a reconceptualization of women's productive and reproduc-tive labor—"If the work of lactation is valued as productive work, not the duty of a housewife, then conditions for its successful integration with other activities must be arranged" (*Beyond* 75)—but she implies that because of the physical exigencies of breastfeeding, infant care will continue to fall to women. On the other hand, it does anyway, as the quotation above and a look around us indicate.[32] Like other breastfeeding advocates, Van Esterik is skeptical of any purported freedom that emerges through the mediation of technology and "male-dominated modes of production," especially when it depends on the disembodiment of the mother in conjunction with the devaluation of her roles (*Beyond* 76). Linda Blum notes this problem in the current advocacy emphasis on breast pumping (*At the Breast* 52–62). Significantly, Van Esterik does not see the decline in breastfeeding as a result of individual choice; nor does she understand infant feeding decisions to be private. Rather, she understands shifts in infant feeding patterns to be the result of divergent causes that can be identified through studying "poverty environments, the empowerment (or lack of empowerment) of women, the medicalization of infant feeding, and the commoditization of infant foods" (*Beyond* 15–20; see also 193–94). Thus, Van Esterik would take issue with Law's claim that "Infant feeding . . . should be regarded as . . . a form of social labor whose division is open for negotiation, not as an extension of biological reproduction" (442), because she would argue that *lactation* is a form of social labor whose division is not open for negotiation *because it is an extension of biological reproduction,* but which would probably force a form of social negotiation to occur if women were able to press their demands as breastfeeding mothers.

Pam Carter argues that the women in her study didn't experience breast-feeding in the manner that Van Esterik claims it empowers women (encouraging self-reliance, for example, or enhancing women's networks). Yet Van Esterik articulates a somewhat utopian framework that promotes breast-feeding in the context of what it, as a socially valued maternal practice, has the potential to do to other social structures, rather than what breastfeeding in the context of its social invisibility or denigration is actually like. The idea here is that if breastfeeding were properly understood and valued, these social changes would have to take place, and these changes would improve women's lives and the lives of their children. After all, Van Esterik's own research demonstrates that infant feeding is a fully enculturated activity. Carter's argument assumes that Van Esterik means that breastfeeding itself accomplishes positive changes for women in a political sense. Although successful breastfeeding will help women feel more confident about their ability to provide for their children, a key advantage in Van Esterik's schema, it seems clear to me that the overall argument in *Beyond the Breast-Bottle Controversy* is to show how breastfeeding fits into a more woman-centered perspective on development and maternal-child health than currently exists, precisely to counteract "forms of social control which are expressed through infant feeding regimes at any particular period" (Carter 196).

Feminist breastfeeding advocates, like Penny Van Esterik, argue that breastfeeding cannot be promoted unless it is also supported socially. Such social support would mean entitlement policies directed toward mothers, rather than the gender-neutral policies that currently exist in the United States[33]; clearly, this opposition falls along the lines of the familiar "equality versus difference" debate. Linda Blum tries to show, however, that breast-feeding as a maternal practice, at least in the United States, defies such easy categorization as a practice of "difference": "In the contemporary United States, we can no longer map the bottle on to equality, and the breast, to difference. Advice to rely on breast pumps is now ubiquitous, and because so many mothers reenter the workplace within a few weeks or months of giving birth (or face other reasons to be apart from their babies), this causes signif-icant blurring of equal and different, of bottle and breast, of technology and nature, and finally, of medical and maternalist visions" (199–200). While she writes that originally she conceptualized the answer to the problem of breastfeeding as "resources for women to genuinely choose interludes of difference, policies for equality and difference" (196), through the writing of *At the Breast* she came to the conclusion that

> To nurse our babies at the breast may offer a way to revalue our bodies and force a public reevaluation of caregiving—*or*—at the same time, it may represent acquiescence to dominant regimes of self-sacrifice, overwork, and surveillance. It can blur into a disembodied regime and threaten an overriding sense of failure. Bottlefeeding can thus be empowering, a refusal to be tied to our biology, to always be marked by gender and race, to always be vulnerable to oversexualization. But, at the same time, it can represent capitulation to inhumane public and workplace demands, to compulsory heterosexuality, to letting external forces interpret our embodied choices. (198–99; emphasis in original)

Blum's understanding of the fluidity of meanings of breastfeeding is based on a postmodern sensibility concerning meaning and the way particular practices serve as conduits for seemingly unrelated discourses: "Breastfeed-ing does not have inherent truth, but meanings determined out of power relations, various disciplining practices, and conflicting needs and interests, which are inherently political" (200); "infant feeding questions are about citizenship, national and global politics" (201). Carter also ends up affirm-ing fluidity in the meanings of breastfeeding; throughout *Feminism, Breasts and Breast-Feeding* she is insistent that breastfeeding not become the truth of womanhood. In criticizing Penny Van Esterik, Carter writes, "The difficulty is that she attributes to breast-feeding a 'truth' of the self which she argues is in itself empowering to women" (196).

Instead of a postmodern focus on fluidity, Van Esterik addresses the "cultural models" of breastfeeding and bottle feeding as "general purpose models that apply to multiple domains of life" (200). It is important to present these models in depth, because examining them demonstrates the significance of a global analysis, rather than one that splits off First World mothers from their Third World counterparts. In addition, Van Esterik's attention to ecological issues suggests another significant way that biological discourses need to be taken account of when considering infant feeding issues.

> *Breastfeeding Model.* The breastfeeding model develops from the model of renewable resources. As a renewable resource, breastfeeding operates on the satiation principle stressing nonmeasurable criteria like satisfaction. In this model, as demand increases, supply increases. Time orientation is to cyclical, recurrent rhythms, reinforcing the continuity between the reproductive phases of pregnancy, birth, lactation, and weaning. Breastfeeding is an individualized process; breastmilk [*sic*] is a living, changing product adapted to the age of the child and the microenvironment of the mother. The primary social links formed are highly personalized links between mother and infant, or more rarely between another female adult and an infant. Most significant, in the breastfeeding model the infant is active and in control of the process. It is thus a newborn's first experience of empowerment.
>
> *Bottle Feeding Model.* The bottle feeding model develops from the use of nonrenewable resources. Bottle feeding operates on the scarcity principle, reinforcing the idea of limited good and the fact that resources can be used up. As demand increases, supply decreases, resulting in a stress on quantity and measurement. Time, too, must be measured and divided into components, sequences, and schedules. Infant formula, the most appropriate breastmilk substitute, is a standardized product, constantly being improved in an effort to replicate human milk. The process of bottle feeding encourages the formation of generalized social links, as bottle feeding can be accomplished by males or females, adults or children. During bottle feeding, the infant is passive and controlled by others, providing the newborn's first experience of dependency and creating a consumer from birth. (200–2).

These two models take into account the biological significance of both breast- and bottle feeding. First World accounts that suggest the biological case for breastfeeding is more defensible in the developing world than in the West imply that the developed world has transcended the physicality of embodied motherhood. Any such transcendence that seems to exist depends heavily upon available medical treatments and a technological approach to the body; this fact is obscured in arguments concerning expected childhood illness and demonstrates a lack of attention to inequities in access to health care in the developed world. Such arguments, made by Blum and Law, also neglect to interrogate infant formula itself through an ecological paradigm. The separation of biology from the social impoverishes their conclusions, as they are unable to advocate for social change with anything other than an explicitly political argument.[34] But as Van Esterik points out, "Unlike infant formula and bottle feeding, which utilize nonrenewable resources, breastfeeding only requires investing in the health of the mother. Although breastfeeding is essentially a conservative mammalian function, it requires radical social structural transformations to succeed. These include changes in the division of labor, more equitable distribution of income and resources, and higher priorities on maternal and child welfare" (210). Breastfeeding advocates like Penny Van Esterik believe that social change *for women* can occur on the basis of biological discourses about breastfeeding, as long as they are articulated within feminist frameworks ("Breastfeeding and Feminism" S48). I think that such a view is more compelling and, in America, will succeed far better than Blum's "coalitions of 'disreputable' and 'denigrated' mothers who can seize maternalism and force its moral authority to speak for them" (198). It is hard to see what kind of discursive ground will support such coalitions and the rights such mothers will demand. The traditionalist perspectives of La Leche League that Blum criticizes, their "romantic sentimental views" of motherhood, are effective for at least some portions of the U.S. population (and in the international arena) because they work as a common, culturally popular discourse to link with breastfeeding advocacy. They also operate as a buffer for the more scientifically-oriented discourses of medical breastfeeding advocacy.

Van Esterik's model overestimates the infant's control of the breastfeeding experience, given the fact that the mother generally engages in highly enculturated practices of lactation (see Panter-Brick). Nevertheless, biological perspectives may provide significant leverage in demanding women's political and social right to breastfeed. Access to health care and medical resources has been part of civil rights struggles in the contemporary period. The difficulty is that biological perspectives on breastfeeding have been produced in the context of scientific motherhood, so that discourses about breastfeeding as an embodied maternal practice with health benefits have been articulated in the context of the physician's authority to regulate infant feeding. Thus, the specific biological benefits of breastfeeding are recognized at precisely the point in the modern period when mothers themselves have little public authority over infant nurture and child rearing (see Jones).

In the next section I examine the statistics on breastfeeding that I brought up in the introduction to *Mother's Milk,* in order to demonstrate how biomedical discourses might be articulated in the context of a feminist health activist approach to breastfeeding advocacy. Health activism is not foreign to the women's movement, although it's not as prominent as it once was.

Through the overtly political orientation of health activism, breastfeeding advocacy can demonstrate how a biological understanding of the body need not preclude culturalist interpretations.

Health Activism, Health Disparities, and Women's Rights

In the introduction to this book, I discussed the history of the medicalization of infant feeding, including breastfeeding, in the twentieth century. Throughout the text I have criticized medical representations of women and mothers, and the scientific discourses about motherhood that medicine relies on for some of its recent theories concerning breastfeeding. Yet in this chapter I have been arguing that biomedical discourses about breastfeeding's health benefits cannot be disregarded in favor of a feminist perspective that focuses exclusively on political and ideological issues. Maternity, in my view, deserves to be understood as an embodied experience, and the unique embodiment of lactation should not be conceptualized as merely one kind of nutrition delivery system. Biological discourses about maternal embodiment help us to focus on those aspects of maternal practice that cannot be shared equally with men; attention to them should be a crucial part of feminist attempts to reconfigure social and economic structures to accommodate mothers as members of civic society.

Attention to biomedical information does not have to suggest an acquiescence to medicalization. Van Esterik writes,

> Medicalization of infant feeding refers to expropriation by health professionals of the power of mothers and other caretakers to determine the best feeding pattern of infants for maintaining maximum health. There follows from this definition no judgment as to how medicalization of infant feeding relates to infant morbidity and mortality—only an argument that what was in the past largely the concern of mothers and women is increasingly part of the medical domain. (*Beyond* 112)

In the last three decades, the women's health movement has tried to return to women information and knowledge about their bodies that have been appropriated by medicine as an institution. In the introduction to *Our Bodies, Ourselves: For the New Century,* Jane Pincus states that one of the goals of this bible of the women's health movement is "providing women with tools to enable all of us to take charge of our health and lives" (22). Feminist health activism challenges the medicalization of everyday practices by reappropriating the biomedical perspective and politicizing it. In this sense, La Leche League represents a form of feminist health activism because as an organization League has offered biomedical information about breastfeeding to women in order to help them manage their own experiences and interact more knowledgeably with their health care providers. A health activist perspective is thus one way to retain the significance of biological knowledge about breastfeeding in the context of a political approach to mothering.

The feminist critics contend that breastfeeding promotion, based on a medical model, stigmatizes the life choices of poor women and women of color, and treats their decisions as irrational (as opposed to being responsive to their circumstances and worldviews). Van Esterik agrees, in part, with this analysis:

> Breastfeeding promotion campaigns are ethically complex in that they infer that medical practitioners and institutions have the right to try and influence a mother's private decision about how to feed her infant. In the biomedical model, physicians have a responsibility for health education and public health, while the community should be the passive recipient of services and advice from health professionals.... This approach to educating mothers about how to feed their infants may easily slip into moralizing and blaming mothers for their infant feeding decisions. (*Beyond* 150)

Health activists respond to this issue by encouraging communities and individuals to develop health goals and practices that are based on biomedical information but not subject to the authority of professional health care providers. Again, La Leche League serves as an important example: as stated in the *Leader Handbook*, the leader's role is to empower mothers to pursue their own breastfeeding goals. Much of the leader's responses to an individual mother are geared toward helping the mother clarify those goals and offering her information about how to achieve them (Sachetti 12).

How might a health activist perspective approach the ethnoracial disparities in breastfeeding initiation and duration? For a long period, in the early to middle twentieth century, poor, working-class, and black women were the *most* likely to breastfeed, while wealthier white women were abandoning the practice in favor of "scientific" bottle feeding. Current statistics on breastfeeding initiation and duration, which show that older, educated, and wealthier white women are among those most likely to breastfeed, demonstrate that the reversal of the decline in breastfeeding that has occurred since the late 1960s also reverses this earlier paradigm. It is not simply the case that middle- and upper-class white women are the first to follow trends in expert medical advice about infant feeding because they know more about such trends, or are better at following such advice. Rather, as Linda Blum argues, the material circumstances of white middle- and upper-class women's lives mean that they are more likely to experience such advice as appropriate and achievable. In other words, they are more likely to experience the advice as fitting in with both their worldview and their capabilities as mothers. Even so, fewer than 35 percent of *all* American mothers currently breastfeed their babies for six months, and fewer than 20 percent breastfeed for a year, the minimum period recommended by the American Academy of Pediatrics (please see the discussion on current statistics in the introduction). Public health initiatives seek to raise the rates of initiation and duration of breastfeeding for all ethnoracial groups, but generally offer education and counseling as the main efforts in this regard—precisely the kind of promotion that Van Esterik suggests is "ethically complex" because it is likely to target individual women's choices, rather than broader social institutions and values, for reform.

In her chapter on African-American women in *At the Breast*, Linda Blum argues that black women "take their own independence" by resisting marital norms, "rejecting resonances of the historical legacies that threaten to entrap and define their bodies" (179), and *refusing to breastfeed*. Through her discussion, Blum tries to show that the decisions the black women in her study made about infant feeding and care were rational and reasoned decisions that respond to the particularities of life for African-American families in a racist and class-bound society. In this way, Blum argues against what she sees as a public health framework that represents "poorly made choices by immature or ignorant mothers" and "misunderstands mothers' own stories." While she notes that "public health frameworks ignore that health care itself is racially discriminatory, with Blacks receiving less and worse care than whites overall" (161), Blum claims that the black women in her study had "adequate information" about breastfeeding from their health care providers, but most chose not to breastfeed. Ultimately, Blum argues that "some mothers are better off rejecting breastfeeding—like these Black mothers—than feeling that they have failed at their motherly duty" (161). This argument reflects Blum's view of the public health perspective on breastfeeding—that it is primarily a "motherly duty." It also suggests that there is nothing at stake in infant feeding other than this problem of the mother's subjective feelings. Bottle feeding, as Blum argues further, helped these women cope with the material effects of racism because it allowed others to feed the baby, thereby unburdening the already burdened mother of this aspect of infant care (162).

While it is clear that Blum has been able to articulate a rich understanding of black women's perspectives on breastfeeding and motherhood in her study, it's also possible to suggest that black women are underserved by breastfeeding promotion in the context of their health care. The low rates of breastfeeding within the African-American community, given the medicalized context of infant feeding, fit with black Americans' discriminatory experiences in U.S. medicine in general. In other words, rather than mothers' resistance to white maternal norms, low rates of breastfeeding in the African-American community might indicate *neglect*, or the medical establishment's inability to connect with black women's specific concerns about infant feeding and motherhood. A 1994 study, published in the *American Journal of Public Health*, suggests such a conclusion, as the authors assert that "black women are more likely [than white women] to report *not* receiving" specific advice from their prenatal caregivers about quitting smoking and the dangers of alcohol use. The authors add that the "difference between Blacks and Whites also approached [statistical] significance for breast-feeding" (Kogan et al. 82; emphasis added).

Black women's health advocacy organizations concur, offering vital information to help black women take charge of their own health *and* get appropriate medical attention and care. The National Black Women's Health Project, the most prominent health activist organization for black women, has no links for breastfeeding on its web site, but a new organization, the African-American Breastfeeding Alliance (AABA), has recently formed. The AABA's literature emphasizes the significance of breastfeeding for African-American babies and mothers, as well as the idea that breastfeeding is a way to empower women (*An Easy Guide* 10; *Breastfeeding Education*). The materials also stress that black women may not receive appropriate prenatal advice concerning infant feeding: "Often, we do not receive adequate, or any, information on the importance of breastfeeding" (*An Easy Guide* 10).[35] Significantly, the *Easy Guide to Breastfeeding for African-American Women* indicts the "culture of bottle feeding" for impeding black women's ability to freely choose a method of infant feeding, directly contradicting the formula industry position that offering information about infant formulas is about choice: "We are not given a choice about how we want to feed our babies. We are overloaded with coupons, samples and literature from infant formula companies." The *Guide* goes on to suggest bias in standard breastfeeding promotion materials: "There are . . . many brochures, posters, etc. that show pictures of White and Hispanic women in breastfeeding situations. This lack of culturally sensitive images has greatly influenced a belief that breastfeeding is no longer a part of our community" (9). Here, the AABA materials echo traditional breastfeeding advocacy, in lamenting a lost maternal tradition through cultural influence and suggesting the health benefits of breastfeeding for infants. These same materials also target racism as a cause of the low rates of nursing in the black community.

African-American women have, in the past few years, increased their rates of breastfeeding initiation and duration more than any other studied group, but continue to lag behind white and Hispanic American women significantly. To understand black women's feeding practices, we need to understand their reproductive experiences in more detail. The Fall 2001 issue of the *Journal of the American Medical Women's Association* (JAMWA) focuses on health disparities among women; quick perusal of this issue offers the following information about health factors affecting African-American women's reproductive experiences:

> [Maternal mortality (MM)] has been higher among nonwhite than white women in the United States since 1915 (the first year for which records exist) when the nonwhite/white MM ratio was 1.76. . . . as the 20th century progressed, the gap between races in the United States *grew ever larger,* until by 1990 the MM ratio was more than 4 times higher among black women than among white women. . . . *One can speculate that part of the racial disparity in the United States may be due to poorer quality of care for minorities.* (Maine 190–91; emphasis added)

> Preterm infants suffer death, disability, and other morbidity more frequently than infants born at full gestation. . . . In 1997 and 1998, the U.S. infant mortality (IM) rate was at its lowest recorded point of 7.2 infant deaths per 1000 live births. The IM rate for black infants (14.3) was more than twice that for white infants (6.0), however. . . . In 1999, 17.6% of black infants were preterm, compared to 10.5% of white infants. Black women experience 1.7 times the risk of PTD [preterm delivery] as white women, and the disparity for very preterm births (less than 32 weeks) was even higher, with blacks experiencing 2.6 times the risk of whites (4.2% and 1.5%, respectively). A reduction in black PTD is needed to eliminate the IM disparity. (Hogan et al. 177)

> Bacterial vaginosis is a lower genital tract marker of an upper reproductive tract infection and is associated with an increased risk of PTD. *It is almost 3 times more common among African-American women than white women and could account for as much as 30% of the racial difference in PTD and IM.* It is not known why bacterial vaginosis is more prevalent among African-American women. . . . Screening for and treating bacterial vaginosis is only one prenatal care service that is not consistently delivered. . . . Studies have also shown that black women perceive that they receive lower-quality prenatal care. (Hogan et al. 179; emphasis added)

Just as it would be inappropriate to address the causes of preterm delivery without looking at both disease manifestation *and* social conditions (Hogan et al.), it seems problematical to address the health of women and children in black communities without looking at the social *and* health-related impacts of not breastfeeding. Breastfeeding rates in black communities fit a pattern of inadequate preventive health care, lack of support from providers, lack of community traditions, and high rates of particular conditions that make breastfeeding even more difficult (i.e., preterm delivery). (Breastfeeding rates for preterm infants are significantly lower than the figures for all women, although higher in hospital and at six months than the rate for black women overall [Ross Laboratories]).

Because of these factors, black women may need different kinds of support for breastfeeding, as well as a different approach from advocates. After all, it is clear that black women face a number of specific health risks with pregnancy, and these risks may make their experience through pregnancy, childbirth, and the early postpartum period different from other women's experiences, apart from social and cultural differences. Focusing on reproductive risks like preterm labor or low birth weight infants may make preparing for breastfeeding less of a priority. Lack of a tradition of breastfeeding in the African-American community can compound the social and biomedical difficulties African-American women already face.

Black breastfeeding advocates agree. At the 2001 La Leche League Seminar on Breastfeeding for Physicians and the LLL parenting conference, two African-American speakers advocated forceful promotion of breastfeeding within African-American communities. Neonatologist Michal Young, in "Promoting Breastfeeding in Vulnerable Populations," argued that African-American mothers are ill-served by the 24-hour postpartum hospital stay typically covered by insurance and Medicaid. Without a tradition of breastfeeding in the community, African-American mothers need more immediate support for initiating and continuing with breastfeeding. She stated that "many, many of the mothers believe that formula and breast milk are equal," and that family exposure to and education about breastfeeding have the most positive effect of improving rates of maternal lactation within the black population. Significantly, she addressed the issue of low self-esteem in mothers (also addressed by the AABA), stating that she asks mothers, "Why do you want what is less than best for your baby?" and commenting that "50% of the mothers who get mad at you will try [to breastfeed]."

Both Young and Inga Spurlock, an applied anthropologist who spoke at the LLL parenting conference in 2001, suggested far more assertive approaches to breastfeeding promotion than do most white breastfeeding advocates. For instance, Young said that when she has a formula-fed infant of two months of age come in with a runny nose, she tells the parents that if the baby was breastfed she or he would not have a runny nose. Spurlock similarly stated that physicians and health care providers should never "give up on a mom" suggesting that if the mother is bottle feeding, the health care provider should continue to give her positive information about breastfeeding (since there may be another baby) rather than assume that her choice with one baby will determine all of her subsequent feeding decisions. Neither of these speakers was concerned about inducing guilt in the mother who chooses to bottle feed her child; both implied that their responsibility is to articulate the best possible argument for breastfeeding in a population that could use a significant boost in health outcomes.

Spurlock listed six problems in communities of color that lead to low rates of breastfeeding: lack of a breastfeeding model in these communities, lack of support for decisions to breastfeed, lack of prenatal care generally, lack of knowledge about breastfeeding technique, lack of support for breastfeeding women, and lack of support from health care providers. She argued that obstetricians need to actively support breastfeeding by assuming that it is best and that the mother will need to get support for it. Both Spurlock and Young, in defining the issues pertinent to breastfeeding promotion among African-American women and other communities of color, assumed that breastfeeding is a public health issue and that black women and other women of color are underserved by current methods of breastfeeding promotion and support. Young specifically commented that the current stereotypes of teenage mothers work against promoting breastfeeding in this population. Yet teenagers, she said, "grow fine babies," and have done so historically. Indeed, Arline Geronimus writes, "Research has suggested that older black women [in their 20s and 30s] are *more* likely than teens to smoke, drink, use illicit drugs, be hypertensive, and have dangerously high levels of circulating blood lead during pregnancy, and that they may be *less* likely than teens to breastfeed their infants or bring them to clinics for well-child medical attention, including immunizations" (136; original emphases). Her point, and that of Inga Spurlock and Michal Young, is that to promote healthy be-haviors in specific populations of women, medical practitioners (including breastfeeding advocates) need to address in an informed way the real needs of those populations, and not perceived needs based on "routine obstetric screening protocols that apply maternal age uniformly across populations to assess risk" (Geronimus 136).

Black children who grow up poor might be especially in need of the health advantages of breastfeeding—at the National Breastfeeding Policy Conference, researcher Anne Wright asserted that "the burden of illness as-sociated with the use of formula falls disproportionately on minority infants and those in the lower socioeconomic strata" (40). In a specific example, children in poor inner-city environments experience higher rates of asthma than middle-class children, and "Black race, male gender, and preterm birth are found to be risk factors for asthma regardless of data source" (Miller). Two recent publications, one a review of prospective studies concerning breastfeeding and asthma and the other a population-based study, conclude that breastfeeding is protective against the development of asthma (Dell and To, Gdalevich et al.).[36] But poor children also represent a population most in need of structural social and economic changes in order to be breastfed. For example, black women, like working-class and poor women in general, are likely to work in jobs that do not offer an opportunity to express breast milk and save it for the baby. Because of the historical legacies of their representation as lascivious and oversexed, black women are more at risk for public censure if they breastfeed outside their homes. Patricia Hill Collins has stated that black women cannot afford to be perceived as sexual in their work environments, implying that nursing or pumping on the job would risk that perception. In order to make it possible for black women to reach the goals set out in the *HHS Blueprint for Action on Breastfeeding*—to have 50 percent of mothers breastfeeding at six months, and 25 percent breastfeeding at a year—changes to national maternity and family leave policies will have to be enacted and more effective cultural campaigns to stress the physiological normality of breastfeeding will have to take place. In addition, more effective economic and practical support for all breastfeeding mothers will have to be made available. Blum, Carter, and Law are right to suggest that it is unfair that the burdens of breastfeeding fall so completely on the bodies of already overburdened women, but the answer to this problem is not to promote bottle feeding as an "ideologically resistant" response. Rather, the answer is political action to transform the maternal burdens of all women so that breastfeeding becomes a real option for all women, and especially those women who currently find it most difficult to nurse their infants.[37]

Low rates of breastfeeding in the African-American community fit with blacks' generally discriminatory experience with the U.S. medical institution. They indicate structural neglect as well as community resistance to the norms of middle-class white mothering. By arguing for increased rates of breastfeeding by black mothers, and promoting such efforts with practical support and culturally appropriate materials, breastfeeding advocates can transform their focus on individual mother's choices and practices. At some point, "mother-to-mother" support needs to address the structural impediments to breastfeeding faced by many mothers in the United States and around the world. (Recent publications indicate that breastfeeding advocates are already moving in this direction.[38]) But if breastfeeding advocacy needs to become more feminist, feminists need to acknowledge that biological measures of health are crucial to understanding the significance of breastfeeding in the lives of women and children. The body is not just an ideological construct.

The feminist fear, of course, has been that to focus on the biological body is to court essentialism. In this scenario, to insist on the validity of biomedical arguments for breastfeeding is tantamount to consigning women to domesticity and traditional motherhood. This is why, I think, Linda Blum ends *At the Breast* with a section entitled "Partial Answers, Endless Questions."

The section itself begins, "Can breastfeeding be in women's interests in the twenty-first century? I have shown through these chapters that there is *no one* answer and *no position free of danger*" (198; first emphasis in original, second emphasis added). The dangers she refers to, however, are predominantly ideological—that is, they refer to the meanings of breastfeeding in the social sphere (whether breastfeeding represents a revaluation of female bodies or capitulation to "inhumane public and workplace demands," for example [198–99]). No danger specifically about the body itself, an identified health risk, for example, comes up. The threats are discursive, which is not to say that because they are about political meanings they are insignificant. But while Blum argues against "any assumption of one true, fixed meaning of the maternal body" (199), she doesn't notice that avoiding biological meanings unnecessarily narrows the range of meanings about the body that she can produce.

Black feminist literary critic Deborah McDowell marks a similar impoverishment of cultural studies scholarship on the body. In her afterword to the collection *Recovering the Black Female Body*, McDowell comments that "no set of meditations on 'recovering the body' with black women as its focus can fail to consider perhaps the most resonant and everyday meaning of 'recovery': to regain a state of bodily health and wellness. If the headlines can be trusted, the state of black women's bodies gives great cause for alarm" (309). She goes on to discuss rates of breast cancer and fibroid tumors among African-American women, and writes, "We can quickly lose sight of these material realities, as well as the ever-worsening socioeconomic environmental factors that place black women's health at great risk. The counterpart of these totalitarian abuses on black women's reproductive lives is the outright refusal, on the part of the medical profession, to provide their bodies the serious and specialized attention they deserve" (312–13). Noting that "Black women's children, like black women themselves, are not bodies that matter. They remain vulnerable in a system, the economies of which still operates as the functional equivalent of 'family separation' and which still places all black bodies at risk" (314), McDowell concludes that "the times call for resisting the lure of the ideal body, while mobilizing to keep the real ones alive, lest we be left with ever-dwindling bodies to represent, bodies to recover. These times call for resistance that stretches beyond discursive realms" (331–34).

Focusing on the biological body does not have to be essentialist. Obviously, the biological meaning of breastfeeding in terms of infant and maternal health is not the only meaning that should matter in discussions of the contemporary significance, and effects, of infant feeding practices. But biomedical discourses supporting maternal nursing provide feminists and health activists with a language to press for enhanced attention to needy populations of women and children and to support an expanded under-standing of women's rights. Dismissing the scientific evidence for the health benefits of breastfeeding is a problematic strategy for feminists to engage at this time, when health disparities within the United States continue to widen and women with means are the most likely to be able to breastfeed successfully. As Judith Galtry suggests, in the current American context poor women do not have a real choice in infant feeding method, because breast-feeding is generally possible only for those women with flexible professional careers and/or extensive control over their private arrangements (Galtry "'Sameness' and Suckling" 78). And *that* should be a major concern for feminist scholars and theorists.

Conclusion

The other day, a woman I know told me that she has been educating her doctor about breastfeeding. White and middle class, this mother is typical of other mothers I know in my La Leche League group, although I know her from my synagogue. The project of "educating physicians" is a well-established League anecdote. Being able to educate a physician suggests a certain amount of social power and access to resources. After all, to educate a physician about breastfeeding means that one might have to find another one; in the least it means sticking to what one knows and challenging the doctor's authority over infant feeding.

If the League mothers I know are any indication, then certain middle-class white women are involved in a long-term political battle to transform medical perspectives on infant feeding and support breastfeeding more suc-cessfully. And this is as it should be—they are using their social capital for themselves *and for other women*. In the community I live in, physicians see a wide range of clients, and if some white middle-class women are educating their physicians about breastfeeding, then that education may affect other patients. But to truly enact a feminist revolution around infant feeding, white middle-class mothers need to do more.

They need to understand that their own breastfeeding practices are largely made possible by cultural and economic privilege, and they need to work to extend the privileges that they enjoy personally to the public realm. Feminist activism around breastfeeding and breastfeeding promotion must include action for maternity leaves and specific benefits for mothers. Breastfeed-ing advocacy must pay more attention to the structural impediments to breastfeeding—economic barriers, lack of support from medical personnel, and work/family patterns—that mothers face. Mothers themselves must make the individual decision to breastfeed, but clearly education about the biological benefits of breastfeeding without real social change will only create the "exhortation to breastfeed" that Linda Blum finds so objectionable and that many women chafe against, and rightly so. Mothers must demand their rights to breastfeeding as an ordinary aspect of embodied maternity, just like pregnancy, and they should use the traditions of feminist health activism to press their cause. Mothers can come together across race and class divisions if they press for benefits *for all women* that are currently available to only a few. Breastfeeding activists must stop representing breastfeeding as a gift and articulate its practice as a right.

To admit women into the public sphere on the condition that they give up the physiological uniqueness of maternity to be there is wrong. It is also wrong to suggest that because a few well-resourced women can breastfeed, all women can and therefore should. To press for women's right to breastfeed as an ordinary aspect of embodied maternal practice, we have to argue for equality that accommodates difference, and in political terms that means benefits for mothers and significant changes to the current organization of market work. And we have to stop using the pregnant body as the symbolic marker of female difference, and see lactation as offering both a discursive and biological argument for women's rights as mothers and as human beings. Breastfeeding is a social act that is also part of biological reproduction; it represents the conundrum of sexual difference.

Epilogue: Lactation and Sexual Difference

As Linda Blum notes in *At the Breast: Ideologies of Breastfeeding and Motherhood in the Contemporary United States,* new paradigms for breastfeeding include, paradoxically, the erasure of lactation as an embodied practice of maternity. Popular and medical discourses tout the advantages of breastfeeding as part of a modern maternity that involves paid work, exercise, and travel away from the baby, all facilitated by the technological wonder of the breast pump. Blum writes, "the mother in her body, her pleasures and needs, satisfactions and pains, have been largely erased" (55). Likening this disembodiment to "the erasure of the pregnant maternal body" that occurs in the context of routine obstetrical care—emphasis on fetal monitoring and ultrasound screening for determinative information about the fetus, apart from the mother's reported experiences, for example—Blum implies that maternal disembodiment occurs when technological apparatuses mediate women's experiences of reproduction in ways that ignore the social, political, and material realities of women's lived experience. Thus, the "career-breastfeeding Supermom seems to transcend recalcitrant embodied needs, wants, or desires" (although she probably depends upon poorer women to care for her children and it isn't clear how she gets enough sleep), and laboring women are ignored by birth attendants who track fetal heart rates on the monitor print-out (59–60). Blum links this representation of disembodied motherhood directly to medical discourses of breastfeeding advocacy, noting that the American Academy of Pediatrics 1997 statement concerning breastfeeding "mentions only the need for employers to provide space and time for breast-pumping" without arguing for longer periods of paid maternity leaves. In addition, Blum suggests, "The AAP also might advocate for more on- and near-site nurseries, which are scarce, but instead it stresses the need for health insurance to cover breast-pump rentals and lactation consultant fees" (53).

Biomedical discourses supporting the biological benefit of breastfeeding can thus be appropriated to problematic sociocultural projects—in this case, the assurance, to both women and business leaders, that mothers can do the "best" for their babies while at the same time remaining productive and competent at work. The discourses promoting breast pumping as the optimal practice for working mothers of infants is not merely a repetition of the moral injunctions for maternal nursing in the eighteenth century, but a new formulation of maternal responsibility that suggests that producing breast milk is only one function among many that she is obligated to continue as a modern woman. As Blum points out, however, other ways of promoting breastfeeding are possible: the AAP *chose* to foreground pumping over other models of breastfeeding promotion, such as extended maternity leaves, which are prevalent in industrialized European countries.

Feminist inattention to breastfeeding as a maternal practice has allowed public debates to be dominated by medical practitioners, maternalist breastfeeding advocates, and business interests. Thus, prominent formulations of breastfeeding advocacy have, in the recent past, involved calls for women to stay home with infants and toddlers (this is the traditional La Leche League position), or suggested the breast pump as the technological fix to allow mothers to work outside the home and continue to breastfeed (this is a newer La Leche League position and the one advocated by the AAP).[1] Clearly, such a position places the onus of responsibility on women as mothers and workers, and places the least burden on businesses to accommodate breastfeeding mothers as employees. One result seems to be a split between women committed to a traditional model of embodied motherhood that demands their enclosure within domesticity and modern disembodied mothers who work outside the home on the condition that their maternal practices in the workplace are displaced onto the breast pump (see Blum, *At the Breast*, 57, for an interesting illustration of this idea).

Notwithstanding the recent feminist interest in the body, traditionally feminist theory has been ambivalent about the female body and its meanings. Historically, of course, many arguments about women's inferiority have been predicated on arguments about the inferiority of the female body. In the 1980s, theories that used bodily metaphors to create meanings for sexual difference—I am thinking specifically about the work of French feminists Luce Irigaray and Hélène Cixous—were criticized by some American feminists for being essentialist. Many U.S. feminists felt that these philosophers were creating ontologies of femininity rather than grounding the interpretation of women's lives in material circumstances. Currently, the cultural feminism of the 1970s is under scrutiny for its essentialisms, which are often linked to quasi-biological ideas about women's bodies. Of course, the 1990s ushered a frantic decade of feminist body studies, perhaps as scholars tired of the rarified terms of deconstructionism and French psychoanalysis and sought something more concrete to study. Yet much of feminist body scholarship tends to emphasize the body as a socially constructed product of overlapping cultural discourses, and thus to dematerialize the physical body in favor of a model of corporeal inscription.[2] The body, of course, isn't simply self-evident, but neither is it a blank slate written on by culture.

Biomedical research and related medical practice constitute prominent, culturally significant sources of representations about the body in contemporary society. Their importance will only continue to increase as the biological sciences refine their ability to produce pharmacologically significant substances in the coming years. At a talk during the 2001 La Leche League parenting conference in Chicago, global breastfeeding advocate Ted Greiner commented that researchers were working on producing "human" milk from genetically modified mice; for Greiner, this research program meant that breastfeeding advocates could no longer promote maternal nursing on the basis of breast milk as a substance. It was time, he argued, to promote breastfeeding as an experience.

Feminist intervention in this area is sorely needed.[3] Feminist scholars should confront, challenge, and work with biomedical discourses about female bodies in order to help to shape the public debates that emerge from biomedical research and practice. Yet feminist health activism and scholarship on medical institutions and practices, much of which does both contest and engage biomedicine, continue to pay little attention to breastfeeding. Emphasis is placed on reproductive practices like childbirth and fertility treatments, and on breast cancer and hysterectomies. As is clear from Linda Blum's assessment of the medical promotion of breast pumps as the technological "fix" to help working mothers continue to breastfeed, feminist discourses about mothers' right to work can be appropriated for purposes that may be at odds with feminist goals. But biomedical discourses can also be utilized by feminists to change the terrain of public debates about maternity, women's roles, and women's rights. Disembodying mothers is at best an ambivalent advance for feminism, even if many women find that this is the only way to participate in waged labor and motherhood simultaneously. Biomedical research about the biological benefits of breastfeeding could serve as a basis for arguing for other sorts of provisions for mothers, provisions that acknowledge the unique embodiment of lactation.

Indeed, such an acknowledgment might serve to question traditional models of personhood that imply that adult persons are independent, autonomous beings without encumbrances. Breastfeeding advocates speak of the mother–infant dyad as the proper object for the study of lactation. A nursing mother is physiologically linked to her dependent infant; nursing mothers necessarily have encumbrances that limit their participation in a public sphere that assumes a male model of parenthood—genetic transfer without significant physical impact on the body. What if feminists insisted on the nursing mother as a plausible model for adult autonomy; that is, a model for autonomy that admits of dependence, that accepts the unique provision of nutrition from mother to offspring, that doesn't demand mothers' disembodiment?

These are questions that my study cannot answer but inevitably points toward. In a sense, they are unanswerable right now because there has been so little research on breastfeeding from a perspective that engages biological discourses while insisting on the constructed nature of all experience. In bringing attention to the biological breastfeeding body in this way, I am not arguing that breastfeeding and maternity are not sociocultural practices. Rather, I am suggesting that responsible research on representations of breastfeeding, breastfeeding advocacy, and feminism must attend to biomedical discourses about lactation and the information about the body that those discourses offer. To neglect this dimension of the cultural context of maternity is to participate in the disembodiment of motherhood, since these are the most prominent public representations of the physical significance of nursing that currently exist. Ignoring these discourses has the effect of conceptualizing breastfeeding as an ideological, rather than a material, practice; a practice that has effects in the realm of cultural discourses and social meanings, but not on the physical body. To engage biomedical discourses politically is to make them work *for women* as a statement about mothers' rights to certain forms of embodied maternal experience, and to challenge the presumption that the bodily experiences of maternity (can and should) mean nothing to women's participation in market work and civic life. To be sure, this approach is not without difficulty: there is a fine line between a feminist maternalism that reorients current philosophical conceptions about the body and personhood by using biomedical accounts of maternity against their usual bias toward conservative social views, and a maternalism that simply uses biomedical discourses for traditionalist ends. This is the dilemma of La Leche League, as I discussed in chapter 5. The fine line is, however, what I am proposing to draw; the preceding study traverses that line and attempts to demonstrate the benefit of defining it, in order to argue for breastfeeding as an important subject for feminist analysis and, potentially, an important material practice of sexual difference.

Notes

Introduction

1. In case the reader is curious, reality pretty much followed this script.
2. See Rothman, *In Labor*, and Davis-Floyd, as examples. Other authors who write in this field are Oakley, Kitzinger, and Adams. The Boston Women's Health Book Collective provides a discussion of childbirth that presents feminist perspectives while affirming women's different decisions in birth practice.
3. Adrienne Berney, in her suggestive and interesting dissertation, *Reforming the Maternal Breast*, does a good job in complicating Apple's argument, claiming that cultural transformations in the period 1870–1940 were instrumental in changing infant feeding practices away from breastfeeding and toward the more mechanized and quantifiable practices of bottle feeding. See also Yoshioka.
4. Current figures present an optimistic upturn at the end of the twentieth century. See discussion in the text.
5. There is a growing literature on male lactation. Jared Diamond's work notwithstanding, breastfeeding is still considered to be a physiological function of the female sex. It may be that male lactation will change the scenario I discuss here. See Diamond; also Giles, *Fresh Milk*, 187–99.
6. The current feminist tendency of linking middle-class white women's experiences and practices with the *problems* attendant to such privileged status is an example of what Lisa Ruddick calls "the summoning of the near enemy":

   > People can often become ethically confused because of a particular problem inherent in human dealings, namely, that any virtue has a bad cousin, a failing that closely resembles the virtue and can be mistaken for it—what in Tibetan Buddhism is called the *near enemy*.... For example, let us say that there is such a thing as *decency*, which is a virtue. In the interest of decency, a person could refrain from taking credit for someone else's ideas, or forgo the thrill of humiliating a colleague. A second meaning of the word "decency," though, is adherence to a set of communal norms that are really a screen for class bias or prejudice. Thus in the name of decency, people can be condemned for wishing to read books about sex, or parents can pressure their children into securing a "decent" income and achieving a "decent" middle-class lifestyle.
   >   What current critical theory often does, though, is to *collapse the difference*, making the good thing look bad by calling it the name of its near enemy—saying that anyone who speaks up for decency is imposing an oppressive social norm (B9; emphases in original).

   White middle-class women have become the "near enemy" in much feminist writing, in which their practices are understood to be signs of the negativity of their privilege. Ruddick writes, "With numbing regularity, one finds articles that make cogent and indeed powerful claims about how bourgeois discourses, as they appear in one literary text or another, construct or engender in the reader a commitment to a repressive moralism, or to a particular kind of complacent, sentimental compassion. Yet these articles are usually silent on whether there is any kind of moral intuition or compassion that is not just an oppressive bourgeois illusion" (B9). Instead of this kind of paralyzing analysis, we might try to produce social contexts in which all women have access to some of the privileges (time, resources, status) that allow white middle-class women to practice their mothering in relative ease and social acceptance.
7. "Dry nursing" is a term that refers to feeding infants with animal milks, paps, or gruels. "Hand feeding" is another term that refers to the same practice. Paps are foods made from

mixing flour, water, and milk together. Janet Golden notes, "As bottles became the more common device [for artificial feeding], the term most often used became 'bottle-feeding'" (9).

8. See Golden, and Fildes, *Wet Nursing: A History from Antiquity to the Present*, for general historical discussions of wet nursing.

9. Valerie Lastinger agrees with Perry. In "Re-defining Motherhood: Breastfeeding and the French Enlightenment," she writes, "Although on the surface the revival of maternal nursing had infant survival as its main purpose, one prime consequence was to tie women to the home more securely at a time when women in France were becoming a strong political force." Even though "Maternal nursing had the advantage of both keeping women at home *and improving infants' survival*," she concludes that "Along with Perry . . . , we have to . . . consider that the breastfeeding campaign was part of a broader effort to manage women through motherhood." Lastinger suggests that "for many women the employment of wet-nurses was very successful," although she does not delineate what she means by "success." Presumably she means that the baby survived, although as far as I can tell she does not consider the wet nurse's child in the least.

10. For the paradigmatic theoretical treatise on this topic, see Michel Foucault's "The Politics of Health in the Eighteenth Century," especially page 172. Foucault argues that the medicalization of the family begins in the eighteenth century, as opposed to the historical accounts of breastfeeding in nineteenth-century America that I discuss in this chapter, and links calls for maternal nursing to the mechanism of social control and surveillance through familial regulation of health.

11. Rima Apple's *Mothers and Medicine* also, at the very end, takes account of the biological significance of breastfeeding in comparison to bottle feeding, but is quite circumspect in its conclusions about the health effects of changing infant feeding patterns in the twentieth century. Indeed, my main frustration with this book was that the author seemed overly careful in her attempts to not articulate a stand in relation to one form of infant feeding over another (which is usually what a consideration of biological discourses entails).

12. Pure milk was milk undiluted and devoid of additives. It might also be certified. See Berney 365–69 for a lengthy discussion. See also Wolf 42–73.

13. This process, which Jacquelyn Litt calls "medicalized motherhood," was not continuous, and created deep divides in the experience of motherhood by women of different groups. In *Medicalized Motherhood,* Litt shows that poor and working-class African-American women in the 1930s and 1940s remained largely outside the middle-class frame of scientific motherhood that came to define good mothering in the twentieth century. This perhaps explains why breastfeeding rates among poor white and African-American women declined later than the rates of white middle-class women, and why rates in the former group are currently lower than rates of the latter group now that breastfeeding has been defined as a practice of scientific motherhood.

14. Kumiko Yoshioka argues, in a very interesting paper, that in the early twentieth century, breastfeeding and artificial feeding with modified cow's milk are grouped together against other proprietary infant foods. She concludes that formula feeding and breastfeeding are linked necessarily by a logic that defines one as the impossible ideal that the other aspires to.

15. Much of the discussion of chapter 5 of Haraway's *Modest Witness*, "The Virtual Speculum of the New World Order" (especially the section "The Statistics of Freedom Rights"), concerns these issues. See also "Situated Knowledges."

16. Ideas in this section are drawn from a variety of sources; significantly, Jack Newman's 1995 *Scientific American* article, "How Breast Milk Protects Newborns," was helpful in providing lay language for specific immunological mechanisms.

17. Indeed, breastfeeding folklore suggests using breast milk to cure pink eye (conjunctivitis), a common illness among children in communal day care situations. I can testify to the success of this practice, which also stings less than the traditional eye drops prescribed by physicians. Because breast milk contains both antiviral and antibacterial factors, it can be helpful in eradicating both kinds of pink eye, while prescription drops only work for bacterial conjunctivitis.

18. Ball and Wright state that "Compared with 1,000 infants who were breastfed exclusively for [greater than or equal to] 3 months, the never-breastfed group experienced 60 more episodes of LRI [lower respiratory infection] and 580 more episodes of OM [otitis media, or ear infection] after adjusting for maternal education and smoking. These children also

experienced 1,053 more episodes of gastrointestinal illness. For 1,000 never-breastfed infants, there were [greater than] 609 excess prescriptions and 80 excess hospitalizations, relative to 1,000 infants breastfed exclusively for 3 months" (872).

19. Ball and Wright note that "Studies of the costs associated with formula-feeding are limited by the fact that it is ethically impossible to conduct a randomized, controlled trial of breast-feeding. The best alternative is to carefully select methodologically strong cohort studies that include appropriate data and to adjust for significant covariates, as we have done here" (875).

20. See Fraser (ed.), *The Bell Curve Wars*.

21. The authors also suggest that "the overall pattern of results suggests that no additional positive [intelligence] effects are associated with breastfeeding after 9 months," a position refuted by many breastfeeding advocates (2370).

22. Because of these acknowledged problems in the scientific research, it seems problematic to me that popular breastfeeding advocacy states in unqualified language that breastfeeding will make your baby smarter, as I saw recently on a poster.

23. See Guttman and Zimmerman's article, "Low-Income Mothers' Views on Breastfeeding," for a discussion of factors other than a belief in the benefits of breastfeeding that affect mothers' decisions concerning infant feeding method.

24. There has always been, within American medicine at least, a perception that breastfeeding is more healthful than bottle feeding. What changed beginning in the late nineteenth century was physicians' sense of women's capacity to breastfeed, and their growing acceptance of their ability to monitor bottle fed infants and help them to grow adequately. See Apple, *Mothers and Medicine*.

25. In "The Politics of Health in the Eighteenth Century," Foucault argues that medicalization of infant feeding occurred through the medicalization of the family as the main unit to promote health. It seems to me that the process he analyzes in the eighteenth century reaches a certain critical stage with the development of proprietary infant foods in the nineteenth century (*Power/Knowledge* 166–82).

26. Riordan and Auerbach write that "most health care providers now recognize" the benefits of breastfeeding (22), but the health care workers I have met at La Leche League seminars on breastfeeding for physicians routinely denounce their colleagues' lack of understanding about the mechanics of breastfeeding, and the too-quick reliance on supplementation with formula as an answer to any breastfeeding difficulty. Anecdotal evidence from La Leche League leaders and members supports this view.

27. A recent article in *American Family Physician,* adapted from *Pediatrics,* reports on a study indicating that "less than two-thirds of residents or practitioners knew to advise the mother to continue exclusive breastfeeding" if the mother called in with worries about her milk supply. The study also showed that "only 52% of residents and 64% of pediatricians knew that formula supplementation during the first two weeks of lactation was a cause of breastfeeding failure" (Huffman 1–2). The residents and practitioners studied were pediatric residents and attending physicians.

28. They also suggest contacting La Leche League as a source for breastfeeding advice, specifically noting that physicians often know little about breastfeeding, although in earlier editions of *Our Bodies, Ourselves* they also stated that they did not feel that breastfeeding had to define one's mothering experience.

29. Ironically, it was initially middle- and upper-class women who first gave up nursing as a demographic group, to be followed by poorer women. The trend now is exactly the opposite.

30. For example, knowing that depression and mood disorders are, at least in part, social constructions does not necessarily mean that we won't use Prozac or another psychopharmacological treatment.

31. Dr. Lawrence Gartner informed me, by e-mail, that the Ross Mothers Survey is not a very sophisticated instrument: the survey is "not done with such precision or sampling methods that really allow [it] to be looked upon as scientific data." The Mothers Survey, however, shows up as a source all over the World Wide Web, and it is used by the Department of Health and Human Services as the basis for its *Healthy People 2010 Conference Report* and the *HHS Blueprint for Action on Breastfeeding*. That latter document was published in October 2000 and uses the figures from the 1998 Mothers Survey. I include the figures from the most recent survey, but augment the discussion with the *HHS Blueprint*.

32. Women, Infants, and Children, a federal program providing nutritional support for poor women and children.

33. The attempt to make breastfeeding easier for working mothers does, of course, address the issue of women's roles in contemporary society, but only in order to argue for workplace accommodation of working mothers and not in order to examine the social context that idealizes stay-at-home mothers but doesn't provide the real accommodation of extended maternity leave to all mothers.

34. Exceptions to this mapping include higher rates of breastfeeding in the Pacific and mountain states, and lower rates in the south and east.

Chapter 1

1. My account of this case is drawn from the presentation and discussion about it at the 2000 La Leche League Seminar on Breastfeeding for Physicians, as well as the accounts presented in the New York press following the death of the infant and during the trial. See Tipograph, et al.

2. This information indicates a number of red flags, danger signs that she was at a high risk for breastfeeding failure. The most significant are her previous breast surgery and the fact that the baby was not breastfeeding consistently for the first week and a half of its life.

3. The idea that education makes women unfit for motherhood has a long history in the United States. See Carroll Smith-Rosenberg, *Disorderly Conduct: Visions of Gender in Victorian America*, for discussion of this concept. This notion has been replaced in the twentieth century with the idea that all women need special education to be mothers, and that this education should come from and be practiced under the supervision of physicians or other scientific experts. See Rima Apple, *Mothers and Medicine: A Social History of Infant Feeding, 1890–1950*, for discussion of this development.

4. In 1999 I attended the annual La Leche League Seminar on Breastfeeding for Physicians, in Buena Vista, Florida. Naomi Baumslag, a well-known breastfeeding advocate and medical doctor, gave a talk that essentially revolved around images of dead babies and the horror that these images evoke. Some members of the audience commented that the talk was a bit odd, since she was clearly preaching to the converted. I interpret that response, in part, as referring to the dead babies that proliferated in the slide show. The audience was made up of people for whom the rhetoric of the dead baby was unnecessary, as they were already involved in advocacy for breastfeeding as a way to avoid infant death, especially in the Third World. Thus, the "preaching to the converted" response meant that they didn't feel the need to see more dead babies, as they had been convinced previously of the cause. The dead babies as well as the rhetoric of the presentation and slides were perceived as hyperbolic; audience murmurs suggested many felt the talk should be targeted to other audiences on whom the images had not yet had an effect.

5. In Palmer, *Politics*, the caption reads "Mother of twins. The child with the bottle is a girl—she died the next day. Her twin brother was breastfed. This woman's mother-in-law told her she didn't have enough milk for both children, so she breastfed the boy. She certainly could have fed both, because suckling induces milk production. Even if she could not produce sufficient milk—unlikely as that would be—a better alternative would have been a wet-nurse. Ironically, this could have been the grandmother, a common practice before the advent of bottle-feeding. (UNICEF 1992: *Photo* by Mustaq Khan)" (270).

6. A *Salon* article on the Tabitha Walrond case is entitled "Nursed to Death" (Houppert). Thanks to Donna Lisker for sending me this article.

7. In the late 1990s Kathleen Tyson, an HIV-positive mother stopped antiretroviral treatment (AZT) during her pregnancy and decided to breastfeed her newborn son. The baby was taken from her by the state. For her view of the situation in 1999, see Tyson, "In the Eye of the Storm."

8. The actual rate of HIV transmission from infected mothers to infants through breastfeeding is not known. Most HIV transmission from mother to infant occurs during childbirth, although use of specific drugs can cut the rate of transmission substantially. In the first weeks and months postpartum, newborns cannot be accurately tested for HIV infection because their systems continue to carry their mother's antibodies. It has been suggested that the highest rates of HIV transmission from mother to child occur when breastfeeding does not occur exclusively, i.e., when breast milk is supplemented with formula, other animal milks, or other foods. Breastfeeding advocates often find themselves at odds with AIDS researchers

concerning issues of HIV transmission during breastfeeding. For example, "Very little is known about the impact of not breastfeeding in communities where breastfeeding is the cultural norm, for instance, in Africa. Scant attention has been paid to the social stigma of not breastfeeding, which would immediately identify a woman as HIV-positive, nor to the implications for increased fertility and population growth if the contraceptive effects of breastfeeding were no longer available to African women" (Morrison and Greiner 27). The World Alliance for Breastfeeding Action (WABA) states that "every mother has a right to know her HIV status, and to be fully informed about the risks of alternative infant feeding choices" (WABA Steering Committee). See also Coutsoudis.

9. See also Patricia Hill Collins, *Black Feminist Thought: Knowledge, Consciousness, and the Politics of Empowerment.*

10. See Roberts, *Killing the Black Body: Race, Reproduction, and the Meaning of Liberty,* as well as "The Value of Black Mothers' Work" (in *Critical Race Feminism*).

11. See Maher, "Breast-Feeding and Maternal Depletion."

12. For example, a March 12, 1992, editorial in the *New York Times* begins "In countries like the United States, breast-feeding, though always desirable, doesn't mean the difference between good and poor nutrition—or life and death. But it does in developing countries . . . In all, the United Nations Children's Fund estimates, at least a million infants die every year because they aren't adequately breastfed" ("Breast Milk for the World's Babies"). See also Faul.

13. Black infants, on the other hand, have an infant mortality rate two to three times higher than white infants, are more likely to be born prematurely or with a low birth weight, and have a higher risk of dying of sudden infant death syndrome (SIDS).

14. It's unclear if Mr. Helliker has any data to support his causal claim here.

15. See Riordan and Auerbach, p. 64.

16. In a 1996 article for the *Philadelphia Inquirer,* Natalie Pompilio notes that "When legislation in Virginia declared that breast-feeding did not constitute indecent exposure, for example, officials said they feared hordes of *topless women* flocking to the beaches, either nursing or pretending to" (emphasis added). In addition, see Collins, *Black Feminist Thought,* for a discussion of the "controlling images" of black women in contemporary culture (67–90). She identifies the Jezebel as the "whore, or sexually aggressive woman . . . [whose function it] was to relegate all Black women to the category of sexually aggressive women" (77).

17. Given the resurgence of breastfeeding under the sign of scientific motherhood, in the context of medical research to extol the values of breastfeeding, there emerges a conflict between the "respectability" of bottle feeding in relation to the mother's body and the expectation that mothers should comply with new recommendations of the American Academy of Pediatrics to breastfeed their infants for at least a year.

18. And in hindsight, I don't know precisely what I said, since I didn't write down my question. I do know that I prefaced my question with the statement "I am writing a book about breastfeeding and feminism," and it may have been that statement that provoked the hostility from Collins. In her view, I was really writing about (and out of) white feminism and breastfeeding, and she clearly thought that I was engaging the terms of the breast–bottle controversy to denigrate black women's infant feeding choices.

19. All quotations from this session were transcribed by the author (who was also in attendance) from tapes made available by the seminar organizers. "Ums" and "ahs" have been excised from the comments, although grammatical idiosyncrasies remain. In addition, the names of audience members who made comments have been left out of the discussion, although I have included the names of presenters.

20. The 1999 La Leche League International Parenting conference was called "Breastfeeding: Wisdom from the Past—Gold Standard for the Future."

21. In response to the suggestion that physicians get credentials in breastfeeding medicine, Lawrence Gartner, moderator of the seminar and a longstanding promoter of breastfeeding within the American Academy of Pediatrics and the newly formed Academy of Breastfeeding Medicine, said, "I don't think that we should make the basic knowledge into a specialty, because I think every physician—I mean this is something that involves such a broad spectrum of our medical practice, you can't limit to a few; it's not like neurosurgeons or other areas, it's got to be a broad spectrum. I think we do need experts and I think in this room we have a number of people who are really experts in the field of breastfeeding who are the educators, the researchers, and people like that who are the Ph.D. level of knowledge and maybe they

should be credentialed, maybe that's not a bad idea just to give them some credibility through a title, but I think the great majority of people, all the physicians really, do need to have some basic knowledge."

22. Mothers writing in to La Leche League's *New Beginnings* magazine often discuss public or familial pressures to feed with formula, while Peggy Robin's *When Breastfeeding Is Not an Option* (formerly *Bottle Feeding without Guilt*) begins with an extended discussion of how mothers who feed with formula experience frequent public criticisms of that practice.

23. Katha Pollitt, in "A Bronx Tale," comments, "This is family-values America, where mothers and only mothers are held responsible for their children's well-being, even as fathers decamp and communities and social services fall apart. . . . You need a lot of information and a lot of support, and we're not living in villages where these things are part of the social fabric, where breast-feeding is part of life and every woman is able to instruct new mothers." See also Ann Crittendon, *The Price of Motherhood: Why the Most Important Job in the World Is Still the Least Valued*. For a perspective on black women's mothering in a racist society, see Dorothy Roberts, "The Value of Black Mothers' Work."

24. Susan Tipograph stated, "In terms of the breastfeeding advice that Tabitha [unclear syllable]– this was a kid who was really inspired. She read stuff; I mean she had the *Time/Life* book on babies. . . . And unfortunately she read some of the literature, that I took a look at the package, and I read some of the literature that's given out in these packages, and I'm sure it's very helpful to 99 percent of the women who it's given out to, but it's really unhelpful and potentially dangerous to the one or two or three percent of women who are either at risk or who have breastfeeding problems, because it says—I believe in cheerleading breastfeeding also, but you can't cheerlead in a way that's gonna deny women who are, have potential problems, particularly women who don't have access to unlimited medical care, or lactation counselors, or who wouldn't know La Leche if they fell over it, or they don't have a telephone in any case."

25. With regard to Tabitha Walrond's mother, who had breastfed Tabitha, Susan Tipograph said, "And, you know, they lived in one room, her, the mother, Tabitha, and the baby all slept together, so the, on some level, the same reasons why Tabitha wouldn't have noticed the weight loss apply to the mother as well, although, I had friends when I took this case and I told them the story they all, their responses were all that they should put Tabitha's mother in jail. I mean, there was a way in which she got blamed also, and I do certainly think she was more responsible than her child, because she was older and better educated, but I think she suffered from the same sort of feeling, [a] sense of both excitement and being thrilled about having a grandchild but feeling helpless and overpowered by a system that didn't seem to really sort of give a damn about them."

26. "Up to a point, [Anthony Bosco, a juror] said, he could give credence to testimony from lactation experts that breast-feeding mothers with insufficient milk frequently do not notice an infant's weight loss because they see the baby every day. But Mr. Bosco, a reservations manager at a midtown hotel, said the emaciated condition of the baby in the photographs appeared too severe to miss" (Bernstein, "Bronx Woman Convicted," B1).

27. Katha Pollitt comments, "Tipograph told me she received many letters from such women [well-off, well-educated women] with stories much like Walrond's. The difference is that those women had private pediatricians, and their babies' problems were caught in time— although sometimes only just."

Being regularly seen by a doctor, the assumption of current well-baby provisions in health insurance, of course, is a very contemporary view of infant care, and it became normalized in the context of increasing expectation of infant and child survival. Although infant mortality rates in the United States are higher than those in most other developed countries, many more infants currently survive into adulthood than in previous historical eras. Much of the improvement in infant mortality results from improved sanitation and higher standards of living (Apple, *Mothers and Medicine*). An interesting fictional representation of infant death due to failure to thrive is presented in Mary Austin's *A Woman of Genius* (originally published in 1912). The protagonist gives birth to a "delicate baby": "My baby, too, poor little man, was feeble from birth, a bottle baby; the best that could have been done would hardly have been a chance for him" (79); "To this day I cannot come across any notices of the more competent methods for the care of delicate children, without a remembering pang" (80). The grandmother at first dominates with her assumption of superior knowledge about infant care, and the mother feels she cannot supersede with her more modern notions, gained through *reading*: "I made a fight for him, tried to interpose such scraps of better knowledge as had come to me through reading, but they made no headway against my mother's confidential, 'Well, I ought to know, I've buried five,' and against Forester [her brother] . . . who overbore with ridicule my suggestion that he should be fed at regular hours, for which I never forgave him" (79). Later, the grandmother is more solicitous of the mother's situation, when it is clear that the baby will die. The baby died at about nine months of age, clearly "failing to thrive."

In Austin's representation, the mother has a premonition that the baby is failing, but in fact cannot really see it—she is instead enveloped in exhaustion and uncertainty. The grandmother comes to visit, and *sees*: "She was quite excited . . . and then as soon as she had sight of the child, I saw her checked and startled inquiry travel from me to Tommy and back to the child's meagre little features, and a new and amazing tenderness in all her manner to me" (82). Failure to thrive was never a welcomed outcome for infants, but when infant mortality was much higher it was, perhaps, a more expected outcome. Note in this representation conflicts between regulated and unregulated feedings, and between traditional and modern (educated) maternal knowledge. What's ironic, of course, is the mother's sense that greater regulation might have saved her infant son, when contemporary biomedical research has repudiated this early-twentieth-century faith in mechanistic approaches to infant care.

With regard to expectations about infant death, anthropologist Nancy Scheper-Hughes writes, "I argue that in the absence of a firm grounding for the expectancy of child survival, maternal thinking and practice are grounded in a set of assumptions . . . that contribute even further to an environment that is dangerous, even antagonistic, to new life" (20). She elaborates, "[I]n many Third World countries mired in a relatively crude form of dependent capitalism and still characterized by a high mortality and a high, untamed fertility, the naturalness of infant and child mortality has yet to be questioned, and parents may understand a baby's life as a provisional and undependable thing—a candle whose flame is as likely to flicker and go out as to burn brightly and continuously. There, child death may be viewed less as a tragedy than as a predictable and relatively minor misfortune, one to be accepted with equanimity and resignation as an unalterable fact of human existence" (275).

28. There is also the issue of overseeing failure to thrive—mothers used to media images of big babies or not familiar with the different growth patterns of breastfed babies, worrying about smaller or slower growing infants who are perfectly healthy. My first child was a big baby at birth (over eight pounds) and continued in the 90th percentile for height and weight well into her second year. She was 19 pounds at 6 months and 24 at a year. She was built like a tank—solid and heavy. Her younger brother, Sam, was bigger at birth (over nine pounds) although he looked spindly, being longer. In the first few months after birth he slipped between the 10th and 25th percentiles for weight, while reaching the 75th percentile for height. He gained steadily in that pattern, which means that he was (and is) tall and thin. He weighed 19 pounds at a year of age and a bit over 24 pounds when he was two (that is, he weighed at two years what my daughter weighed at one). Because of the comparison with my daughter, I worried about him and pestered the doctor: Is he gaining enough weight? Is there a problem? My family practice physician, bless his heart, always said "He's on the charts and he's growing consistently. Don't worry." Thus the height and weight charts posed a problem for me—his height and weight seemed disproportionate, compared to Rachel's solid march at the top of the curve—but the charts also provided comforting information: he was on the charts and his numbers stayed roughly in the same relation to each other over time. These charts helped me to put aside my maternal worries over his well-being—to see a thin infant and not a starving one. Yet when I look at photographs now, I think, "He looks fatter than I remember him." This makes me think that my own perceptions were overly affected by my perception of what a normal baby should look like. (I should note here that standard growth charts for infants and children are based on bottle-feeding norms. There are situations in which breastfed infants are off the charts but nevertheless healthy.)

29. Susan Tipograph made this point as well about Tyler Walrond: "Now I understand in England they have a name for this syndrome, which is called happy to starve. This was a child who seemed happy to starve."

30. Of course, the bottle-feeding mother would also, presumably, see her baby pretty often.

31. In this case, the baby died at five weeks of age and there was specific evidence that the mother, Tatania Cheeks, had been turned away from a hospital for a scheduled appointment

for the infant at one week postpartum because she didn't have enough money to pay for the visit. There was no such clear evidence in the Walrond case, although the defendant claimed that she had made attempts to make an appointment for the child. Presumably, there was no evidence that she had *tried* to do so, while Tatania Cheeks had an appointment on the books that she was not allowed to attend.

32. Nancy Scheper-Hughes makes similar comments about the physical status of dying and dead babies in the favelas of northeastern Brazil, in *Death without Weeping*.

33. Thanks to Amy Nichols for pointing this out to me.

34. See also Small, p. 219, for a discussion of differential growth and size of Latino babies.

35. This information comes directly after information about how much weight an infant should gain (4–8 ounces a week after the first three weeks of life). Yet it is also preceded by the following sentence: "Family characteristics and the baby's individual makeup need to be considered" (La Leche League, *The Womanly Art*, 6th ed., 74). Tabitha's mother reportedly told her that she was a small baby.

36. Sollinger writes, "The focus on mind rendered white illegitimate pregnancy essentially asexual. White women got pregnant without husbands due to higher order, psychological causes.... Without the benefit of cultural institutions as mediators, the sex behavior of black females was constructed as a natural expression, once again, of biological urges" (61).

37. In another stereotype, black women are often represented as welfare cheats, having babies to get on welfare and receive a monthly check. In the context of this view, a black woman would have to be crazy to let her child die. In the trial, the prosecution argued that Tabitha Walrond neglected her child in order to get back at the father for his abandonment of her while she was pregnant (they broke up, and he began seeing another woman, who also became pregnant by him). Thus, their argument hinged on her being crazy, but in a vindictive sense.

38. Deep breast pain during nursing can also indicate a thrush infection or, if the pain continues when the baby is not nursing, mastitis (bacterial breast infection). See Giles, *Fresh Milk*, pp. 83–99 for a discussion of breast pain while nursing and of bleeding nipples.

39. This means that the milk-producing tissue of the breast does not develop during pregnancy, indicating that the breast tissue does not respond to the changing hormonal conditions of pregnancy and nursing, and will probably not produce enough milk.

40. Indeed, Susan Tipograph suggests that "if it happens to Tabitha Walrond, it will happen to other women. And certainly, the other women, who are, who are converts. I mean women, poor women, and women of color, are the women who most should be breastfeeding. These are the women who believe that in order to, to be viewed as being good mothers for their children they have to spend money that they don't have to buy, to buy formula. And let me tell you, when they see pictures day after day in the media in New York of a young black women being prosecuted for breastfeeding and killing her child, I can't tell you how many women are gonna be discouraged from breastfeeding: far more than are gonna be frightened from doing something by watching a piece on *20/20* which raises, which raises problems."

41. Susan Tipograph, in her presentation to the Seminar on Breastfeeding, claimed that Tyler Walrond did exhibit the signs indicated in the guidebooks, such as the designated number of wet and soiled diapers per day.

42. Ginney Fowler, Dan Mosser, and Laura Tze all provided me with videotapes of these programs.

43. The *Chicago Hope* episode, "The Breast and the Brightest," begins with the following scene, an early morning staff meeting at the hospital:

White Male Chief of Staff: We can't start without Diane. There are items on the agenda which directly affect her.
White Female Neurologist: Well it's not like her to be late. Shall we page her?
Black Male Pediatrician: Did already.
Black Male Emergency Room Physician: Can we at least talk about this Baby-Friendly nonsense?
Black Male Pediatrician: What nonsense? It's a contract stating that the hospital feels that breastfeeding is best for the baby.
White Female Neurologist: Forcing women to breastfeed? It's a little Orwellian.
Black Male Pediatrician: They're not forced, they're encouraged.
Black Male ER Physician: But we're not allowed to send them home with formula. That seems like pretty heavy encouragement.

Black Male Pediatrician: Are you challenging the obvious health benefits of breastfeeding?

Black Male ER Physician: I'm not challenging anything.

White Male Orthopedist: Where's the contract for the dad to sign stating that he won't beat the crap out of the kid?

White Male Neurologist: Phillip, I think your meeting has begun.

[At this point, the white female cardiology surgeon makes an announcement that she is going to be participating in NASA training for a space mission to pursue some medical experiments.]

White Male Chief of Staff: Will someone please page Diane again?

The scene then cuts to Diane (white female internist and sometimes ER physician), in the bathroom, pumping her breasts. The first shot is of a Medela Lactina Plus, and the camera follows the tubing up to Diane, who is sitting on a toilet pumping one breast while talking on a cell phone to her husband, who is having some trouble calming the baby. Her beeper goes off, and while she checks it, she does not call back. The scene ends as she sings a children's song to the baby over the cell phone.

Later in the show, the mother of the dead baby indicates that she was complying with the Baby-Friendly contract that she signed, and the parents sue the hospital due to the Baby-Friendly contract.

The Baby-Friendly Hospital Initiative is not even a contract that the hospital makes with WHO or UNICEF. Birth facilities in the United States send a letter of intent to become Baby-Friendly to Baby-Friendly USA, whereupon they receive a Certificate of Intent, which is given out without verification. To be certified as Baby-Friendly, the facility must undergo an on-site assessment of its protocols and practices regarding infant feeding, breastfeeding education for patients and staff, and maternity care. Thus, being Baby-Friendly is a *designation* that follows from hospital policies and practices, rather than a binding contract that the hospital signs and then must force itself to adhere to. See Baby-Friendly USA.

44. Step 6 may cause some confusion. According to Laura Ingvall, RN, lactation counselor at Baby-Friendly USA, *mothers* can feed their infants with formula at hospitals designated as Baby-Friendly. The mother's choice would be noted in the infant's chart, at which point formula feeding becomes the de facto medically indicated method of infant feeding for that baby. Once indicated, nurses could feed the baby formula as well. Baby-Friendly hospitals simply have policies in place to promote and support breastfeeding, and they do away with policies or practices that tacitly support bottle feeding, such as sending mothers home with packets of free formula (personal communication, 13 Feb. 2001).

45. In late 2001, a case of infant death began making its way through the courts, and the newspapers, in Washington, DC. The child was a seven-month-old baby born to a black mother already supervised by social service agencies for possible negligent care of other offspring. The mother claims she fed the baby formula on a regular schedule but that he did not gain weight. Interestingly, in published accounts of this case, infant feeding method is not an issue, unlike the Tabitha Walrond case, where breastfeeding and infant death were conceptually linked. See Higham and Horwitz, and Santana.

46. The fact that she is concentrating on many so-called optimizing practices of motherhood—black and white toys are thought to stimulate brain development, for example—demonstrates this mother's middle-class status.

47. Diane, the breastfeeding doctor, is adamant about her right to work when she is questioned by the chief of staff about whether she is ready to come back, but her neighbor tells her that she herself "couldn't do that" [go to work] because she'd miss all that time with her baby.

48. See Roberts, *Killing the Black Body,* for a discussion of this issue.

Chapter 2

1. Both Katherine Dettwyler and Lawrence Gartner confirmed this point to me in personal communications over electronic mail.

2. Antoinette Brown Blackwell argued, in *The Sexes throughout Nature,* that since women provide "primary nutrition" to their young, men's "biological role" was to provide secondary nutrition to the entire family. In other words, Blackwell believed that if women had to nurse then men should do the marketing and cooking.

3. The idea that the child receives maternal qualities along with the milk is an old one, and is especially prominent in advice literature concerning choosing a wet nurse. See Fildes, *Wet Nursing*. Katherine Dettwyler suggests that nursing older toddlers and children might be more visible if many mothers didn't choose to do so privately; of course, such a choice is clearly influenced by the censure of public culture. See Dettwyler, "A Time to Wean," 57–58.

4. As D'Emilio does when he writes, "Human sexual desire need no longer be harnessed to reproductive imperatives, to procreation; its expression has increasingly entered the realm of choice. Lesbians and homosexuals most clearly embody this split, since our gay relationships stand entirely outside a procreative framework. The acceptance of our erotic choices ultimately depends on the degree to which society is willing to affirm sexual expression as a form of play, positive and life-enhancing. Our movement may have begun as the struggle of a 'minority,' but what we should now be trying to 'liberate' is an aspect of the personal lives of all people—sexual expression" (175). This elevation of sexual expression over reproduction as the meaning of sexuality—play not procreation—is utopian in its scope: certainly human sexual desire is in the realm of choice only for certain individuals in particular circumstances. Throughout the world, most women experience most of their adult lives in some maternal condition or role.

5. Oddly enough, Eisenberg, Murkoff, and Hathaway's popular *What to Expect When You're Expecting* includes the following comment, as part of a response to the ostensible question "Ever since the baby was born I just don't feel very interested in sex": "If you are breastfeeding, this may unconsciously be satisfying your sexual needs" (404). This might suggest that popular culture accepts the notion of maternal sexuality, although on closer analysis I would note that the idea that nursing *unconsciously* satisfies the sexual needs of the mother clears her of any suspect sexual sensibility (which would have to be conscious). After all, she can't control what goes on unconsciously. As the rest of the passage goes on to suggest modes of reconnecting sexually with one's (male) spouse, the impact of the idea that a nursing mother gains sexual satisfaction from breastfeeding disappears; and after all, since it was unconscious, she doesn't really know about it *or experience it* as sexuality per se. This is, in Rossi's terms, sexual pleasure in service of the species.

6. See also Dettwyler, "Promoting Breastfeeding or Promoting Guilt?"

7. At the 1999 La Leche League International conference, a WIC (Women, Infants, and Children) counselor group from Texas presented a poster display of their recent program to promote breastfeeding among WIC mothers, which involved education *plus* peer counselors. The woman I spoke with emphasized the significance of peer counselors to successful breastfeeding with this population of women.

8. Dr. Michael Green confirmed this point to me in a conversation at Hershey Medical Center, the Penn State Medical College, in July 2002.

Chapter 3

1. Formula manufacturers are required to state in their materials that breast milk is the superior form of infant food, or best for baby. Pregnancy and infant care guidebooks will usually provide that view as well, although, as I will show, in a variety of ways.

2. I am interested in what women looking for information about infant care and feeding would find on the shelves of their local bookstores. Although there are a number of specific guides for breastfeeding, I will not examine these in this chapter, since I want to analyze representational contexts that are not committed to one form of feeding over another in order to interrogate the structure of the comparison between the two. In addition, I include an analysis of promotional literature sent to mothers by formula companies. These companies get mothers' names and addresses when they sign up for childbirth education classes at hospitals, buy prescription prenatal vitamins, visit certain OB/GYN offices or clinics, or have their babies in a hospital (which about 99 percent of American mothers do (Davis-Floyd 186n).

3. Adrienne Berney develops this idea, although not in alignment with Foucaultian thinking, in *Reforming the Maternal Breast*. There she discusses how social ideals valuing mechanization and the realignment of wives with husbands in the companionate ideal of marriage served to culturally validate mothers' increasing separation from children. For Foucault, see *The History of Sexuality* and *The Care of the Self*.

4. This view is made very clear in a web page published by the U.S. Food and Drug Administration: "Infant Formula: Second Best but Good Enough." See Stehlin.

5. Katherine Dettwyler, in "Beauty and the Breast: The Cultural Context of Breastfeeding in the United States," provides an important initial analysis of these issues.

6. It may seem odd to argue that breastfeeding doesn't fit into American ideals of infant care, given that all women (except those who are HIV-positive) are encouraged to breastfeed, in infant care guides and by health care practitioners. However, one of the points of this chapter is to demonstrate that, at least in these representations, breastfeeding ends up seeming anomalous and difficult, and thus out of step with dominant values.

7. At a party in summer 2001, I was speaking with a woman who was at the tail end of her pregnancy. In talking with her about my research, she was surprised to hear me speak about a bottle-feeding culture. It was her impression, she said, that breastfeeding was really promoted by the hospital and local physicians. One reason why she felt this way, I think, is that most women in her circle of white, middle-class women (like me) breastfed. In addition, the local La Leche League group is very strong and two leaders are also lactation consultants at the local hospital. In many ways, my small university town is very breastfeeding friendly. It is also very white and middle class, with a highly professional citizenry. It is easy, I have found, to think of one's own immediate context as the norm.

8. A number of interesting studies examine the effects of discharge packs (the "goodies" mothers receive upon leaving the hospital after the birth of a baby, routinely supplied by formula manufacturers) on breastfeeding rates and infant feeding choices. See Dungy et al., Bliss et al., and Frank et al.

9. There are, interestingly, a number of pictures of mother–infant co-sleeping in the Mead Johnson materials. This may be an attempt to represent maternal-infant closeness without breastfeeding images.

10. Anecdotally, the "nesting instinct" that many mothers experience in the early stages of labor can encourage a flurry of home activity. My childbirth education teacher reported that she regrouted the tile in her bathroom during the early stages of labor with one of her children. I made cheese cake during the early stages of labor with my second child. But the representation in the Mead Johnson materials serves to diminish the real pain that many women experience with labor, and to suggest that the new mother's main function is to continue to care for her family. It seems to me primarily comical that many women sense an urge to do things around the house—cook, clean—when they are in labor, and I believe that such energy should not be represented as routine or expected. On the other hand, it's nice to have an alternative to the one-contraction-and-we're-going-to-the-hospital representations offered in most popular television shows and films.

11. I cannot find where I learned this fact.

12. Ironically, I did have to supplement when Sam was eleven months old and just starting full-time day care. He bit me hard enough to cause my nipple to bleed, and pumping was impossibly painful. I came to the center at noon to nurse him, but he had formula—some of those cans of Similac I had received after his birth—in the morning and early afternoons. The rest I gave to a friend who had stopped nursing at about five months.

13. In both the Mead Johnson and Ross materials, most of the mothers and babies presented are white, although there are a number of African-American mothers and babies, and a few Asian mothers and babies. All the pictures use models, so they are probably not of actual mother and baby pairs.

14. Many breastfeeding advocates feel that this is an important element of breastfeeding promotion—assuring the mother that even if she needs to be separated from the child she can provide breast milk for it. In her 2001 presentation to the La Leche League Seminar on Breastfeeding for Physicians, neonatalogist Michal Young supported this position in addressing the issue of promoting breastfeeding among young African-American mothers.

15. This book was originally published, to much ballyhoo, as *Bottlefeeding without Guilt,* but when I tried to purchase it in 1999, the same ISBN turned up *When Breastfeeding Is Not An Option: A Reassuring Guide for Loving Parents.* Most of the text is a diatribe against the horribly stressful breastfeeding culture that makes bottle-feeding moms feel guilty, and the author argues that breastfeeding is oversold.

16. Given the complex relation that most American women have with their bodies, it's not surprising that so many women choose against nursing. There are, of course, other reasons

why women choose against nursing, including (perhaps most significantly) structural inequities in the split between work and family that burden women with the majority of child care even when they work outside the home. In this chapter I am trying to analyze those specific aspects of pregnancy and infant care guides that influence women's choices not to nurse, and while working comes up as an obstacle to nursing in a few of these texts, the most obvious problems that nursing presents in these representations concern the maternal body.

17. At Books-A-Million, there is an entire set of shelves devoted to *What to Expect* books. *What to Expect When You're Expecting* is listed as number 176 on Amazon.com's list of bestsellers (November 2001), even though many of the readers' reviews are negative.

18. Even Stoppard's breastfeeding-positive discussion has a section titled "Breast versus Bottle."

19. See Iris Marion Young's interesting essay, "Breasted Experience: The Look and the Feeling," for a discussion of the sexuality/motherhood divide. Her representation of breastfeeding attempts to overcome this dichotomy, but only achieves, in my view, a reiteration of it, by representing certain forms of relaxed and sensual nursing as metaphorical intercourse between baby and mother.

20. See also Davis-Floyd about regulating women into a technological gestalt.

21. According to DeLoache and Gottlieb, "over 50 million copies of the seven editions of Benjamin Spock's *Baby and Child Care* have been sold since 1946—second only to the Bible" (20).

22. Lawrence notes that adequate nutrition is available in so-called junk foods, and that "it has been shown that malnourished women make adequate milk at the expense of body stores" (267–68).

23. See Gabrielle Palmer's *The Politics of Breastfeeding* for an extended list of "Artificial Feeding Mishaps" (306–12), which include excess aluminum levels and vitamin deficiencies. Palmer also points out that the 1982 FDA "quality control regulations" concerning formula manufacturing were not heralded by parents' groups seeking redress after their infants were damaged by faulty formulas: "FORMULA and other parents' groups have filed a lawsuit charging that the Reagan administration has violated the Infant Formula Act of 1980 by leaving the specifics of quality control up to the manufacturers. Lynn Pilot commented that the supposedly explicit regulations did not even rise to the level of the Food and Drug Administration's rules for cold remedies, yet were dealing with an infant's sole source of nutrition" (242). The Food and Drug Administration (FDA) continues to allow formula companies to regulate their own products: "The safety and nutritional quality of infant formulas are ensured by requiring that manufacturers follow specific procedures in manufacturing infant formulas. In fact, there is a law—known as the Infant Formula Act—which gives FDA special authority to create and enforce standards for commercial infant formulas. Manufactures must analyze each batch of formula to check nutrient levels and make safety checks. They must then test samples to make sure the product remains in good condition while it is on the market shelf. Infant formulas must also have codes on their containers to identify each batch and manufacturers must keep very detailed records of production and analysis" ("Overview of Infant Formulas").

    See also Blum, *At the Breast*, for a discussion of PBBs and PCBs in human breast milk in Michigan in the 1970s (94–95).

24. See Blum, *At the Breast*, for a discussion of the decision of nurses at a public health clinic not to provide as much breastfeeding information and support to "mothers facing difficult circumstances," so that they "not be overloaded with guilt" when breastfeeding didn't work out for them. Blum writes, "One insightfully commented that they risked patronizing working-class mothers either way, whether they advised them to breastfeed *or* if they backed off from information they routinely provided to more privileged mothers" (122; original emphasis).

25. Of course, there used to be choice available to well-off women, but it was the choice of which woman, mother or wet-nurse, rather than which milk. See Golden.

26. Berney calls breastfeeding on a schedule "rationalized" breastfeeding.

27. After my daughter was born, I met frequently with two mothers who had been in my childbirth education class. Our daughters were all around the same age. We met for companionship and to trade ideas about mothering. When the babies were about two months old, I became aware that the other mothers were attempting to space out their infants' nursing sessions (all of us were breastfeeding), mainly by trying to entertain fussing babies with play and stimulation. It never occurred to me to do so—the *first* thing I did when my daughter fussed was to see if she wanted to nurse. When I asked the other women why they tried to space out the feedings, usually to make the interval between feedings at least

three hours, they both replied that they thought it appropriate to do so, that it was better for the baby to have a more defined feeding routine. This anecdotal evidence suggests the cultural embeddedness of the notion of spaced feedings as the proper way to feed a baby.

28. Kahn suggests that agricultural time is natural, but surely its name belies that idea. Agriculture, as well as industry, is a product of human manipulation of what is understood as nature.

29. However, see Catherine Panter-Brick's discussion of breastfeeding in rural Nepal, where two different tribal groups have developed different feeding patterns and infant care expectations because of the differing kinds of work that they do. In both cases, mothers leave their nursing children for specific periods. The kind of work they do and the women's involvement in household work affects the patterns of breastfeeding and weaning in each community, but both groups continue to breastfeed predominantly.

30. Jacquelyn Litt relates the story of a mother whose child refused to eat according to the doctor's expectations (58–60). This Jewish mother's son refused to eat and only wanted his bottle, so she would lay him on a table and pretend to offer him the bottle, only to cram food into his mouth when he opened it up. She expresses considerable frustration at his resistance to proper eating habits, and conveys the sense of her own responsibility to enforce certain eating habits on her children.

31. At La Leche League meetings, mothers often articulate confusion over their infants' behaviors. Much of the meeting time is taken up with members offering information about their own babies, in order to share strategies and interpretations (for example, a baby who wants to nurse more frequently than advice books suggest is normal does not need a bottle for extra nutrition, but is building up its mother's milk supply or seeking nurturance through suckling).

32. A friend of mine who had her baby in the 1980s told me about visits to a doctor who always asked how often the baby nursed. Since she didn't count, and the baby nursed a lot, she began making up numbers. In her view, the doctor had a specific idea about how many nursing sessions were appropriate and how the number should diminish with time.

Chapter 4

1. Although a baby can never be allergic to the breast milk itself, factors in the mother's diet will make their way into the milk and can cause allergic responses in the baby. A main culprit is casein, the protein in cow's milk. Breastfeeding mothers with very fussy babies may be advised to eliminate milk from their diets in order to assess the infant's response. At the 2001 Seminar on Breastfeeding for Physicians, sponsored by La Leche League, a family practice doctor presented a case in which a breastfed baby who was failing to thrive was found to have severe and wide-ranging food allergies to elements in the mother's diet. The infant's true failure to thrive became manifest after he was weaned to formula; he was weaned because he was having difficulty nursing and was not gaining weight adequately. A restrictive elimination diet might have helped this mother nurse her infant more successfully, as he was later found to be allergic to many elements in a typical American diet. Cases of actual allergic sensitivity like this are rare, however, although many infants seem to be sensitive to dairy products and wheat in the mother's diet.

2. Since Rachel had taken bottles of expressed breast milk so well, I had thought I could be gone two days a week to teach and attend meetings, leaving him with my husband and some pumped milk in my absence.

3. *High need baby* is a term I first encountered in William and Martha Sears's *The Baby Book*. They use it to describe, in positive terms, an infant who demands a lot of personal attention from caretakers, often refusing to be alone (to sleep) and requiring more stimulation than other babies. *The Baby Book* specifically uses the term *high need baby* to replace the negative terms *fussy* and *colicky*. According to William and Martha Sears, high need baby features include: being supersensitive, not liking to be put down, not being a self-soother, wanting to nurse all the time, awakening frequently, being unsatisfiable and unpredictable, being hyperactive (in a non-clinical sense), being draining on caretakers, being uncuddly, and being demanding (340–41). Sam exhibited many of these features, although I called him fussy and demanding rather than high need.

4. Büskens borrows the term *intensive mothering* from Sharon Hays.

5. As I demonstrated in the last chapter, demand feeding is promoted in infant care advice literature, but usually includes the idea that infants will develop their own schedules.

For the record, my mother-in-law never criticized my breastfeeding or child-rearing practices, although many women at La Leche League meetings did express exasperation at the attitudes and interference of their husband's mothers. My own mother was equally supportive. Pediatric support for bottle-feeding norms was often subtle: when my newborn son was back in the hospital for an unspecified infection with fever, the hospital pediatrician, who was very attentive and caring and who very well may have saved Sam's life, commented to me that when Sam was feeling better I could begin to lengthen out the time between feedings in order to establish a schedule. At the time, Sam was six days old. A few days earlier, the family practice physician (standing in while my doctor was away), who didn't catch Sam's impending illness during a routine post-hospital checkup, told me that while demand feeding was all very well and good, most mothers found scheduled feedings to be easier. I ignored both doctors' suggestions, primarily because I knew better, but also because I was at the time engorged and needed to nurse Sam as often as possible to relieve my own discomfort. It is clear to me now that to have followed their advice would have been to risk cessation of my own milk supply.

Also, while in retrospect I can label my maternal practices as intensive, many women in my La Leche League group would not have agreed with me, since I worked full-time while my child was an infant and arranged paid care for him when I was not available. See Hays for an extensive description of intensive mothering.

6. What's interesting about the idea of natural weaning is that it isn't necessarily really natural, even in the conception of La Leche League. As Diane Bengson puts it in *How Weaning Happens* (a La Leche League publication), "Natural weaning means allowing the child to outgrow nursing on his own timetable.... However, this doesn't mean the mother has no influence on the process. Natural weaning incorporates the natural limit-setting that babies need as they grow into toddlers. A mother who is practicing natural weaning views weaning as a developmental skill, and lovingly guides her child as he learns the skills that replace nursing" (3).

7. One friend of mine, at a La Leche League meeting, commented that she was waking up a half hour early in order to nurse her three-year-old daughter before taking her to day care; she had to wake the child up in order to have the time to nurse. The mother was currently considering weaning, since the nursing seemed to happen only because she put it into the daily schedule and she really wanted the extra sleep. In thinking about weaning, she said, "I try to consider what I would be doing if I were living in the Stone Age." The incongruity of the thought and her dilemma seems amusing, but represents the real decisions of women who establish extended nursing as a priority in their lives and then have difficulty finding discourses to use in terminating the experience. The child weaned soon after, in what the mother described as child-led weaning.

8. For example, Randy Thornhill and Craig T. Palmer's *A Natural History of Rape*.

9. Marc Lappé's *Evolutionary Medicine* is more concerned with how humans have affected the evolution of microorganisms, thereby producing virulent strains of dangerous bacteria and viruses.

Significantly, Carol M. Worthman writes, in a chapter entitled "Evolutionary Perspectives on the Onset of Puberty," that "evolutionary thinking is emphatically not about social Darwinism—that things are as they must be.... By emphasizing the centrality of resource distribution to understanding human development, health, and behavior, evolutionary analysis focuses our attention on the necessity for social change to effect change in development and health. Instead of confirming the status quo, an evolutionary perspective provides a deeper reason for critically analyzing resource distribution or maldistribution and its consequences....

"Second, an evolutionary perspective is popularly associated with species-universal, shared features, and some fear that it promotes a deterministic, invariant view of human nature. This analysis has shown that, to the contrary, an adaptationist, evolutionary view also leads us to an understanding of the causes of our differences and reveals that those causes lie in the dynamic between individual and context that cross-cuts biological and social-ecological domains" (155–56). In presenting evidence and analysis concerning the wide variation in human entry into puberty, especially as evident in the wide variation of menarche across the globe, Worthman argues that humans evolved a potential to respond to specific ecological conditions by hurrying or delaying puberty. This approach to studying human diversity is not popularly linked to evolutionary theory.

10. Jules Law offers another critique of evolutionary advocacy for breastfeeding practices, arguing that the uses of evolutionary theory are contradictory, in that species-specific arguments are used sometimes, while at other times analogies to other mammalian lactational experience are made (435).

11. Thanks to Martha McCaughey for suggesting this wording to me.

12. Jenny Shuster, personal communication, Blacksburg, VA. 19 July 1999.

13. Howard Kushner, personal communication, San Diego, CA. 29 October 1999. Because they often occur in texts written for general audiences, the stories of evolution and of the influence of Pleistocene lifestyles on contemporary human functioning don't alert the reader to the complexities of evolutionary theory left out of the accounts. Indeed, these stories don't even gesture broadly toward the current controversies between those Stephen Jay Gould called the Darwinian fundamentalists (who believe that natural selection and only natural selection is at work in evolutionary adaptation) and the group Gould belonged to, the pluralists (who argue that natural selection is the most important but not the only mechanism at work in evolutionary development). That fact wouldn't be an issue, except that evolutionary psychology and the evolutionary discourses articulated in the service of breastfeeding advocacy are clearly situated in the Darwinian fundamentalist camp, and thus rely on a set of claims that are contested within scientific communities today.

In *Becoming Human: Evolution and Human Uniqueness*, Ian Tattersall argues that the "discipline of evolutionary psychology, essentially sociobiology as applied to our species, purports to explain vast amounts of human behavior by reference to our genetic heritage, implying that, in a very concrete way, we are prisoners of our evolutionary past" (203). Evolutionary psychology is the discipline that tries to identify "mental adaptations" in order to determine how specific behavioral traits apparent in contemporary society evolved over the millennia that Stone Age hominids occupied the African savanna. As Richard Morris writes in his primer of evolutionary controversies, evolutionary psychologists believe that "if we want to understand why human beings behave the way they do, we should look for specialized brain modules that induce them to do things and then try to understand why such behavior would have been advantageous in a hunter-gatherer society" (171). Evolutionary psychologists tend to downplay or repudiate the anthropological emphasis on culture as the strong determinant in human behavior, seeking universals that can be linked back to Stone Age lifestyles. This demonstrates a key difference from previous evolutionary thinkers who sought to reform human behavior by using Darwinian theory. For turn-of-the-twentieth-century feminist evolutionist Charlotte Perkins Gilman, for example, evolution meant variation and adaptation; evolutionary theory was a way to think through reforms that would correct social institutions that remained stuck in outdated traditions. Cultural stasis was the drag that human evolution could break from. Now, much of evolutionary psychology seems to want to rationalize seemingly problematic contemporary social behavior through justificatory explanations grounded in evolutionary perspectives. Randy Thornhill and Craig T. Palmer's *A Natural History of Rape* is a case in point, as it argues that rape (conceptualized as men raping women) is an evolved adaptation for insuring male reproductive success. (Charlotte Perkins Gilman is turning over in her grave.)

Tattersall identifies reductionism as one key problem with evolutionary psychology, which he links to the fundamentalist position that all adaptations represent specific selections (204). Indeed, the pluralist camp argues that some traits have evolved as what Gould called spandrels and Tattersall suggests are exaptations, or "features that originally arose in one context but were later co-opted for use in another" (Tattersall 108). Morris describes spandrels as "traits that are not molded by natural selection. The traits exist because they are a by-product of something else. This does not mean that these traits are not useful. Once a spandrel exists, natural selection may modify it in some useful way.... Gould has cited the human ability to read and write as an example of a spandrel. Natural selection caused our brains to become big, he says, 'for a small set of reasons having to do with what is good about brains on the African savannas.' But once they become big, human brains were able to do numerous different things that had nothing to do with the reasons natural selection caused them to grow larger in the first place" (84). Morris identifies paleontologist Elisabeth Vrba as the originator of the term *exaptation* used by Tattersall (84).

In addition, evolutionary psychology argues that because the development of human societies since the agricultural revolution has been so short (about 10,000 years), we can't imagine that humans are currently adapted to the environments of non–hunter-gatherer societies (the majority of peoples in the world today). But, as Tattersall suggests, this implies that evolution has stopped, primarily because the fundamentalists believe in long, slow, gradual adaptation. The pluralists argue for what Gould termed punctuated equilibrium, which describes short bursts of evolutionary adaptation in relation to the emergence of new species, in comparison to long periods of stasis with little evolutionary change. Even if we can't claim any specific evolutionary adaptation in the period since the agricultural revolution—admittedly a very short period of time in evolutionary terms—we can suggest, as Tattersall does, that adaptation itself is a feature of humans and thus must be accounted for in any claims about the hold of the past on our behavior today:

> In their search for mental adaptations, evolutionary psychologists are fond of referring to the "ancestral environment" in which our own behavioral adaptations evolved. How or where we live today is irrelevant, they say, because industrial or even agricultural lifestyles are such *recent* phenomena. For keys to our mental adaptations, we must look to our hunting-gathering past. . . . [But], even if our knowledge of the evolutionary process teaches us that our species has to have originated in a single local area, and thus in a fairly specific environment, our *success* has had to do with our remarkable ability to move out from that environment and displace our competitors from all other human habitats. Evidently what we innately are has little do with specific adaptation to any particular environment, whether social, geographical, technological, or ecological. (205; emphasis in original)

In addition, Stephen Palumbi, in *The Evolution Explosion: How Humans Cause Rapid Evolutionary Change,* suggests that contrary to popular belief, humans continue to evolve, especially in areas of the world where medicine and technology haven't had the success in mitigating hardship that they have had in the United States (207–30). Sarah Blaffer Hrdy states, "But natural selection didn't stop dead in its tracks when the Pleistocene ended. We are kidding ourselves if we think so. A mother today, whether in New York, Tokyo, or Dacca, is not just a gatherer caught in a shopping mall without her digging stick. We are subtly and not so subtly different from our Pleistocene ancestors in ways that have been transmitted genetically as well as through multiple parental effects between generations" (105), adding, "We are at once relics of Pleistocene foragers *and* altered specimens. . . . Whenever humans find themselves living under novel conditions, there are new opportunities for selection to act" (106; emphasis in original). In subsequent sections she documents how rapid selection for genes can be, using the examples of cystic fibrosis (a single copy of the gene confers resistance to typhoid fever), sickle-cell anemia (a single copy of the gene confers resistance to malaria), cow's milk tolerance among adults (an adaptation to dairy in populations that herd cattle), and the possibility that rapid selection may be occurring with respect to AIDS and HIV (107–8).

14.   Sarah Blaffer Hrdy writes, "The unfortunate and much misused expression 'survival of the fittest' to paraphrase this phenomenon [natural selection] was not introduced by Darwin but by his prolific and widely read contemporary, the social philosopher Herbert Spencer. To Spencer, survival of the fittest meant 'survival of the best and most deserving. . . . For him, evolution meant *progress*" (13; emphasis in original). Hrdy states that Darwin believed that "individuals that are *best* adapted to their current environment survive and reproduce" (13; emphasis added), but it is clear that *adequate* adaptation for reproduction and successful parenting of the next generation is all that is necessary for a given organism to survive through natural selection. Adaptation depends completely upon the given environment in which an organism finds itself, and "No adaptation continues to be selected for outside the circumstances that happen to favor it" (13).

15.   The need to specify how much breast milk a breastfed baby actually ingests arises from faulty research that has, historically, not distinguished between full and partial breastfeeding, and breastfeeding on demand or scheduled (and thus restrictive) breastfeeding.

16.   This is not to suggest that physicians were not interested in breastfeeding before the twentieth century. On the contrary, many physicians were interested in advising women about infant feeding practices in past historical eras. See Valerie Fildes, *Breasts, Bottles, and Babies,* for discussions of pre-twentieth-century doctors' views of adequate breast milk and the best methods of choosing a midwife. However, both Rima Apple and Janet Golden

have demonstrated the increasing influence of physicians on women's choices and practices having to do with lactation in nineteenth- and twentieth-century America.

17. This is a coauthored article, but the different sections of the article are attributed to specific authors. The conclusion is not attributed to any one author, and thus I understand it to represent the common conclusions of all the listed authors.

   The American Academy of Pediatrics, in a policy statement concerning SIDS and the infant sleep environment, specifically states that "no epidemiologic evidence exists that bed sharing is protective against SIDS," even though "some behavioral studies have demonstrated that infants have more arousals and less slow-wave sleep during bed sharing" ("Changing Concepts of Sudden Infant Death Syndrome").

18. At the 1999 La Leche League Seminar on Breastfeeding for Physicians, and again in his presentation at the 2001 seminar, James McKenna suggested that babies that sleep alone are maladaptive. The comment was meant to be humorous, turning the tables on the normative expectations of parents and sleep researchers, but was also meant to seriously question received ideas about the so-called good babies who sleep a lot on their own.

19. For specific arguments about the purported dangers of co-sleeping, or sleep sharing, see Consumer Products Safety Commission, "CPSC Warns Against Placing Babies in Adult Beds" and Drago and Dannenberg's influential *Pediatrics* article, "Infant Mechanical Suffocation Deaths in the United States, 1980–1997."

20. See Michal Young.

21. James McKenna's work is very complex and interesting, and, as an anthropologist, he is interested in cultural and ideological issues attendant to perceptions of proper sleep, both in terms of proper biological sleep patterns and in terms of proper sleep arrangement of family members. My critique is not meant to detract from the significance of his work to resituate normative American views of infant–parent bedsharing (or co-sleeping) in terms of dominant cultural ideologies. His work contesting the Consumer Products Safety Commission's 1999 statement against co-sleeping and bedsharing is politically very important: that statement suggested that all co-sleeping was dangerous and explicitly said that infants should only sleep in cribs (designed for infant safety). Such a statement is not only based on questionable evidence (as McKenna suggested, in the Drago and Dannenberg article, on which the CPSC's report was based, the infant deaths that occurred in an adult bed but had no specific cause were considered to have been influenced by the environment, but the infant deaths that occurred in a crib were thought to be SIDS, that is, of undeterminable cause ["Never Sleep with Your Baby?"]), but sets a federal standard for maternal behavior that is every bit as problematic as the notion that formula is appropriate for all infants. McKenna's work sets out to broaden women's choices in maternal behavior (he says that while he's passionate about bedsharing advocacy, he never advises specific parents where members of *their* family should sleep; that, he says, is up to them). His talk, "Never Sleep with Your Baby?" detailed a complex anthropological view of both infant sleep and sleep researchers.

22. While volunteering at the "Breastfeeding Rest Stop" at the New River Valley Fair in Dublin, Virginia, July 2001, I noticed a poster someone had tacked up on the tent. While I forget the exact wording, the gist of the message was "If you breastfeed your child, she will be *smarter, healthier, and have sweeter smelling diapers.*" Breastfeeding, of course, doesn't guarantee such results, except perhaps the last, since the benefits can only be measured across populations and not on an individualized basis.

23. Of course, infants in impoverished Third World contexts remain susceptible to the same virulent killers they always have been: gastrointestinal illness, malaria, cholera. Infants in most of these contexts are particularly at risk if they are fed formula, since they depend on the immunological properties of breast milk to insure survival: researchers and activists aren't worried that such infants will develop juvenile diabetes or Crohn's disease as a result of bottle feeding; they are concerned that bottle-fed infants in the Third World won't live to their first birthday.

24. At the La Leche League Seminars on Breastfeeding for Physicians that I have attended, physicians and other attendees tend to greet with glee any statistics demonstrating benefits for breastfeeding or deficits for formula use. The commitment to breastfeeding seems to precede the evidence for its beneficial effects; thus, while the studies reported are designed to produce honest results, the desire of the participants is always to see breastfeeding demonstrably superior to formula.

25. Hrdy does suggest that Bowlby was correct in identifying infants' needs for secure attachment to develop healthily, and she argues that he was correct in identifying the difficulty of finding people to care for one's children as a prime problem in women working outside the home (495–96). She implies that he should have been more objective about his personal views.

26. I continue to see this story as psychological manipulation, given Nisa's previous description of her desires to continue to nurse, yet Shostak does not offer this interpretation, either in *Nisa* or *Return to Nisa*.

27. Marjorie Shostak died in 1996 from a metasticized breast cancer.

28. In the *HHS Blueprint for Action on Breastfeeding*, Hispanic women are shown to breastfeed almost in the same percentages as white women, and in a slightly higher percentage at one year (19 percent to white women's 17 percent). The reasons for such similarity are unclear, and go uncommented upon in the document, which focuses on the health disparities of Native American and African-American women with respect to breastfeeding in the dominant white population. These figures are relatively recent (October 2000), and there is little discussion of them in the general medical and social literature on lactation in the United States.

29. WIC (Women, Infants, and Children) provides supplemental formula; according to Michal Young, about a two to three week supply each month. Mothers are responsible for providing the remaining formula. Relative safety in formula feeding means that formula feeding is not perceived by most medical personnel to increase infant mortality risks.

30. Dettwyler also ignores the historical fact that social concepts of childhood and adolescence are not fixed in biology, although biological rationales are now used to define these periods. Thanks to Marian Mollin for emphasizing this point to me.

31. "Hamilton derived simple mathematical expressions predicting that altruism should evolve whenever the cost to the giver (which he designated C) was less than the fitness benefits (B) obtained by helping another individual who was related by r, a term designating the proportion of genes these two individuals shared by common descent" (Hrdy 63).

32. See Valerie Fildes, *Breasts, Bottles, and Babies,* for historical evidence of feeding vessels throughout history.

Chapter 5

1. For a discussion of social pressure to wean early, see Dettwyler "Beauty and the Breast" and "A Time to Wean." La Leche League philosophy includes the following principles:
   * Mothering through breastfeeding is the most natural and effective way of understanding and satisfying the needs of the baby.
   * Mother and baby need to be together early and often to establish a satisfying relationship and an adequate milk supply.
   * In the early years the baby has an intense need to be with his mother which is as basic as his need for food.
   * Breast milk is the superior infant food.
   * For the healthy, full-term baby, breast milk is the only food necessary until the baby shows signs of needing solids, about the middle of the first year after birth.
   * Ideally the breastfeeding relationship will continue until the baby outgrows the need.
   * Alert and active participation by the mother in childbirth is a help in getting breastfeeding off to a good start.
   * Breastfeeding is enhanced and the nursing couple sustained by the loving support, help, and companionship of the baby's father. A father's unique relationship with his baby is an important element in the child's development from early infancy.
   * Good nutrition means eating a well-balanced and varied diet of foods in as close to their natural state as possible.
   * From infancy on, children need loving guidance which reflects acceptance of their capabilities and sensitivity to their feelings. (La Leche League, "La Leche League Philosophy")

2. Physicians, nurses, and others may become certified as IBCLC. Many lactation consultants have no medical degree (such as an M.D. or an R.N.).

3. League mothers go through a complex and lengthy process to become leaders. See Lowman,

The LLLove Story, and Cahill, *Seven Voices, One Dream,* for discussions of how leader applications evolved in the organization.

4. See Lauri Umansky's *Motherhood Reconceived: Feminism and the Legacies of the Sixties* for an extensive discussion of feminist ideas about motherhood from the late 1960s to the early 1980s.

5. Linda Blum suggests that La Leche League's emphasis on *individual* mother-to-mother support constrains its maternalism. See Blum, *At the Breast,* and Blum and Vandewater.

6. This book was originally published as *Bottlefeeding without Guilt,* which is now no longer available. Both books have the same ISBN number. It caused an uproar in my La Leche League group when it appeared in 1998.

7. At League conferences, discussions of maternity leave legislation are usually met with almost universal approval, however. The distinction is what LLL can support as an international organization to promote breastfeeding, and what individual members can support politically.

8. It is interesting as well that while feminists tend to highlight how white and middle class LLL is, as an example of its exclusivity, elitism, and lack of social consciousness, feminists themselves have been targeted for the same problems.

9. So we have Susan Chira, in *A Mother's Place: Choosing Work and Family without Guilt or Blame,* arguing that a half hour at bedtime with children is enough to "give [one mother] a sense of intimacy and assurance that is evident every time I have seen her with her children" (165)—in other words, that a half hour is enough to be a good mother. Concerning another mother who is an investment banker, Chira writes, "bath and bedtime are crucial hours. She has told her employers that she is committed to getting home in time for these rituals" (164). I'm not claiming that these women aren't good mothers, but that the whole thrust of Chira's book is to argue that they are, when it seems to me patently clear that to ask anyone to work beyond the time a child needs to go to bed is to be asking too much of the worker.

   For an excellent discussion of "Feminism and the Motherhood Wars" in relation to La Leche League, see Julia DeJager Ward.

10. Julia DeJager Ward makes the same argument (173–89).

11. Cahill suggests that Mary White, Marian Tompson, and Edwina Froehlich wrote most of the first edition of the manual, with the others contributing (92). Lowman states that Mary White, Edwina Froehlich, and Mary Ann Cahill wrote the "Course by Mail," with the others "offering suggestions and criticisms" (24). Subsequent editions were also joint efforts. See the third edition, pages 342–43.

12. See Lowman's *The LLLove Story* for a lengthy discussion of the creation of *The Womanly Art of Breastfeeding.*

13. This benefit of breastfeeding would have been very important for the founding mothers of LLL, all of whom were Catholic. Between the seven of them there were over fifty children, and two of the women had ten or more children.

14. While the discourse of childbirth as part of woman's "natural function" may seem off-putting, the emphasis on unmedicated childbirth in League practice is pragmatically motivated. Many women giving birth in the 1950s were knocked out completely and first shown their babies hours after birth. The babies often had difficulty nursing because the drugs used during labor and delivery persisted in their systems. A number of the founding mothers had home births, and were adamant about women remaining aware of the experience. In *The LLLove Story,* Mary White recounts her second delivery: "I did have a natural delivery, although I think I made the doctor very nervous. *He had never worked on a conscious mother before, and didn't know quite how to manage it*" (Lowman 88; emphasis added).

15. "Going home as soon as possible" had a different meaning in the late 1950s, when mothers often spent longer than a week in the hospital following the birth of a baby, than now, when women are pushed out the door 24 hours after a normal vaginal birth and 48 hours after a cesarean.

16. Conflict between the maternity nursing staff and individual doctors at a given hospital is a common occurrence. When I gave birth to Rachel at Chicago's Lying In Hospital (affiliated with the University of Chicago), the labor and delivery nurse would not allow me to drink any water until my midwife arrived and okayed the request. With a small midwifery service, the nursing staff was more accustomed to the rules set down by most of the obstetricians—no water, only ice chips, in the event that a surgical birth would be necessary.

17. "Kangaroo care" describes care for premature infants that places them on their mother's chest instead of in an incubator in order to stabilize their vital signs and help them to develop.

18. *The LLLove Story* includes a selection of photographs from the League's pamphlet on breastfeeding, for many years titled "Why Nurse Your Baby?" From the 1960s through the early 1970s, with the exception of founder Betty Wagner and a black woman (Harriety J. Murray), all the women on the cover of the pamphlet are referred to in the book by their husband's names: "Mrs. Robert Troch, Mrs. F. Rachford, Mrs. John Welch," etc. One other black woman is identified as Mrs. Joseph Hardin; the rest of the women are white. In the pamphlet covers presented from 1974 to 1976, the six mothers photographed are identified by their own names; five are white and one is black.

19. Julia DeJager Ward speaks of breastfeeding as a "learned art" (161).

20. For the record, many feminists' argument against League ideology is that most women *have* to work. Both sides of this dispute are, to my mind, missing the point, since any discussion that doesn't include women's *right to work* and to contribute to society through their work will easily devolve into questions concerning whether or not a given woman really has to work and what social provisions can be generated to keep her home.

21. See Hausman, 95–109, for a discussion of the development of the idea of "gender identity" in the late 1950s and 1960s.

22. See Stearns for a discussion of breastfeeding as work that can only be done by the mother (323).

23. It's not clear to me why six months is understood to be an adequate period for maternity leave, since many infants at six months are still breastfeeding as their main source of nutrition. It may be a completely conventional (that is, arbitrary) period of time, like the idea that one year is optimal minimum length of time for breastfeeding (see American Academy of Pediatrics' 1997 policy statement on breastfeeding).

24. See Donna Haraway's discussion of Scheper-Hughes (*Modest Witness* 210).

25. See also Galtry, "Suckling and Silence" and " 'Sameness' and Suckling."

26. For example, one LLL leader in my local group consistently lamented the poor state of child care in the area (and in the country at large). "What about the children?" she would ask. While I initially understood this as a knee-jerk argument against day care, this woman was expressing heartfelt concern about children's experiences in less than optimal circumstances. Having put both my children in the local day care system for years, and having been lucky enough to enroll them in two of the best day care centers in the area (if measured in terms of staff development, quality of the facilities, and staff attention to children's needs), I better understand the significance of her question. Understood as a genuine concern, this question is about current economic and familial circumstances—not a statement against nonmaternal child care, but a statement of concern for circumstances that force families to make choices that may not be in their children's best interests. What about the children? is a question about a society that seems to consider their needs insignificant, especially in relation to changing social values about welfare and poor mothers. When feminists hear the question What about the children? they may be frustrated with the lack of attention to women's needs and desires, but ignoring the question or repudiating it as a legitimate question risks ignoring mothers' concerns and children's needs.

27. See La Leche League, "LLLUSA: What Is LLLUSA?"

28. Recently LLL began a new venture in hope of developing a workable structure. Called the "Chaordic Initiative," it is discussed briefly on their web site. See Lowman and Cahill for discussions of their needs, early and often, for reorganization.

29. LLL did not even participate in the Nestlé boycott, presumably as part of its policy not to mix causes (Blum, *At the Breast*, 44–45).

Chapter 6

1. "Prolonged jaundice or elevated bilirubin is thought to be caused by a combination of three factors: a substance in most mothers' milk that increases intestinal absorption of bilirubin, individual variations in the baby's ability to process bilirubin, and the inadequacy of feeding in the early days." Mothers whose babies have prolonged jaundice may want to have the infants tested in order to "rule out causes of pathological jaundice," but in most cases continued breastfeeding, if the baby is growing adequately, will suffice to eliminate

the excess bilirubin (*The Breastfeeding Answer Book* 226). Interestingly, a series of studies have shown that mothers of babies diagnosed with jaundice are more likely to give up breastfeeding than mothers of babies who were not diagnosed with jaundice; they were also more likely to "judge their infant's minor illnesses as serious and to have taken the child to an emergency room" and their infants were more likely to have experienced feeding problems (*The Breastfeeding Answer Book* 222). Supplementing feedings with formula will often put breastfeeding at risk, especially before the mother's milk supply is fully established. There is also the implication, in protocols for jaundice management that suggest supplementation, that the mother's breast milk is harmful to her baby (*The Breastfeeding Answer Book* 233–34).

2.   "Less frequent bowel movements are normal in an older breastfed baby. Some have bowel movements only once a week without signs of constipation" (*The Breastfeeding Answer Book* 123).

3.   Some women with large babies have difficulty giving birth vaginally. Yet I can't count the number of times I've heard a new mother's story about "having" to be induced because the baby was "too large"; the end of those narratives is (far too often) a cesarean-section delivery. Even the Department of Health and Human Services seeks to decrease the number of nonemergency C-sections in the United States; see *Healthy People 2010*.

4.   Thanks to Martha McCaughey for suggesting the language here. Eisenstein does mention lactation a few times in the text, but does not sustain a conversation about it. Instead, it is mentioned in passing, and usually as part of a list (pregnancy, childbirth, lactation, for example).

5.   And all I wanted to do was to exclaim, No, they are the *woman's* responsibility!

6.   Here I am thinking of the influential work of American feminist Catherine MacKinnon, as well as the popularity, at least in the 1980s and 1990s, of French feminist writers like Luce Irigaray and Hélène Cixous, whose focus on "feminine difference" was explicitly about the sexuality of sexual difference.

7.   Some feminists have argued for a view of breastfeeding as part of maternal and/or female sexuality—see Sichtermann and Iris Marion Young, as well as the discussion in chapter 2.

8.   Studies have shown that training for pediatricians does not lead to increased knowledge about the management of breastfeeding (Huffman).

9.   This is not to say that breastfeeding advocates don't try to educate others about breastfeeding, and to gain rights for women by arguing for extended maternity leaves and nursing breaks for working mothers. But the discourse of breastfeeding advocacy is education about the health benefits of breastfeeding—why, for example, employers benefit when the babies of employees are breastfed—and does not concern women's rights.

10. This is clearly not an exhaustive list, although throughout this book I hope to have mentioned, at some point, most of the existing feminist scholarship on breastfeeding.

11. An example similar to Stearns's article would be Tiina Vares' "Feminist Women Talk about Breastfeeding."

12. This distinguishes this newly emerging field from the work on La Leche League that I discussed in the preceding chapter. Many of the feminist essays on La Leche League were addressed primarily to a disciplinary audience and had as their purpose the affirmation or negation of a particular disciplinary model (concerning, for example, how voluntaristic groups reproduce themselves or police perceived inappropriate behaviors).

     Some very interesting new scholarship is being produced by Australian feminist theorists. I learned about the work of Fiona Giles and Alison Bartlett too late to incorporate a discussion of it in the main portion of this book, but direct the reader to their nuanced and theoretically deft approaches to breastfeeding as both experience and representation.

13. Teresa Ebert, in a short discussion in her *Ludic Feminism, and After: Postmodernism, Desire, and Labor in Late Capitalism*, mirrors this strategy, but from a solidly Marxist position. After critiquing Nancy Hartsock as an essentialist, she suggests that "lactation and breastfeeding are being revalorized in advanced capitalist countries, especially among the middle and upper middle classes," an effort that is "complicit with the political status quo" which endeavors "to recall women from the labor force and [to] reinstate domesticity, the traditional family and the regime of the social as composed of specific bodies" (238–39). In making these claims, Ebert writes that "these [medical] studies validating breast feeding—and the corporeal of the subjectivity of the mother—are appearing at a time of considerable unemployment and corporate attempts to downsize the labor force" (238). Later, she argues that "Contrary to the scientific as well as the romanticized claims for breast feeding among the middle and upper

middle classes, especially in overdeveloped countries, breast milk is neither self-evidently perceived as healthy nor universally recognized as a 'river of life'" (240). Thus, her argument uses concurrent trends—corporate downsizing and breastfeeding promotion—to make a causal argument against breastfeeding as an ideological activity dependent on the economic mode of production for its meaning and bent on domesticating women. At its core, the argument repudiates scientific evidence by treating it as epiphenomenal to political economy. She notes that "it is not women's bodies that redeem alienating production but rather the exploitative relations of production in capitalism that produce women's alienation from their bodies" (241). This latter point is echoed in Law's work as he argues against the idea that women's bodies should make up for shortfalls in the health care system (commenting on the bumper sticker "Affordable healthcare begins with breastfeeding").

14. Carter, for example, highlights the exhausting burden of breastfeeding for working-class women (50). Education campaigns neglect the physical experience of breastfeeding on the mother, she maintains, implying that bottle feeding reduces the mother's domestic workload because it doesn't tax her body physically and can be outsourced to other family members.

    Shulamith Firestone argued in *The Dialectic of Sex* that pregnancy was an embodied burden on women that should be avoided, but, aside from Marge Piercy in *Woman on the Edge of Time*, few feminists went along with Firestone's vociferous denunciations of the reproductive functions of the female body.

15. Thanks to Martha McCaughey for pointing out this specific example to me.

16. Immunity in children continues to develop and strengthen until about the age of six (Dettwyler, "A Time to Wean").

17. This is a particularly important issue for feminist politics concerning reproduction and reproductive technologies. As the potential viability of fetuses to exist outside the womb continues to move back earlier into pregnancy, there is an increasing tendency to see the fetus as an infant enclosed in the mother's womb, and thus a separable entity. This shift in thinking coincides with fetal medicine, its own specialty, which tends to perceive the fetus as always already an antagonist to and within the mother's body.

18. See Galtry, "Suckling and Silence," 16, for a similar discussion.

19. For example, in "Biocultural Perspectives on Breastfeeding," Patricia Stuart-Macadam writes "Breast milk is not a magic potion, not a panacea for all human ills. It is a vital, dynamic substance that can transmit both beneficial (such as immunoglobins and nutrients) and detrimental (such as nicotine and alcohol) substances to the infant. The benefits of breastfeeding or the disadvantages of formula feeding for mothers and infants no doubt vary depending upon the individual, family, ethnic group, living situation, environment, and time period.... Not being breastfed will probably not have as much impact on healthy infants without genetic predisposition to serious disease born into a good environment.... However, for infants born with some genetic defect or genetic predisposition to serious or chronic disease, or into a disadvantaged or unhygienic environment, breastfeeding can confer critical advantages" (27). This seems a particularly measured account of the possible beneficial effect on the infant of being breastfed.

20. Carter does not consider this issue.

21. The arguments about IQ in relation to infant feeding are a case in point. That breastfeeding makes smarter babies is a common claim in breastfeeding promotion campaigns. The *HHS Blueprint for Action on Breastfeeding* makes equivocal statements with regard to this issue (11). Feminist scholars point out that increasing IQ by breastfeeding is part of the middle-class optimizing aspect of intensive mothering (e.g., Blum, *At the Breast*, 50), but Katherine Dettwyler, anthropologist and mother of a developmentally disabled child, has suggested that the potential IQ benefit from breastfeeding would be *most* significant for those children who, like her son, have very low IQs. As she put it, a seven-point increase from the upper-60s to the mid-70s could mean the difference between being able to live independently as an adult or being dependent on others for one's entire life (personal communication, July 1999).

    In addition, it is unclear what Linda Blum considers a serious health risk to be, and what she considers the threshold for "thriving." The verb *to thrive* means to grow vigorously or flourish, but she uses it to mean that most formula-fed babies grow big and grow up—most growth charts, in any event, are based on formula-fed norms, so breastfed babies often seem as if they aren't growing fast enough. The scientific evidence that Blum herself cites suggests that formula-fed infants get sick more often, lag behind breastfed babies in cognitive measures, and may be more susceptible to chronic illness. That's hardly "thriving" in comparison to breastfed infants.

22. It is very difficult to design double blind studies to demonstrate clear health benefits to any nutritional practice.

23. Carter argues, "feminist strategy as regards infant feeding can be rooted in resistance to dominant discourses" (31).

24. Carter resists such an easy conceptualization of resistance: "feminists cannot simply celebrate bottle feeding amongst working class women. Although bottle feeding can be used as part of resistance to complex demands regarding mothering, it is important to recognize that it is a form of resistance which often emerges from relatively little control over resources and sometimes from poorer health. Some of the conditions which shape infant feeding practices and experiences are clearly undesirable" (226).

25. Riordan and Auerbach provide a more balanced approach to breastfeeding promotion: "The promotion efforts outlined in this chapter are needed because, to some degree in most countries (and in particular in industrialized ones), the most important requirement is missing: acceptance by society of the need for a mother and child to be together and the right of the breastfeeding dyad to participate in social, civic, and commercial activities outside the home. For many women, the ultimate barrier to breastfeeding is not sore nipples, nighttime nursing, or employment outside the home. It is the disapproval they encounter for 'wasting' their education and career skills by staying home with their breastfeeding infants or for being considered disruptive or even obscene for taking their breastfeeding infant with them to work or worship, perhaps to a city council or parent-teacher meeting, or simply to a restaurant or to a park. A goal for women should be to empower all mothers so that they are able to attend to all their duties, maternal as well as civic, religious, and professional" (22–23).

26. Dettwyler herself criticized Vanessa Maher's views to me in a private conversation.

27. I first came across Vanessa Maher's work while evaluating Martha Ward's *A World Full of Women*, an anthropologically oriented Introduction to Women's Studies textbook, for classroom use. Ward spends considerable space describing and defending Maher's maternal depletion thesis, which argues that women's health can be severely compromised through prolonged lactation when they do not receive adequate resources to sustain such a practice, and ends up arguing that "breasts and bottles are equally cultural" (81). Fair enough. However Ward, unlike Maher, never admits that there are any biological consequences to these differing cultural feeding practices. As in the sources discussed above, the perceived status of any biological benefit to breastfeeding is key in articulating its cultural significance.

28. Carter's book was published the same year as Dettwyler's major publications.

29. She writes, "Objective scientific proof does not always exist on the determinants of breastfeeding, but there is certainly adequate proof to defend the superiority of breastfeeding over artificial feeding" (Van Esterik, *Beyond,* 143).

30. Van Esterik discusses conflicts between a research approach and activist advocacy (*Beyond the Breast-Bottle Controversy* 20–27). Interestingly, both Law and Blum include Van Esterik in their lists of works cited, although both refer to her research in the briefest possible manner. Blum uses her book to support a factual claim about La Leche League noninvolvement in the Nestlé boycott, and Law includes her in a footnote that concerns Pam Carter's 1995 treatment of Van Esterik's research (Blum 93; Law 435n).

31. Some feminists might argue that the high rate of cesarean sections is an indication of encroaching disembodiment for women in childbirth.

32. Judith Galtry comments that "in countries with relatively low rates of breastfeeding, such as the United States, there is no indication that bottle feeding, whether of infant formula or expressed breastmilk [*sic*], has resulted in a high incidence of shared parenting arrangements" (" 'Sameness' and Suckling" 86 n42).

33. Provisions such as the Family Medical Leave Act (FMLA) and current laws mandating pregnancy coverage as a disability if similar disabilities are covered for men are examples of gender-neutral policies that address women's "difference" in reproductive function and roles.

34. Blum concludes that breastfeeding might be understood and experienced as a resistance to capitalism and a revaluation of embodied maternal experience, but it can't always be perceived this way. She argues that "we cannot assume some true, positive meaning, some purity of experience, in the maternal body or at the breast" (198). While her analysis does not preclude alternative material interpretations of breastfeeding, in denigrating biological

arguments she ends up without any rationale to frame an argument for breastfeeding, outside of the idea that it might "offer a way to revalue our bodies and force a public reevaluation of caregiving" (198). Blum also misinterprets the views of feminist breastfeeding advocates like Gabrielle Palmer and Penny Van Esterik, who believe, she says, "that there is one true meaning [of breastfeeding], outside of these dilemmas and paradoxes. This truth may be an ultimate rejection of patriarchal capitalism" (199). Van Esterik, as we have seen, takes a much more complex view of the situation. What distinguishes Blum from Van Esterik is the latter's perspective on the biological body in an ecological and social context.

35. See Kogan et al. This 1994 study indicates that "approximately 50% [of all women] received no prenatal information on breastfeeding" (86).

36. Certainly, as Jules Law points out, decreasing the pollution in inner cities would help rates of asthma among the children that grow up in them. This argument is not meant to suggest that other sorts of public health measures should be neglected in order to support breastfeeding as a beneficial practice. Indeed, only when more mothers are able to breastfeed will we be able to measure more accurately how much urban pollution contributes to the development of asthma in children.

37. As of 2001, the only groups of women to come close to the *Blueprint*'s goals are college educated women (44.1 percent breastfeeding at a six months and 23.4 percent at a year) and women aged 35 and older (44 percent breastfeeding at six months and 24.8 percent breastfeeding at a year). Women who live in the Pacific region of the United States also have high rates of breastfeeding (41.2 percent at six months and 26.2 percent at a year). See Ross *Mothers Survey*.

38. See, for example, the May/June 2000 issue of the *Journal of Midwifery and Women's Health*.

Epilogue

1. The *HHS Blueprint for Action on Breastfeeding* follows a similar line to the AAP, advocating for pumping breaks and hospital-grade breast pumps at worksites, but not for day care centers or extended maternity leaves (16).

2. Kate Hayles discusses this concept in her article "The Materiality of Informatics."

3. Australian feminist writers Alison Bartlett and Fiona Giles are rectifying this neglect, as is New Zealand economist Judith Galtry. It may be that feminist work on breastfeeding in Australia and New Zealand is more advanced than that in the United States because breastfeeding rates are higher in those countries, thus making more salient the public consequences of feminist silence on the issue. For interesting theoretical considerations, see especially Bartlett's "Scandalous Practices and Political Performances: Breastfeeding in the City" and "Thinking Through Breasts: Writing Maternity."

   For an example of the culture of breastfeeding promotion in Australia, see the Australian Breastfeeding Association's Media Releases web page, which has a discussion of a controversial public service announcement promoting breastfeeding. In the short video clip, available on the web site, a mother plays with and nurses her baby, who then looks over her shoulder and says, to the camera, "Get ahead in life. Suck up to the boss." The controversy concerns whether young children should be able to view the PSA. From an American perspective, the controversy is comical, given that it's not possible that it would even be made in the United States, let alone disseminated for public consumption.

Works Cited

Adams, Alice E. *Reproducing the Womb: Images of Childbirth in Science, Feminist Theory, and Literature.* Ithaca: Cornell University Press, 1994.

African-American Breastfeeding Alliance. *An Easy Guide to Breastfeeding for African-American Women.* Pamphlet. Joppa, MD: African-American Breastfeeding Alliance, nd.

———. *Breastfeeding Myths.* Pamphlet. Joppa, MD: African-American Breastfeeding Alliance, nd.

———. *Breastfeeding Education, Resources & Support.* Pamphlet. Joppa, MD: African-American Breastfeeding Alliance, nd.

American Academy of Pediatrics. "Breastfeeding and the Use of Human Milk." *Pediatrics* 100 (December 1997): 1035–39. <*http://www.aap.org/policy/re9729.html*>. 10 June 1998.

American Academy of Pediatrics Task Force on Infant Sleep Position and Sudden Infant Death Syndrome. "Changing Concepts of Sudden Infant Death Syndrome: Implications for Infant Sleeping Environment and Sleep Position (RE9946)." *Pediatrics* 105 (March 2000): 650–56. <*http://www.aap.org/policy/re9946.html*>. 12 Dec. 2001.

American SIDS Institute. "Annual Rates of SIDS." <*http://www.sids.org/annualrates2.htm*>. 13 Feb. 2001.

Andrews, Florence Kellner. "Controlling Motherhood: Observations on the Culture of La Leche League." *Canadian Review of Sociology and Anthropology* 28.1 (1991): 84–98.

Apple, Rima D. "Constructing Mothers: Scientific Mothers in the Nineteenth and Twentieth Centuries." *Mothers and Motherhood: Readings in American History.* Ed. Rima D. Apple and Janet Golden. Columbus: Ohio State University Press, 1997. 90–110. [Reprinted from *Social History of Medicine* 8 (1995): 161–78.]

———. *Mothers and Medicine: A Social History of Infant Feeding, 1890–1950.* Wisconsin Publications in the History of Science and Medicine. Number 7. Madison: University Wisconsin Press, 1987.

Austin, Mary. *Earth Horizon, Autobiography.* New York: The Literary Guild, 1932.

———. *A Woman of Genius.* Garden City, NY: Doubleday, 1912; Reprint, Old Westbury, NY: Feminist Press, 1985.

Australian Breastfeeding Association. Media Releases. "Breastfeeding Ad Restricted." 18 Mar. 2002. <*http://www.breastfeeding.asn.au/mediareleases/media.html#140302*> 30 Sept. 2002.

Baby-Friendly USA. "Baby-Friendly USA Presents the Baby-Friendly Hospital Initiative." Pamphlet.

Ball, Thomas M., and Anne L. Wright. "Health Care Costs of Formula-Feeding in the First Year of Life." *Pediatrics* 103 (April 1999): supplement 870–76.

Balsamo, Franca, Gisella De Mari, Vanessa Maher, and Rosalba Serini. "Production and Pleasure: Research on Breast-Feeding in Turin." *The Anthropology of Breast-Feeding.* Ed. Vanessa Maher. Oxford, UK: Berg, 1992. 59–90.

Barthes, Roland. *Mythologies.* Trans. Annette Lavers. New York: Hill & Wang, 1972.

Bartlett, Alison. "Scandalous Practices and Political Performances: Breastfeeding in the City." *Continuum: Journal of Media and Cultural Studies* 16.1 (2002): 111–21.

———. "Thinking Through Breasts: Writing Maternity." *Feminist Theory* 1.2 (2000): 173–88.

Baskerville, Diane. "Breastfeeding without Limits: Making It Easier for All Mothers and Babies to Continue Breastfeeding." Pamphlet. Libertyville, IL: Hollister, Inc., 1999.

Baumslag, Naomi, and Dia L. Michels. *Milk, Money, and Madness: The Culture and Politics of Breastfeeding.* Westport, CT: Bergin & Garvey, 1995.

Bem, Sandra Lipsitz. *The Lenses of Gender: Transforming the Debate on Sexual Inequality.* New Haven, CT: Yale University Press, 1993.

Bengson, Diane. *How Weaning Happens.* Schaumburg, IL: La Leche League International, 1999.

Bergman, Nils. "Kangaroo Mother Care: Restoring the Original Paradigm for Infant Care and Feeding." La Leche League International 29th Annual Seminar on Breastfeeding for Physicians: Breastfeeding for Health: Looking to the Future, Mindful of the Past. Chicago, IL, 7 July 2001.

Berney, Adrienne. *Reforming the Maternal Breast: Infant Feeding and American Culture, 1870–1940.* Dissertation. University of Delaware, 1998.

Bernstein, Nina. "Bronx Woman Convicted in Starving of Her Breast-Fed Son." *New York Times* 20 May 1999: B1.

———. "Mother Charged with Starving Baby Tells of Frantic Effort to Save Him." *New York Times* 19 May 1999: B5.

———. "Mother Convicted in Infant's Starvation Death Gets 5 Years' Probation." *New York Times* 9 Sept. 1999: B3.

———. "New York Faults Hospital for Denying Checkup to Baby Who Starved." *New York Times* 26 October 1998: B1.

———. "Prosecutor Drops Charges in Case of Infant's Death." *New York Times* 16 July 1998: B3.

———. "Trial Begins for Mother in Breast-Fed Infant's Starvation Death." *New York Times* 28 Apr. 1999: B7.

BFHI News. UNICEF. March/April 1999.

Blackwell, Antoinette Brown. *The Sexes throughout Nature.* Westport, CT: Hyperion, 1976.

Bliss, Mary Campbell, Joy Wilkie, Curt Acredolo, Susan Berman, and Kathleen Phillips Tebb. "The Effect of Discharge Packet Formula and Breast Pumps on Breastfeeding Duration and Choice of Infant Feeding Method." *Birth* 24.2 (June 1997): 90–97.

Blocker, Anne K. *Baby Basics: A Guide for New Parents.* Minneapolis: Chronimed Publishing, 1997.

Blum, Linda M. *At the Breast: Ideologies of Breastfeeding and Motherhood in the Contemporary United States.* Boston: Beacon, 1999.

———. "Mothers, Babies, and Breastfeeding in Late Capitalist America: The Shifting Contexts of Feminist Theory." *Feminist Studies* 19 (Summer 1993): 291–311.

Blum, Linda M., and Elizabeth A. Vandewater. " 'Mother to Mother': A Maternalist Organization in Late Capitalist America." *Social Problems* 40 (August 1993): 285–301.

Bobel, Christina G. "Bounded Liberation: A Focused Study of La Leche League International." *Gender and Society* 15.1 (February 2001): 130–51.

Bogdan, Janet Carlisle. "Childbirth in America, 1650–1990." *Women, Health, and Medicine in America, A Historical Handbook.* Ed. Rima D. Apple. New York: Garland, 1990. 101–20.

Boston Women's Health Book Collective. *Our Bodies, Ourselves: For the New Century.* 3rd ed. New York: Simon & Schuster/Touchstone, 1998.

"Breast and the Brightest, The." Dir. Martha Mitchell. *Chicago Hope.* CBS. WDBJ, Roanoke. 21 Oct. 1998.

"Breast-Feeding as Manslaughter." Editorial. *New York Times* 16 Mar. 1999: A26.

"Breast Milk for the World's Babies." Editorial. *New York Times* 12 Mar. 1992: A22.

Büskens, Petra. "The Impossibility of 'Natural Parenting' for Modern Mothers: On Social Structure and the Formation of Habit." *Journal of the Association for Research on Mothering* 3.1 (Spring/Summer 2001): 75–86.

Bykowski, Nancy Jo. "The Editor's Note: Beds and Babies." *New Beginnings* 17.1 (January-February 2000): np.

Cahill, Mary Ann. *Seven Voices, One Dream.* Schaumburg, IL: La Leche League International, 2001.

Carter, Pam. *Feminism, Breasts and Breast-Feeding.* New York: St. Martin's, 1995.

Chira, Susan. *A Mother's Place: Choosing Work and Family without Guilt or Blame.* New York: HarperCollins, 1998.

Chodorow, Nancy. *The Reproduction of Mothering: Psychoanalysis and the Sociology of Gender.* Berkeley: University of California Press, 1978.

Cohn, D'Vera. "Percentage of New Mothers in Workplace Fell Last Year." *Washington Post* 18 Oct. 2001: A2.

Collins, Patricia Hill. "Reproducing Race, Reproducing Nation: Black Women and the Politics of Motherhood." Lecture. Blacksburg, VA, 24 March 1998.

———. *Black Feminist Thought: Knowledge, Consciousness, and the Politics of Empowerment.* New York: Routledge, 1990.

Consumer Products Safety Commission. "CPSC Warns Against Placing Babies in Adult Beds." Washington, DC: U.S. Consumer Products Safety Commission, n.d.

Contratto, Susan Weisskopf. "Maternal Sexuality and Asexual Motherhood." *Women: Sex and Sexuality.* Ed. Catharine R. Stimpson and Ethel Spector Person. Chicago: University of Chicago Press, 1980. 224–40.

Coutsoudis, Anna. "Promotion of Exclusive Breastfeeding in the Face of the HIV Pandemic." *Lancet* 356 (Nov. 2000): 1620.

Crittendon, Ann. *The Price of Motherhood: Why the Most Important Job in the World Is Still the Least Valued.* New York: Henry Holt/Metropolitan Books, 2001.

Dally, Ann. *Inventing Motherhood: The Consequences of an Ideal.* London: Burnett Books, 1982.

Davis-Floyd, Robbie. "The Role of Obstetrical Rituals in the Resolution of Cultural Anomaly." *Social Science and Medicine* 31 (1990): 175–89.

Dell, S., and T. To. "Breastfeeding and Asthma in Young Children: Findings from a Population-Based Study." *Archives of Pediatrics and Adolescent Medicine* 155.11 (Nov. 2001): 1261–65.

DeLoache, Judy, and Alma Gottlieb. *A World of Babies: Imagined Childcare Guides for Seven Societies.* Cambridge, UK: Cambridge University Press, 2000.

D'Emilio, John. "Capitalism and Gay Identity." *The Gender Sexuality Reader.* Ed. Roger Lancaster and Micaela di Leonardo. New York: Routledge, 1997. 169–78.

Department of Health and Human Services. *Healthy People 2010: Conference Edition—Volumes I and II.* Washington, DC: U.S. Department of Health and Human Services, Public Health Service, 2000.

Department of Health and Human Services Office on Women's Health. *HHS Blueprint for Action on Breastfeeding.* Washington, DC: U.S. Department of Health and Human Services, 2000.

Dettwyler, Katherine A. "A Time to Wean: The Hominid Blueprint for the Natural Age of Weaning in Modern Human Populations." *Breastfeeding: Biocultural Perspectives.* Ed. Patricia Stuart-Macadam and Katherine A. Dettwyler. New York: Aldine de Gruyter, 1995. 39–74.

———. "Beauty and the Breast: The Cultural Context of Breastfeeding in the United States." *Breastfeeding: Biocultural Perspectives.* 167–215.

———. "Evolutionary Medicine and Breastfeeding: Implications for Research and Pediatric Advice." The David Skomp Distinguished Lectures in Anthropology, 1998–99. Indiana University, Department of Anthropology. Lecture, Nov. 19, 1998, 1–54.

———. "Promoting Breastfeeding or Promoting Guilt?" La Leche League International 16th International Conference: Breastfeeding: Wisdom from the Past, Gold Standard for the Future. Lake Buena Vista, FL, 5 July 1999.

———. "Tricks of the Trade: Infant Formula Companies in the United States." La Leche League International 27th Annual Seminar on Breastfeeding for Physicians: Breastfeeding: Protecting the Future. Lake Buena Vista, FL, 2 July 1999.

Dewey, Kathryn G., Jane Heinig, and Laurie A. Nommsen-Rivers. "Differences in Morbidity between Breast-Fed and Formula-Fed Infants." *The Journal of Pediatrics* 126.5 Part 1 (1995): 696–702.

Diamond, Jared. "Father's Milk." *Discover* 16.2 (1995): 82–87.

Drago, Dorothy A., and Andrew L. Dannenberg. "Infant Mechanical Suffocation Deaths in the United States, 1980–1997." *Pediatrics* 103.5 (1999). <*http://www.pediatrics.org/cgi/content/full/103/5/e59*>. 27 Nov. 2001.

Drane, D. L., and J. A. Logemann. "A Critical Evaluation of the Evidence on the Association between Type of Infant Feeding Method and Cognitive Development." *Paediatric and Perinatal Epidemiology* 14 (2000): 349–56. Abstract. <*http://www.blackwell-synergy.com/Journals*>. 11 Nov. 2001.

Dungy, Claibourne I., Jay Christensen-Szalanski, Mary Laosch, and Daniel Russell. "Effect of Discharge Samples on Duration of Breast-Feeding." *Pediatrics* 90 (August 1992): 233–37.

Ebert, Teresa. *Ludic Feminism, and After: Postmodernism, Desire, and Labor in Late Capitalism.* Critical Perspectives on Women and Gender. Ann Arbor: University of Michigan Press, 1996.

Eisenberg, Arlene, Heidi E. Murkoff, and Sandee E. Hathaway. *What to Expect When You're Expecting.* 2d ed. New York: Workman, 1991.

Eisenstein, Zillah R. *The Female Body and the Law.* Berkeley: University of California Press, 1988.

Elias, Marilyn. "Nurse for Full Year, Moms Urged." *USA Today* 2 Dec. 1997: A1.

Eyer, Diane. *Mother-Infant Bonding: A Scientific Fiction.* New Haven, CT: Yale University Press, 1992.

Faul, Michelle. "Improper Formula Feeding Spreads Malnutrition, Death in Third World." *Los Angeles Times* 19 May 1991: A3.

Feinbloom, Richard I. *Pregnancy, Birth, and the Early Months: A Complete Guide.* 2d ed. Reading, MA: Addison-Wesley, 1993.

Fildes, Valerie. *Breasts, Bottles, and Babies: A History of Infant Feeding.* Edinburgh: Edinburgh University Press, 1986.

———. "The Culture and Biology of Breastfeeding: An Historical Review of Western Europe." *Breastfeeding: Biocultural Perspectives.* Ed. Patricia Stuart-Macadam and Katherine A. Dettwyler. New York: Aldine de Gruyter, 1995. 101–26.

———. *Wet Nursing: A History from Antiquity to the Present.* Oxford: Basil Blackwell, 1988.

Firestone, Shulamith. *The Dialectic of Sex: The Case for Feminist Revolution.* New York: William Morrow, 1970.

Food and Drug Administration. "Overview of Infant Formulas." August 1997. <*http://www.cfsan. fda.gov/~dms/ds-inf.html*>. 19 Nov. 2001.

Foucault, Michel. *The Care of the Self. The History of Sexuality, Volume III.* Trans. Robert Hurley. New York: Random House, 1986.

———. *The History of Sexuality, Volume I: An Introduction.* Trans. Robert Hurley. New York: Random House, 1978.

———. *Power/Knowledge: Selected Interviews and Other Writings, 1972–1977.* Ed. Colin Gordon. New York: Pantheon, 1980.

Frank, Deborah A., Stephen J. Wirtz, James R. Sorenson, and Timothy Heeren. "Commercial Discharge Packs and Breastfeeding Counseling: Effects on Infant-Feeding Practices in a Randomized Trial." *Pediatrics* 80 (December 1987): 845–54.

Fraser, Steve, ed. *The Bell Curve Wars: Race, Intelligence, and the Future of America.* New York: Basic Books, 1995.

Freed, Gary. "Breast-Feeding Education of Obstetrics-Gynecology Residents and Practitioners." Abstract. *Journal of the American Medical Association* 276.9 (Sept 4, 1996): 662F. Infotrac: Expanded Academic Index. 5 October 2001.

Gabriel, Ayala, K. Ruben Gabriel, and Ruth A. Lawrence. "Cultural Values and Biomedical Knowledge: Choices in Infant Feeding." *Social Science and Medicine* 23 (1986): 501–9.

Galtry, Judith. "Extending the 'Bright Line': Feminism, Breastfeeding, and the Workplace in the United States." *Gender & Society* 14 (Apr. 2000): 295–317.

———. " 'Sameness' and Suckling: Infant Feeding, Feminism, and a Changing Labour Market." *Women's Studies Journal* 13 (Autumn 1997): 65–88.

———. "Suckling and Silence in the USA: The Costs and Benefits of Breastfeeding." *Feminist Economics* 3.3 (1997): 1–24.

Garcilazo, Miguel, and Virginia Breen. "Held in Son's Starvation Death." *New York Daily News* 1 October 1997: Suburban 1.

Gartner, Lawrence. Letter to the editor. *The Wall Street Journal.* 16 August 1994: A16.

Gdalevich, M., D. Mimouni, and M. Mimouni. "Breast-Feeding and the Risk of Bronchial Asthma in Childhood: A Systematic Review with Meta-Analysis of Prospective Studies." *Journal of Pediatrics* 139.2 (August 2001): 261–66.

Geronimus, Arline. "Understanding and Eliminating Racial Inequalities in Women's Health in the United States: The Role of the Weathering Conceptual Framework." *Journal of the American Medical Women's Association* 56.4 (Fall 2001): 133–37.

Giles, Fiona. "Fountains of Love and Loveliness: In Praise of the Dripping Wet Breast." *Journal of the Association for Research on Mothering* 4.1 (Spring/Summer 2002): 7–18.

———. *Fresh Milk.* New York: Simon & Schuster, 2003.

Gilman, Charlotte Perkins. *Women and Economics: The Economic Factor between Men and Women as a Factor in Social Evolution.* New York: Harper & Row, 1966.

Golden, Janet. *A Social History of Wet Nursing in America: From Breast to Bottle.* Cambridge History of Medicine. Cambridge, UK: Cambridge University Press, 1996.

Gordon, Jane. " 'Choosing' to Breastfeed: Some Feminist Questions." *Resources for Feminist Research/Documentation sur la Recherche Feministe.* 18.2 (June 1989): 10–12.

Gorham, Deborah, and Florence Kellner Andrews. "The La Leche League: A Feminist Perspective." *Delivering Motherhood: Maternal Ideologies and Practices in the 19th and 20th Centuries.* Ed. Katherine Arnup, Andrée Lévesque, and Ruth Roach Pierson. London: Routledge, 1990. 238–69.

Grant, Julia. *Raising Baby by the Book.* New Haven, CT: Yale University Press, 1998.

Greiner, Ted. "A Return to Promoting Breastfeeding as an Experience." La Leche League International 17th International Conference: A Kaleidoscope of Friends, Family, and Cultures. Chicago, IL, 8 July 2001.

Grosz, Elizabeth. *Volatile Bodies: Toward a Corporeal Feminism.* Bloomington: Indiana University Press, 1994.

Guttman, Nutrit, and Deena R. Zimmerman. "Low-Income Mothers' Views on Breastfeeding." *Social Science and Medicine* 50 (May 2000): 1457–73.

Haraway, Donna J. *ModestWitness@SecondMillennium.Female_Man©_Meets_Onco Mouse^{TM}.* New York: Routledge, 1997.

———. "Situated Knowledges: The Science Question in Feminism and the Privilege of Partial Perspective." *Simians, Cyborgs, and Women.* New York: Routledge, 1991. 183–201.

Hastrup, Kirsten. "A Question of Reason: Breast-Feeding Patterns in Seventeenth- and Eighteenth-Century Iceland." *The Anthropology of Breast-Feeding: Natural Law or Social Construct.* Ed. Vanessa Maher. Oxford, UK: Berg, 1992. 91–132.

Hausman, Bernice L. *Changing Sex: Transsexualism, Technology, and the Idea of Gender.* Durham: Duke University Press, 1995.

Hayles, N. Katherine. "The Materiality of Informatics." *Configurations* 1 (1993): 147–70.

Hays, Sharon. *The Cultural Contradictions of Motherhood.* New Haven: Yale University Press, 1996.

Heilbrun, Carolyn. *The Creation of Patriarchy.* Oxford: Oxford University Press, 1986.

Heinig, Jane M, and Kathryn G. Dewey. "Health Advantages of Breast Feeding for Infants: A Critical Review." *Nutrition Research Reviews* 9 (1996): 89–110.

Helliker, Keith. "Dying for Milk." *Wall Street Journal* 22 July 1994: A1, A4.

Higham, Scott, and Sari Horwitz. "Starvation Killed Baby under D.C. Protection; Caseworker Didn't See Family for 7 Months." *Washington Post* 1 December 2001: B1.

Hogan, Vijaya K., Jessie L. Richardson, Cynthia D. Ferre, Tonji Durant, and Martha Boisseau. "A Public Health Framework for Addressing Black and White Disparities in Preterm Delivery." *Journal of the American Medical Women's Association* 56.4 (Fall 2001): 177–81.

Houppert, Karen. "Nursed to Death." *Salon.* 21 May 2000. <*http://www.salon.com/mwt/feature/1999/05/21/nursing*>. 26 May 2000.

Howard, Cynthia, Fred Howard, Ruth Lawrence, Elena Andresen, Elisabeth DeBlieck, and Michael Weitzman. "Office Prenatal Formula Advertising and Its Effect on Breast-Feeding Patterns." *Obstetrics and Gynecology* 95 (2000): 296–303.

Howard, Fred. "Why Women Should Breastfeed for Their Own Health." La Leche League International 28th Annual Seminar on Breastfeeding for Physicians. Hilton Head Island, SC, 21 July 2000.

Hrdy, Sarah Blaffer. *Mother Nature: A History of Mothers, Infants, and Natural Selection.* New York: Pantheon, 1999.

Hubbard, Ruth. *The Politics of Women's Biology.* New Brunswick: Rutgers University Press, 1990.

Huffman, Grace Brooke. "Physician Knowledge about Breast Feeding." *American Family Physician* 53.3 (February 1996): 957–8. Adapted from *Pediatrics* 96 (1995): 490–94. Infotrac: Expanded Academic Index. 5 October 2001.

Hutcherson, Hilda. *Having Your Baby: A Guide for African American Women.* New York: Ballantine, 1997.

Jacobus, Mary. "Incorruptible Milk: Breast-Feeding and the French Revolution." *Rebel Daughters.* Ed. Sara E. Meltzer and Leslie W. Rabine. New York: Oxford University Press, 1992. 54–75.

Jelliffe, Derrick B., and E. F. Patrice Jelliffe. *Human Milk in the Modern World: Psychosocial, Nutritional, and Economic Significance.* Oxford, UK: Oxford University Press, 1978.

Johnson, Maria Miro. "Conspiracy Debate on Breast-Feeding Article." *Providence Journal-Bulletin* 14 Sept. 1994: 6C.

Jones, Kathleen W. "Motherhood." *The Family in America: An Encyclopedia.* Joseph M. Hawes and Elizabeth F. Shores, eds. Santa Barbara, CA: ABC-CLIO, 2001. 701-14.

Kahn, Robbie Pfeufer. "Women and Time in Childbirth and During Lactation." *Taking Our Time: Feminist Perspectives on Temporality.* Ed. Frieda Johles Forman with Caoran Sowton. Athene Series. Oxford: Pergamon, 1988. 20–36.

Kitzinger, Sheila. *Breastfeeding Your Baby.* Rev. ed. New York: Alfred A. Knopf-Borzoi, 1998.

———. *The Experience of Childbirth.* New York: Taplinger, 1972.

Klaus, Marshall. "Perinatal Care in the 21st Century: Evidence that Supports Changing the Management for Both Mother and Baby." La Leche League International 27th Annual Seminar on Breastfeeding for Physicians: Breastfeeding: Protecting the Future. Lake Buena Vista, FL, 2 July 1999.

———. "Perinatal Care in the 21st Century: Evidence that Supports Changing the Management for Both Mother and Baby." *Report of the National Breastfeeding Policy Conference.* Ed. Wendy Slusser, Linda Lange, and Sarah Thomas. Los Angeles: UCLA Center for Healthier Children, Families, and Communities Breastfeeding Resource Program, In Cooperation with the U.S. Dept. of Health and Human Services, Health Resources and Services Administration, Maternal and Child Health Bureau, 1998. 20–26.

Kogan, Michael D., Milton Kotechuck, Greg R. Alexander, and Wayne E. Johnson. "Racial Disparities in Reported Prenatal Care Advice from Health Care Providers." *American Journal of Public Health* 84.1 (January 1994): 82–88.

La Leche League International. "A Brief History of La Leche League International." 13 Feb. 2001. <*http://www.lalecheleague.org/LLLIhistory.html*> . 29 Nov. 2001.

———. "CBS's Chicago Hope Airs Inaccurate Information about the Baby-Friendly Hospital Initiative." 26 Nov. 1999. <*http://www.lalecheleague.org/Release/bfhi.html*> . Accessed 26 July 2000.

———. "La Leche League International Offers Clarification on Misinformation Presented on Television Show." 16 Feb. 2000. <*http://www.lalecheleague.org/Release/law-n-order.html*>. 26 July 2000.

———. "La Leche League International Offers Support for Mothers Concerning Dehydration and Inadequate Milk Supply." 26 Nov. 1999. <*http://www.lalecheleague.org/Release/hopr.html*>. 26 July 2000.

———. "La Leche League Philosophy." 13 Feb. 2001. <*http://www.lalecheleague.org/philosophy.html*>. 28 Nov. 2001.

———. "LLLUSA: What Is LLLUSA?" Online: Internet. 13 Nov. 2001. <*http://www.lllusa.org/lllusa/background.html*> 29 Nov. 2001.

———. *The Womanly Art of Breastfeeding.* 3rd ed. Franklin Park, IL: La Leche League International, 1981.

———. *The Womanly Art of Breastfeeding.* 4th ed. Franklin Park, IL: La Leche League International, 1987.

———. *The Womanly Art of Breastfeeding.* 5th ed. New York: Plume, 1991.

———. *The Womanly Art of Breastfeeding.* 6th ed. Schaumburg, IL: La Leche League International, 1997.

La Leche League of Franklin Park. *The Womanly Art of Breastfeeding.* Franklin Park, IL: La Leche League of Franklin Park, 1958.

———. *The Womanly Art of Breastfeeding.* 2nd ed. Franklin Park, IL: La Leche League International, 1963.

Ladd-Tayler, Molly, and Lauri Umansky, eds. *"Bad" Mothers: The Politics of Blame in Twentieth-Century America.* New York: New York University Press, 1998.

———. Introduction. *"Bad" Mothers: The Politics of Blame in Twentieth-Century America.* 1–28.

Lappé, Marc. *Evolutionary Medicine: Rethinking the Origins of Disease.* San Francisco: Sierra Club Books, 1994.

Larson, Signe, and Kevin Osborn. *The Complete Idiot's Guide to Bringing Up Baby.* New York: Simon & Schuster Macmillan/Alpha Books, 1997.

Lastinger, Valerie. "Re-Defining Motherhood: Breast-Feeding and the French Enlightenment." *Women's Studies* 25 (Nov. 1996): 603–17. Online: Infotrac.

Law, Jules. "The Politics of Breastfeeding: Assessing Risk, Dividing Labor." *Signs* 25 (Winter 2000): 407–50.

Lawrence, Ruth. "Breastfeeding Advantages with a Focus on Child Development." *Report of the National Breastfeeding Policy Conference.* Ed. Wendy Slusser, Linda Lange, and Sarah Thomas. Los Angeles : UCLA Center for Healthier Children, Families, and Communities Breastfeeding Program, in cooperation with the U.S. Dept. of Health and Human Services, Health Resources and Services Administration, Maternal and Child Health Bureau, 1998. 27–36.

———. *Breastfeeding: A Guide for the Medical Profession.* 4th ed. St. Louis: Mosby, 1994.

———. Letter to the editor. *Wall Street Journal* 16 August 1994: A16.

———. "Major Difficulties in Promoting Breastfeeding: US Perspectives." *Programmes to Promote Breastfeeding.* Ed. Derrick B. Jellife and E. F. Patrice Jelliffe. Oxford, UK: Oxford University Press, 1988. 267–71.

Leach, Penelope. *Your Baby and Child: From Birth to Age Five.* 3rd ed. New York: Alfred A. Knopf, 1997.

Leavitt, Judith Walzer. "Birthing and Anesthesia: The Debate over Twilight Sleep." *Mothers and Motherhood: Readings in American History.* Ed. Rima D. Apple and Janet Golden. Columbus: Ohio State University Press, 1997. 242–58.

Lerner, Gerda. *The Creation of Patriarchy.* New York: Oxford University Press, 1986.

Lindsey, Linda L. *Gender Roles: A Sociological Perspective.* 2nd ed. Englewood Cliffs: Prentice Hall, 1994.

Litt, Jacquelyn S., *Medicalized Motherhood: Perspectives from the Lives of African-American and Jewish Women.* New Brunswick: Rutgers University Press, 2000.

Lopata, Helena Z., and Barrie Thorne. "On the Term 'Sex Roles.'" *Signs* 3 (1978): 718–21.

Lowman, Kaye. *The LLLove Story: The History of La Leche League's Founding.* Schaumburg, IL: La Leche League International, 1978.

MacKeen, Dawn. "When a Breast-Fed Infant Dies from Malnutrition, Is the Mother to Blame?" *Salon.* 16 June 1998. <*http://www.salon.com/mwt/not/1998/06/16hot.html*>. 26 May 1999.

Maclean, Heather. *Women's Experience of Breast Feeding.* Toronto: University of Toronto Press, 1990.

Maher, Vanessa, ed. *The Anthropology of Breast-Feeding: Natural Law or Social Construct.* Oxford, UK: Berg, 1992.

———. "Breast-Feeding and Maternal Depletion: Natural Law or Cultural Arrangements?" *The Anthropology of Breast-Feeding.* Ed. Vanessa Maher. 151–80.

———. "Breast-Feeding in Cross-cultural Perspective: Paradoxes and Proposals." *The Anthropology of Breast-Feeding.* Ed. Vanessa Maher. 1–36.

McDowell, Deborah E. "Afterword: Recovery Missions: Imagining Body Ideals." *Recovering the Black Body: Self-Representations by Black Women.* Ed. Michael Bennett and Vanessa D. Dickerson. New Brunswick: Rutgers University Press, 2001. 296–317.

McKenna, James. "Never Sleep with Your Baby?" La Leche League International 29th Annual Seminar on Breastfeeding for Physicians: Breastfeeding for Health: Looking to the Future, Mindful of the Past. Chicago, IL, 6 July 2001.

———. "The Dance of the Sugar Plum Fairy: Sleeping Patterns of the Breastfeeding Dyad." La Leche League International 27th Annual Seminar on Breastfeeding for Physicians: Breastfeeding: Protecting the Future. Lake Buena Vista, FL, 2 July 1999.

McKenna, James, Evelyn B. Thoman, Thomas F. Anders, Abraham Sadeh, Vicki L. Schechtman, and Steven F. Glotzbach. "Infant-Parent Co-Sleeping in an Evolutionary Perspective: Implications for Understanding Infant Sleep Development and the Sudden Infant Death Syndrome." *Pediatric Review* 16.3 (1993): 263–82.

McKenna, James, Sarah Mosko, and Chris Richard. "Breast-Feeding and Mother-Infant Cosleeping in Relation to SIDS Prevention." *Evolutionary Medicine.* Ed. Wenda R. Trevathan, E. O. Smith, and James J. McKenna. New York: Oxford University Press, 1999. 53–74.

Merrill, Elizabeth Bryant. "Learning How to Mother: An Ethnographic Investigation of an Urban Breastfeeding Group." *Anthropology and Education Quarterly* 18 (September 1987): 222–40.

Michie, Helena, and Naomi Cahn. *Confinements: Fertility and Infertility in Contemporary Culture.* New Brunswick, NJ: Rutgers University Press, 1997.

Millard, Ann V. "The Place of the Clock in Pediatric Advice: Rationales, Cultural Themes, and Impediments to Breastfeeding." *Social Science and Medicine* 31.2 (1990): 211–21.

Miller, J. E. "Predictors of Asthma in Young Children: Does Reporting Source Affect Our Conclusions?" *American Journal of Epidemiology* 154.3 (August 2001): 245–50.

Mohrbacher, Nancy, and Julie Stock. *The Breastfeeding Answer Book.* Rev. ed. Schaumburg, IL: La Leche League International, 1997.

Morris, Richard. *The Evolutionists: The Struggle for Darwin's Soul.* New York: W. H. Freeman, 2001.

Morrison, Pamela, and Ted Greiner. "Infant Feeding Choices for HIV-Positive Mothers." *Breastfeeding Abstracts* 19 (May 2000): 27–28.

Mortensen, Erik Lykke, Kim Fleischer Michaelson, Stephanie A. Sanders, and June Machover Reinisch. "The Association between Duration of Breastfeeding and Adult Intelligence." *Journal of the American Medical Association* 287 (8 May 2002): 2365–71.

"Mother's Milk." Dir. Richard Dobbs. *Law and Order.* NBC. WSLS, Roanoke. 9 Feb. 2000.

National Black Women's Health Project. "Vision Statement." *Still Lifting, Still Climbing: African American Women's Contemporary Activism.* Ed. Kimberly Springer. New York: New York University Press, 1999. 37.

Neifert, Marianne. *Dr. Mom's Guide to Breastfeeding.* New York: Dutton NAL-Plume, 1998.

———. Letter to the editor. *Wall Street Journal* 16 August 1994: A16.

Newman, Jack. "How Breast Milk Protects Newborns." *Scientific American* 273.6 (Dec. 1995): 76–79.

Newton, Niles. *Maternal Emotions.* New York: Paul B. Hoeber, Medical Book Department of Harper & Brothers, 1955.

Oakley, Ann. *Essays on Women, Medicine and Health.* Edinburgh, UK: Edinburgh University Press, 1993.

Ortner, Sherry. "Is Female to Male as Nature Is to Culture?" *Woman, Culture and Society.* Ed. Michelle Rosaldo and Louise Lamphere. Stanford, CA: Stanford University Press, 1974. 67–87. Reprinted in *Women in Culture: A Women's Studies Anthology.* Ed. Lucinda Joy Peach. Malden, MA: Blackwell, 1998. 23–45.

"Overview of Infant Formulas." U.S. Food and Drug Administration, Center for Food Safety and Applied Nutrition, Office of Special Nutritionals. August 1997. <*http://vm.cfsan.fda.gov/ ~dms/ds-inf.html*> 16 August 2002.

Palmer, Gabrielle. *The Politics of Breastfeeding.* 2nd ed. London: HarperCollins/Pandora, 1993.

Palmer, Gabrielle, and Saskia Kemp. "Breastfeeding Promotion and the Role of the Professional Midwife." *Baby Friendly Mother Friendly.* Ed. Susan F. Murray. London: Mosby, 1996. 1–23.

Palumbi, Stephen R. *The Evolution Explosion: How Humans Cause Rapid Evolutionary Change.* New York: Norton, 2001.

Panter-Brick, Catherine. "Working Mothers in Rural Nepal." *The Anthropology of Breast-Feeding: Natural Law or Social Construct.* Ed. Vanessa Maher. Oxford, UK: Berg, 1992. 133–50.

Perry, Ruth. "Colonizing the Breast: Sexuality and Maternity in Eighteenth-Century England." *Journal of the History of Sexuality* 2 (1991): 204–34.

Piercy, Marge. *Woman on the Edge of Time.* New York: Alfred A. Knopf, 1976.

Pincus, Jane. Introduction. *Our Bodies, Ourselves: For a New Century.* 3rd ed. The Boston Women's Health Book Collective. New York: Simon & Schuster/Touchstone, 1998. 21–23.

Pollitt, Katha. "A Bronx Tale." *The Nation* 268 (14 June 1999): 11.

Pompilio, Natalie. "In New Jersey, Second Thoughts on Breast-Feeding." *Philadelphia Inquirer* 18 November 1996: C1.

Pryor, Karen, and Gale Pryor. *Nursing Your Baby.* New York: Pocket Books, 1991.

Riordan, Jan, and Kathleen G. Auerbach. *Breastfeeding and Human Lactation.* 2nd ed. Boston: Jones & Bartlett, 1999.

Roberts, Dorothy. *Killing the Black Body: Race, Reproduction, and the Meaning of Liberty.* New York: Random House, 1997.

———. "The Value of Black Mothers' Work." *Critical Race Feminism: A Reader.* Ed. Adrian Katherine Wing. New York: New York University Press, 1997. 312–16.

Robin, Peggy. *When Breastfeeding Is Not an Option: A Reassuring Guide for Loving Parents.* Rocklin, CA: Prima Publishing, 1998.

Rossi, Alice. "Maternalism, Sexuality, and the New Feminism." *Contemporary Sexual Behavior: Critical Issues in the 1970s.* Ed. Joseph Zubin and John Money. Baltimore: Johns Hopkins University Press, 1973. 146–74.

Ross Products Division, Abbot Laboratories. "Mothers Survey." Unpublished survey data.

Rothman, Barbara Katz. "Beyond Mothers and Fathers: Ideology in a Patriarchal Society." *Mothering: Ideology, Experience, Agency.* Ed. Evelyn Nakano Glenn, Grace Chang, and Linda Rennie Forcey. New York: Routledge, 1994. 139–57.

———. *In Labor: Women and Power in the Birthplace.* New York: Norton, 1982.

Ruddick, Lisa. "The Near Enemy of the Humanities Is Professionalism." *Chronicle of Higher Education* 23 Nov. 2001: B7–9.

Russett, Cynthia Eagle. *Sexual Science: Victorian Constructions of Womanhood.* Cambridge, MA: Harvard University Press, 1989.

Sachetti, Dor, ed. *Leader's Handbook.* Rev. ed. Schaumburg, IL: La Leche League International, 1998.

Santana, Arthur. "Parents Charged with Murder in Baby's Death; 2-Month-Old Died of Starvation While under Watch of D.C. Protection System." *Washington Post* 5 Dec. 2001: B1.

Scheper-Hughes, Nancy. *Death without Weeping: The Violence of Everyday Life in Brazil.* Berkeley: University of California Press, 1992.

Schiebinger, Londa. *Nature's Body: Gender in the Making of Modern Science.* Boston: Beacon, 1993.

Sears, William, and Martha Sears. *The Baby Book: Everything You Need to Know about Your Baby— From Birth to Age Two.* Boston: Little, Brown, 1993.

Sherif, Carolyn Wood. "Needed Concepts in the Study of Gender Identity." *Psychology of Women Quarterly* 6.4 (Summer 1982): 375–98.

Shostak, Marjorie. *Nisa, the Life and Words of a !Kung Woman.* New York: Random House/Vintage, 1981.

———. *Return to Nisa.* Cambridge, MA: Harvard University Press, 2000.

Sichtermann, Barbara. "The Lost Eroticism of the Breasts." *Femininity: The Politics of the Personal.* Trans. John Whitlam. Ed. Helga Geyer-Ryan. Minneapolis: University of Minnesota Press, 1986. 55–68.

Simpkin, Penny, Janet Whalley, and Ann Keppler. *Pregnancy, Childbirth, and the Newborn: The Complete Guide.* Deephaven, MN: Meadowbrook Press, 1991.

Small, Meredith F. *Our Babies, Ourselves: How Biology and Culture Shape the Way We Parent.* New York: Doubleday/Anchor, 1998.

Smith-Rosenberg, Carroll. *Disorderly Conduct: Visions of Gender in Victorian America.* New York: Oxford University Press, 1986.

Snitow, Ann. "A Gender Diary." *Conflicts in Feminism.* Ed. Marianne Hirsch and Evelyn Fox Keller. New York: Routledge, 1990. 9–43.

Sollinger, Rickie. *Wake Up Little Susie: Single Pregnancy and Race before Roe v. Wade.* 2d ed. New York: Routledge, 2000.

Spock, Benjamin, and Steven J. Parker. *Dr. Spock's Baby and Child Care.* 7th ed. New York: Pocket Books, 1998.

Spurlock, Inga. "Promoting Breastfeeding among Women of Color." La Leche League International 17th International Conference: A Kaleidoscope of Friends, Family, and Cultures. Chicago, IL, 8 July 2001.

Starr, Paul. Review of Ann Crittendon's *The Price of Motherhood. New York Times Book Review* (Feb. 11, 2001): 9.

———. *The Social Transformation of American Medicine.* New York: Basic Books, 1982.

Stearns, Cindy A. "Breastfeeding and the Good Maternal Body." *Gender and Society* 13 (June 1999): 308–25.

Stehlin, Isadora B. "Infant Formula: Second Best but Good Enough." FDA Consumer Magazine. June 1996. <*http://www.fda.gov/fdac/features/596_baby.html*> 23 Sept. 2002.

Stoppard, Mirriam. *The Breast Book.* New York: DK Publishing, 1996.

Stuart-Macadam, Patricia, "Biocultural Perspectives on Breastfeeding. *Breastfeeding: Biocultural Perspectives.* Ed. Patricia Stuart-Macadam and Katherine A. Dettwyler, 1–37.

Stuart-Macadam, Patricia, and Katherine A. Dettwyler, eds. *Breastfeeding: Biocultural Perspectives.* New York: Aldine de Gruyter, 1995.

Sussman, George D. *Selling Mothers' Milk: The Wet-Nursing Business in France, 1715–1914.* Urbana: University of Illinois Press, 1982.

Swarns, Rachel L. "Mother Who May Have Fed Her Son Improperly Is Charged in His Death." *New York Times* 1 October 1997: B3.

Tattersall, Ian. *Becoming Human: Evolution and Human Uniqueness.* San Diego: Harcourt Brace, 1998.

Thompson, Becky. *A Hunger So Wide and So Deep: A Multicultural View of Women's Eating Problems.* Minneapolis: University of Minnesota Press, 1994.

Thornhill, Randy, and Craig T. Palmer. *A Natural History of Rape: The Biological Bases of Sexual Coercion.* Cambridge, MA: MIT Press, 2000.

Timbo, Babgaleh, Sean Altekruse, Marica Headrick, and Karl Klontz. "Breastfeeding among Black Mothers: Evidence Supporting the Need for Prenatal Intervention." *Journal for the Society of Pediatric Nurses.* 1.1 (April–June 1996): 35–56. Infotrac, Expanded Academic Index. 5 October 2001.

Tipograph, Susan, Janna Collins, and Lawrence Gartner. "Ethical and Legal Issues that Affect Breastfeeding." La Leche League International 28th Annual Seminar on Breastfeeding for Physicians: A Physician's Perspective on Breastfeeding: Trends, Trials, and Triumphs. Hilton Head, SC, 21 July 2000.

Treichler, Paula. "Feminism, Medicine, and the Meaning of Childbirth." *Body Politics: Women and the Discourses of Science.* Ed. Mary Jacobus, Evelyn Fox Keller, and Sally Shuttleworth. New York: Routledge, 1990. 113–38.

Turner, Brian S. *Regulating Bodies: Essays in Medical Sociology.* London: Routledge, 1992.

Tyson, Kathleen. "In the Eye of the Storm." *Mothering* (May/June 1999): 68–69.

Umansky, Lauri. "Breastfeeding in the 1990s: The Karen Carter Case and the Politics of Maternal Sexuality." *"Bad Mothers": The Politics of Blame in Twentieth-Century America.* Ed. Molly Ladd-Taylor and Lauri Umansky. New York: New York University Press, 1998. 299–309.

————. *Motherhood Reconceived: Feminism and the Legacies of the Sixties.* New York: New York University Press, 1996.

UNICEF. "Breastfeeding: Foundation for a Healthy Future." Pamphlet. nd.

Van Esterik, Penny. *Beyond the Breast-Bottle Controversy.* New Brunswick, NJ: Rutgers University Press, 1989.

————. "Breastfeeding and Feminism." *International Journal of Gynecology and Obstetrics* 47 Supplement (1994): S41–S54.

————. "Lessons From Our Lives: Breastfeeding in a Personal Context." *Journal of Human Lactation* 10.2 (1994): 71–74.

————. "Thank You, Breasts! Breastfeeding as a Feminist Issue." *Ethnographic Feminisms: Essays in Anthropology.* Ed. Sally Cole and Lynne Phillips. Ottawa, ONT: Carleton University Press, 1995. 75–99.

Vares, Tiina. "Feminist Women Talk about Breastfeeding." *Women's Studies Journal* 8.2 (Sept. 1992): 25–41.

WABA Steering Committee. "WABA Position on HIV and Breastfeeding." 6 June 1998. <*http://www.waba.org/br/dechiv.htm*>. 21 Sept. 2000.

Ward, Julia DeJager. *La Leche League: At the Crossroads of Medicine, Feminism, and Religion.* Chapel Hill: University of North Carolina Press, 2000.

Ward, Martha C. *A World Full of Women.* Boston: Allyn & Bacon, 1996.

Weiner, Lynn Y. "Reconstructing Motherhood: The La Leche League in Postwar America." *Journal of American History* 80 (1994): 1357–81. Reprinted in *Mothers and Motherhood: Readings in American History.* Ed. Rima D. Apple and Janet Golden. Columbus: Ohio State University Press, 1997. 362–88.

Whitaker, Elizabeth Dixon. *Measuring Mamma's Milk: Fascism and the Medicalization of Maternity in Italy.* Ann Arbor: University of Michigan Press, 2000.

Williams, Joan. *Unbending Gender: Why Family and Work Conflict and What to Do about It.* New York: Oxford University Press, 2000.

Wolf, Jacqueline H. *Don't Kill Your Baby: Public Health and the Decline of Breastfeeding in the 19th and 20th Centuries.* Columbus: Ohio State University Press, 2001.

World Health Organization. "Fact Sheet." September 1997. <*http://www.who.ch/chd/pub/imci/ fs_180.htm*>. 10 July 1998.

————. *International Code of Marketing of Breast-Milk Substitutes.* Geneva: World Health Organization, 1981.

Worthman, Carol. "Evolutionary Perspectives on the Onset of Puberty." *Evolutionary Medicine.* Ed. Wenda R. Trevathan, E. O. Smith, and James J. McKenna. New York: Oxford University Press, 1999. 135–63.

Wright, Anne L. "Cultures of Breastfeeding in the United States." *Report of the National Breastfeeding Policy Conference.* Ed. Wendy Slusser, Linda Lange, and Sarah Thomas. Los Angeles: UCLA Center for Healthier Children, Families, and Communities Breastfeeding Resource Program, in cooperation with the U.S. Dept. of Health and Human Services, Health Resources and Services Administration, Maternal and Child Health Bureau, 1998. 40–4.

Yalom, Marilyn. *A History of the Breast.* New York: Ballantine, 1997.

Yoshioka, Kumiko. "Maternal Breastfeeding as the Vanishing Point, or What Artificial Feeding Really Substituted For." Society for Literature and Science Conference. Pasadena, CA, 12 Oct. 2002.

Young, Iris Marion. "Breasted Experience: The Look and the Feeling." *Throwing Like a Girl and Other Essays in Feminist Philosophy and Social Theory.* Bloomington: Indiana University Press, 1990. 189–209.

Young, Michal. "Promoting Breastfeeding in Vulnerable Populations." La Leche League International 29th Annual Seminar on Breastfeeding for Physicians: Breastfeeding for Health: Looking to the Future, Mindful of the Past. Chicago, IL, 6 July 2001.

Index